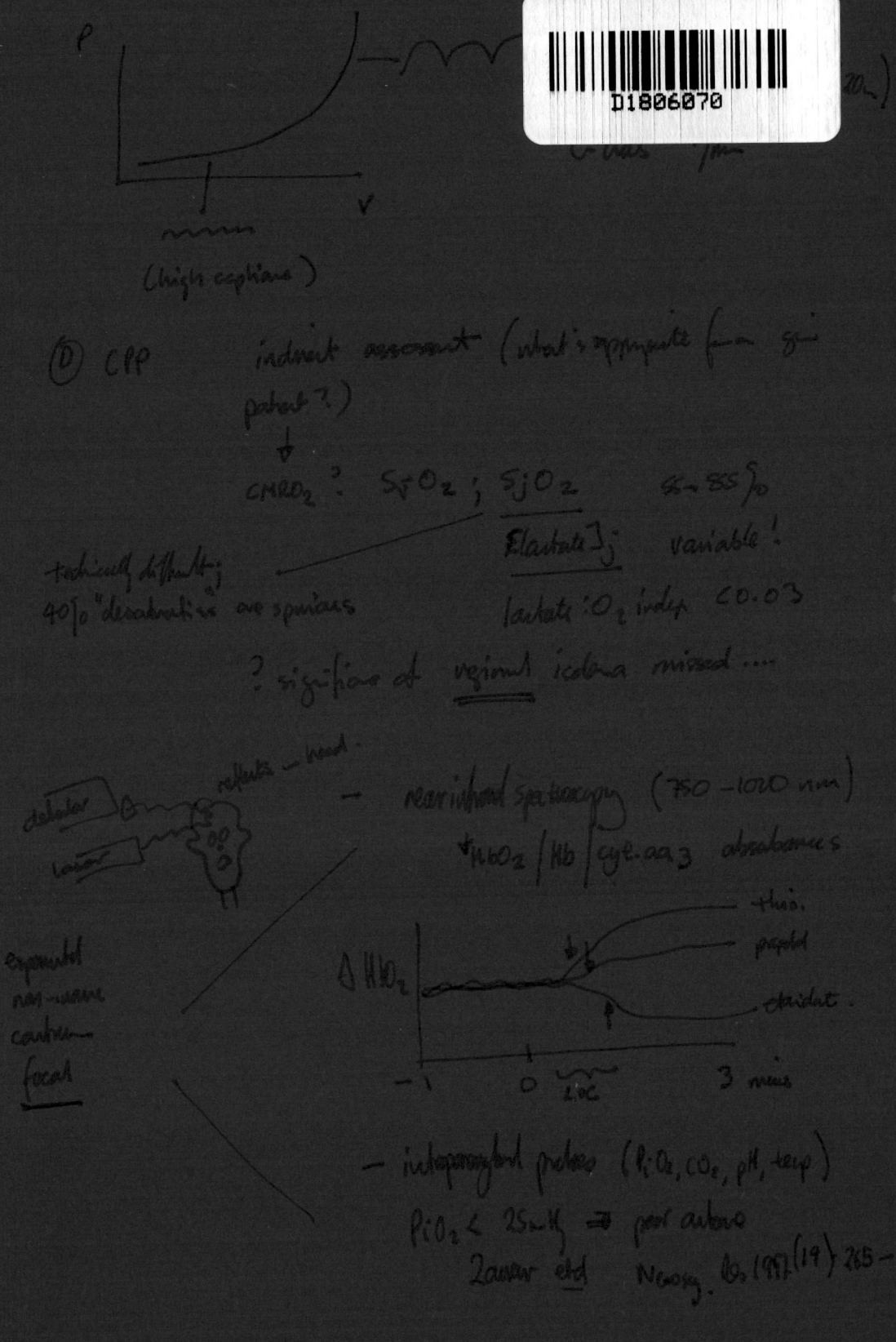

P ... V

(high capitare)

① CPP   indirect assessment (what's appropriate for a given patient?)
↓
$CMRO_2$? SvO_2 ; SjO_2 $\approx$ 55 %

technically difficult;
40% "desaturations are spurious"   [lactate]$_j$ variable!

lactate : O_2 index < 0.03

? significance of regional ischaemia missed ....

detector — reflects — head.

emitter

— near infrared spectroscopy (750 – 1020 nm)
  HbO_2 / Hb / cyt.aa$_3$ absorbances

experimental
non-invasive
continuous
focal

ΔHbO_2 ischaemia
                        normal
                        desiderata.

-1 0   3 mins
        Δ°C

— intraparenchymal probes (P_iO_2, CO_2, pH, temp)
  P_iO_2 < 25 mmHg ⇒ poor outcome
  Zauner et al   Neurol. Res 1997 (19) 265 —

Anaesthesia
and Intensive Care for the
Neurosurgical Patient

Dedicated to our families,
for their forbearance

Anaesthesia and Intensive Care for the Neurosurgical Patient

EDITED BY

FRANK J. M. WALTERS

FRCA
Department of Anaesthesia
Frenchay Hospital
Bristol

G. STUART INGRAM

FRCA
Department of Anaesthesia
The National Hospital for
Neurology and Neurosurgery
London

JIM L. JENKINSON

FRCA
Department of Anaesthesia,
Western General Hospital
Edinburgh

FOREWORD BY

SHEILA M. WILLATTS

SECOND EDITION

OXFORD

BLACKWELL SCIENTIFIC PUBLICATIONS

LONDON EDINBURGH BOSTON

MELBOURNE PARIS BERLIN VIENNA

© 1986, 1994 by
Blackwell Scientific Publications
Editorial Offices:
Osney Mead, Oxford OX2 0EL
25 John Street, London WC1N 2BL
23 Ainslie Place, Edinburgh EH3 6AJ
238 Main Street, Cambridge
   Massachusetts 02142, USA
54 University Street, Carlton
   Victoria 3053, Australia

Other Editorial Offices:
Librairie Arnette SA
1, rue de Lille
75007 Paris
France

Blackwell Wissenschafts-Verlag GmbH
Düsseldorfer Str. 38
D-10707 Berlin
Germany

Blackwell MZV
Feldgasse 13
A-1238 Wien
Austria

First published 1986
Second edition 1994

Set by Setrite Typesetters, Hong Kong
Printed and bound in Great Britain
at the University Press, Cambridge

DISTRIBUTORS

Marston Book Services Ltd
PO Box 87, Oxford OX2 0DT
(*Orders*: Tel: 0865 791155
         Fax: 0865 791927
         Telex: 837515)

USA
Blackwell Scientific Publications, Inc.
238 Main Street
Cambridge, MA 02142
(*Orders*: Tel: 800 759-6102
           617 876-7000)

Canada
Times Mirror Professional Publishing, Ltd
130 Flaska Drive
Markham, Ontario L6G 1B8
(*Orders*: Tel: 800 268-4178
           416 470-6739)

Australia
Blackwell Scientific Publications Pty Ltd
54 University Street
Carlton, Victoria 3053
(*Orders*: Tel: 03 347-5552)

A catalogue record for this title
is available from the British Library

ISBN 0-632-03715-6

Library of Congress
Cataloging in Publication Data

Anaesthesia and intensive care
   for the neurosurgical patient.—2nd ed./
edited by Frank J.M. Walters, Stuart Ingram,
Jim Jenkinson; foreword by Sheila M. Willatts.
      p.   cm.
   Rev. ed of: Anaesthesia and intensive care
for the neurosurgical patient/
Sheila M. Willatts, Frank J.M. Walters.
   Includes bibliographical references
   and index.
   ISBN 0-632-03715-6
   1. Nervous system—Surgery.
   2. Anesthesia in neurology.
   3. Surgical intensive care.
   I. Walters, Frank J.M. II. Ingram, Stuart.
III. Jenkinson, Jim. IV. Willatts, Sheila M.
Anaesthesia and intensive care
for the neurosurgical patient.
   [DNLM: 1 Anesthesia. 2. Intensive
   Care. 3. Nervous System—surgery.
WO 200 A5313 1994]
RD593.A49   1994
617.9'6748—dc20
DNLM/DLC for Library of Congress

Contents

List of contributors

IAN CALDER MB, ChB, DRCOG, FRCA, Department of Anaesthesia, The National Hospital for Neurology and Neurosurgery, Queen Square, London WC1N 3BG

STEVEN CRUICKSHANK MBBS, FRCA, Department of Anaesthesia, Newcastle General Hospital, Westgate Road, Newcastle-upon-Tyne NE4 6BE

MARK DEARDEN MBCHB, FRCA, Department of Anaesthesia, The General Royal Infirmary at Leeds, Great George Street, Leeds LS1 3ER

G. STUART INGRAM MBBS, FRCA, Department of Anaesthesia, The National Hospital for Neurology and Neurosurgery, Queen Square, London WC1N 3BG

JIM L. JENKINSON MB, ChB, FRCA, Department of Anaesthesia, Western General Hospital, Crewe Road, Edinburgh EH4 2XU; Part-time Senior Lecturer in Anaesthesia, University of Edinburgh, Edinburgh EH8 9YL

J.R. DAVID LAYCOCK BM, BCH, MSC, FRCA, Department of Anaesthesia, Southampton General Hospital, Tremona Road, Shirley, Southampton SO9 4XY

ANGELA M. MACKERSIE MB, BS, FRCA, Department of Anaesthesia, The Hospital for Sick Children, Great Ormond Street, London WC1N 3JH

ALEX MANARA MRCP, FRCA, Department of Anaesthesia, Frenchay Hospital, Bristol BS16 1LE

SUSAN MIDGLEY MBCHB, FRCA, Department of Anaesthesia, Victoria Infirmary, Longside, Glasgow G42 9TY

EDWARD MOSS MB, ChB, MD, FRCA, Department of Anaesthesia, The General Royal Infirmary at Leeds, Great George Street, Leeds LS1 3EX

PAUL R. NANDI MRCP, FRCA, Department of Anaesthesia, The National Hospital for Neurology and Neurosurgery, Queen Square, London WC1N 3BG

MIKE NEVIN MD, FRCA, Humphry Davy Department of Anaesthesia, Bristol Royal Infirmary, Marlborough Street, Bristol BS2 8ED

MARTIN SMITH MBBS, FRCA, Department of Anaesthesia, The National Hospital for Neurology and Neurosurgery, Queen Square, London WC1N 3BG

SHEILA M. WILLATTS MRCP, FRCA, Humphry Davy Department of Anaesthesia, Bristol Royal Infirmary, Marlborough Street, Bristol BS2 8ED

FRANK J.M. WALTERS FRCA, Department of Anaesthesia, Frenchay Hospital, Bristol BS16 1LE

Foreword

There can be no doubt that the tremendous advances in neurosurgery and related outcome are in large part attributable to safe, modern anaesthesia and greater understanding of the principles underlying cerebral ischaemia. Advances in cerebral monitoring have led to a change of approach to protecting the damaged brain and it is therefore timely that a second edition of this text has been prepared.

Originally a Bristol book, this second edition is strengthened by having three editors, Frank Walters, Jim Jenkinson and Stuart Ingram, who specialize in neurosurgical anaesthesia and are renowned in the UK for their teaching contributions. Although there is still a local preponderance of authors, a major contribution has been made by experts from all over the country.

The revised format is imaginative and well thought out. It provides an excellent text for those preparing for the FRCA examination as well as those currently practising neurosurgical anaesthesia, who will find in this authoritative book much to stimulate them.

SHEILA M. WILLATTS

Preface to the second edition

As with the first edition we have planned this book so that anaesthetic techniques and problems are described after the scientific fundamentals have been presented. However, by contrast, this edition has been edited by three neuroanaesthetists from different parts of the United Kingdom. We have invited contributors from many centres in addition to our own to draw on the wide range of neuroanaesthetic experience throughout the UK. Authors have been encouraged to include their own views and practice. In new and controversial areas we have incorporated alternative practices where relevant, obtained from enquiries around the country. We have therefore been able to create a textbook of British neuroanaesthetic practice.

The book has been designed as a reference text for trainees preparing for neuroanaesthesia and the final part of the FRCA examination as well as a fuller text for those wishing to specialize and teach in this challenging area of anaesthesia.

FRANK J.M. WALTERS
STUART INGRAM
JIM JENKINSON

Preface to the first edition

The practice of anaesthesia for neurosurgery demands an understanding of the fundamental anatomical, physiological and pharmacological principles governing the brain. Neurosurgery makes specific demands on anaesthetists and surgeons dealing with patients who have particular pathophysiological problems resulting from the disease process. This book aims to introduce the reader to the subject with a detailed review of the basic sciences affecting the brain. The clinical chapters are each begun with a discussion of the pathology and surgical aspects before reviewing the relevant anaesthetic problems.

A clinical textbook has to tread the difficult course between a didactic teaching work and a review which could leave the inexperienced trainee a bit 'at sea'. Therefore we have reviewed the literature, and summarized our own practice, in a way which we hope will be of value to all neurosurgical anaesthetists and their surgical colleagues. This will give the trainee a method with which he can start and new thought for the more experienced practitioner.

SHEILA M. WILLATTS
FRANK J.M. WALTERS

1
Neuroanatomy

SHEILA M. WILLATTS

Introduction

The function of the human nervous system is the acquisition of information about the external environment and its computation to produce integrated responses. The central nervous system (CNS), comprises the brain and spinal cord. The peripheral nervous system comprises 43 pairs of nerves which leave the spinal cord to go to all parts of the body. These contain afferent sensory fibres, conducting impulses to the central nervous system from the periphery and efferent motor fibres conducting in the reverse direction. There are 10 000 million neurones in the CNS, each surrounded by neuroglial cells. Oligodendrocytes form myelin and microglia phagocytose degenerating neurones.

Classification of nerve fibres

In 1943 M.S. Gasser classified nerve fibres in a form which is still useful today.

The sensory system

Detection of mechanical stimuli

Peripheral receptors exist in excitable tissues. Skin receptors can appreciate touch, cold, warmth and pain, and deeper receptors can appreciate pressure and proprioception. There are large numbers of different receptors and end-organs and although end-organs are specialized for one form of sensation, the quality of the sensation does not depend on the stimulus arousing it. Information is transmitted to the CNS by varying the frequency and patterns of action potentials travelling along axons. There is often extensive branching of axons, and single fibres may be said to have a 'peripheral receptive field'.

Table 1.1 Classification of nerve fibres (M.S. Gasser 1943)

Description of nerve fibre	Group		Diameter (in μm)	Conduction velocity (m s^{-1})
Myelinated somatic	A	alpha	20	120
		beta		
		gamma		
		delta	3–4	6–30 (pain fibres)
		epsilon	2	5
Myelinated visceral (preganglionic autonomic)	B		<3	3–15
Unmyelinated somatic	C		<2	0.5–2 (pain fibres)

Adaptation

A sustained, mechanical stimulus produces only a transient response, i.e. there is processing of information at receptor level so that the brain is not constantly informed of an unchanging stimulus. This phenomenon has been highlighted recently during investigations into the perception of breathlessness in asthma. By use of a histamine provocation test for bronchial reactivity, it can be shown that the sensation of dyspnoea was related to pre-existing airflow obstruction (Burdon *et al.* 1982). If resting airflow obstruction was already present patients could tolerate lower forced expiratory volume in 1 s (FEV$_1$) without dyspnoea i.e. breathlessness shows temporal adaptation.

Modalities of cutaneous sensation

There are four main modes of cutaneous sensation; touch, cold, warmth and pain.

Spinal cord pathways

Sensory afferent

Sensory impulses arise in muscles, tendons, joints or by external influences at the skin. Dorsal root sensory ganglia and cranial nerve ganglia comprise

primary neurones whose peripheral processes run from sensory receptors, with spinal nerves, and whose central processes run into the cord.
Some dorsal root fibres, on entering the cord, pass directly to motor
neurones constituting a monosynaptic reflex arc. Others synapse with
cells in the dorsal horn of the grey matter and influence ventral horn
cells on the same side (ipsilateral) by a reflex arc involving several
neurones. The majority, however form synapses with dorsal horn cells,
cells in thoracic nuclei, the base of the dorsal horn or the nuclei gracilis
and cuneatus (second-order sensory neurones).

There are two major sensory systems:

1 The dorsal column, medial lemniscus system which conducts proprioception, fine touch, vibration and some autonomic fibres.

2 The spinothalamic tract which conducts crude touch and pressure in

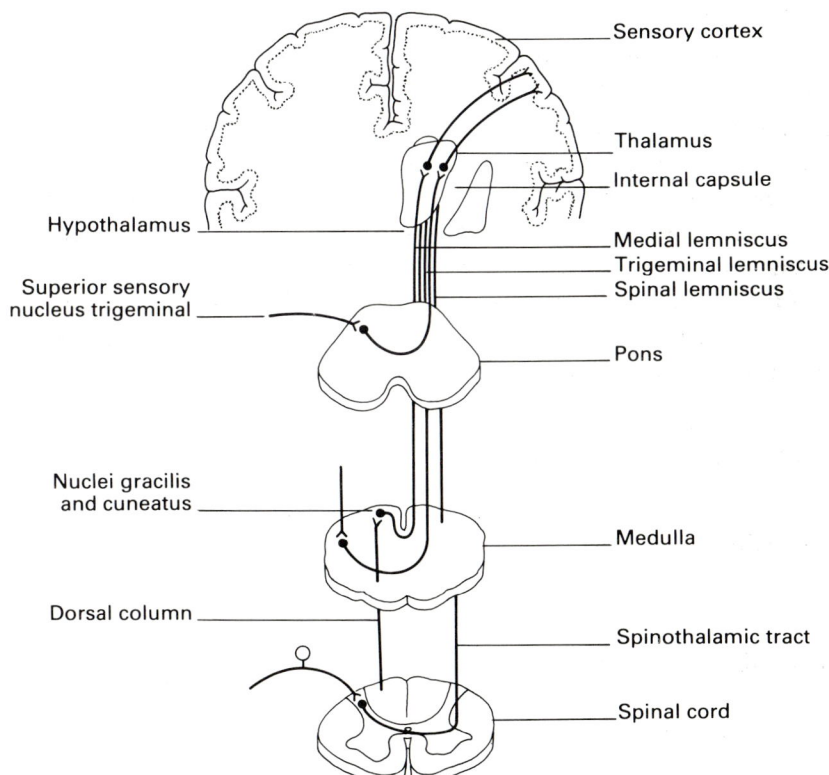

Fig. 1.1 Major somatic afferent pathways.

the anterior spinothalamic tract, and pain and temperature in the lateral spinothalamic tract.

Both these sensory systems decussate (cross over) before they reach the sensory cortex. The dorsal column system decussates in the medulla and the lateral spinothalamic tract crosses close to its site of entry into the cord. In the medulla the two spinothalamic tracts blend to form the spinal lemniscus, which is closely associated with the spinal nucleus of the fifth cranial nerve. In the ventrolateral nucleus of the thalamus sensory fibres synapse with third-order neurones, the fibres of which pass through the posterior end of the internal capsule to the postcentral gyrus of the cerebral cortex. Ultimately therefore somatosensory impulses from one side of the body are represented on the contralateral cerebral cortex only.

There is some central control of sensation. Efferent nerves act at synaptic junctions of the relay nuclei in the ascending pathways, e.g. the dorsal horn, dorsal column and the thalamic nuclei. Such influences may be either facilitatory or inhibitory. The inhibitory mechanism is partly mediated by enkephalins.

The representation of sensation at the postcentral gyrus is shown in Fig. 1.2. Removal of the cerebral cortex results in the thalamus undertaking crude appreciation of sensation. The sensory cortex, however, is responsible for perception of sensation including the full appreciation of

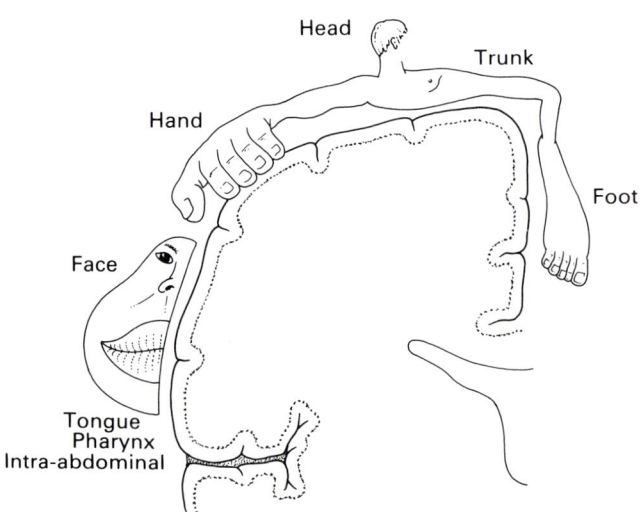

Fig. 1.2 The sensory homunculus.

pain. If this sensory gyrus is completely obliterated, there is impairment but not abolition of sensation, although agnosia and disturbance of body image occur (see below).

Motor efferent

Lower motor neurones (LMN) are those anterior horn cells of the spinal cord grey matter and certain cranial nerve nuclei whose axons innervate voluntary muscle. Upper motor neurones run from the cortex or brainstem to LMNs and comprise the pyramidal and extrapyramidal tracts which are concerned with control of movement.

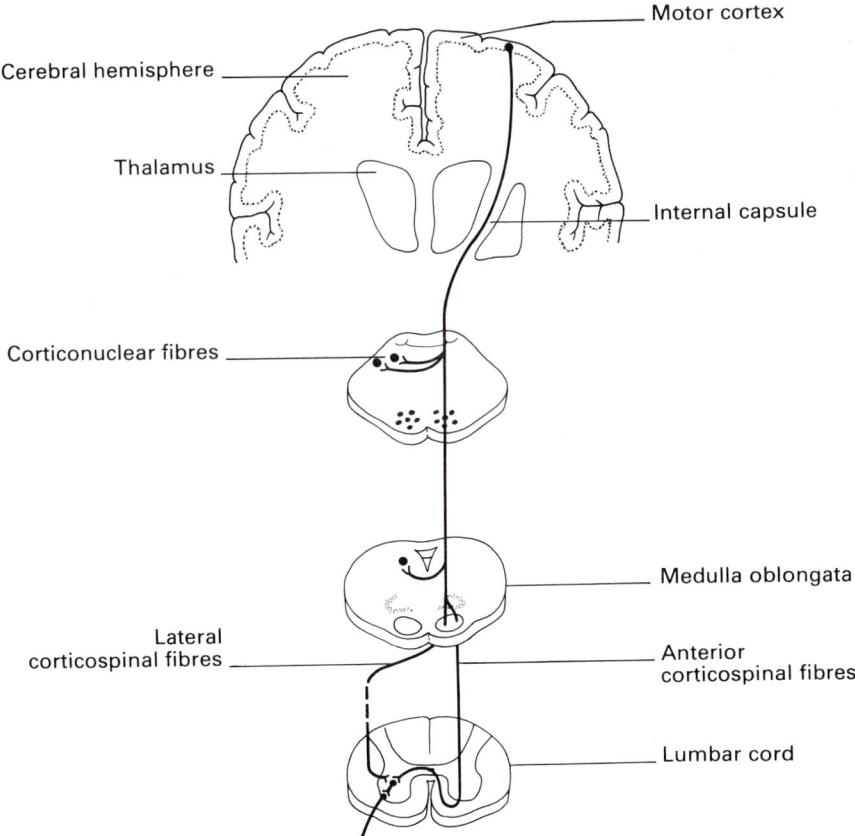

Fig. 1.3 The pyramidal tract.

THE PYRAMIDAL TRACT

This is so named because it forms the pyramid of the medulla. It originates mainly in the precentral gyrus of the cerebral cortex and runs first to cranial nerve nuclei (corticonuclear fibres) and then to the anterior columns of the spinal cord (corticospinal fibres). As these fibres descend from the cortex they traverse the internal capsule in an orderly manner. Most corticonuclear fibres cross the midline in the brainstem terminating in the motor cranial nerve nuclei (third to seventh, ninth and tenth cranial nerves). The main tract, however, then continues through the pons, on the same side, in a dispersed fashion. Fibres then become grouped together in a pyramid on the ventral aspect of the medulla oblongata. In the lower half of the medulla, 90% of fibres cross to the other side to descend in the posterior part of the lateral columns as the lateral pyramidal tract. A few fibres pass down on the same side in the anterior white column as the ventral pyramidal tract. A lesion of pyramidal fibres above the decussation produces a contralateral paralysis of voluntary muscles impairing especially precise movements of the distal aspects of the limbs.

THE EXTRAPYRAMIDAL SYSTEM

This is concerned chiefly with regulation of muscle tone, thus influencing posture and more stereotyped movements. It comprises a series of tracts connecting various areas of the cerebral cortex, subcortical nuclei and brainstem nuclei, thence tracts descend to the lower brainstem and spinal cord to influence LMNs through intermediate neurones.

Descending extrapyramidal tracts include the rubrobulbar and reticulospinal. These accompany the pyramidal tracts to interneurones in the cord. Both systems influence the final common pathways (LMNs) which are also influenced reflexly by sensory impulses.

The net result of extrapyramidal activity is inhibitory, so that lesions in the midbrain nuclei associated with this system may result in increased postural tone and spasticity with uncontrolled tremors or movements. Two other descending pathways influence motor activity: the tectospinal and the vestibulospinal tracts. These two tracts account for the influence of stimuli from the eye and ear on movement. The major ascending and descending tracts in the spinal cord are illustrated in Fig. 1.4.

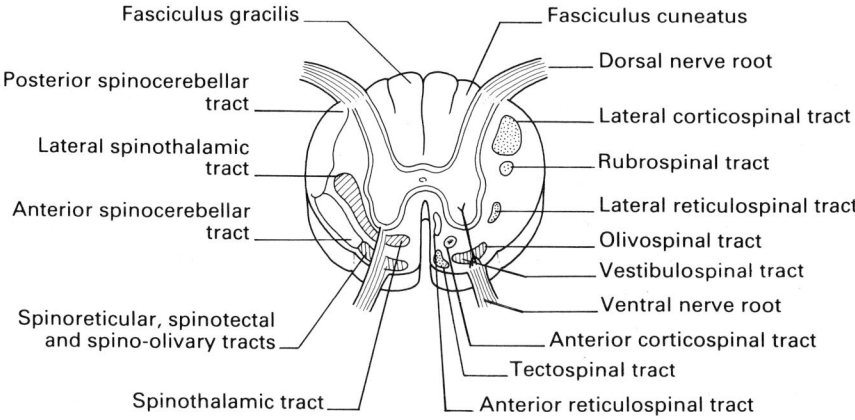

Fig. 1.4 Transverse section of the spinal cord to show major nerve tracts.

Cerebellar pathways

Afferent and efferent pathways traverse the cerebellar peduncles. The afferent pathways contain information from muscle spindles, Golgi tendon organs and other proprioceptors and reach the cerebellum in three main ascending pathways in each half of the spinal cord: the posterior and anterior spinocerebellar tracts and the posterior external arcuate fibres. Efferent fibres from Purkinje cells in the cerebellar cortex ultimately traverse the superior cerebellar peduncles and cross to the opposite side in the lower half of the midbrain, ending mainly in the contralateral red nucleus. They project thence to the cerebral cortex, brainstem, reticular, vestibular and other nuclei.

Autonomic pathways

The autonomic system supplies smooth muscle. It may be divided into sympathetic and parasympathetic, as shown in Fig. 1.5.

THE SYMPATHETIC SYSTEM

This is a two-neurone system. Preganglionic sympathetic efferent fibres have their cells of origin in the lateral horns of the grey matter in segments T1−L2 and fibres leave the cord with motor nerves to voluntary muscle via their ventral nerve root.

Preganglionic fibres generally run to the sympathetic trunk which

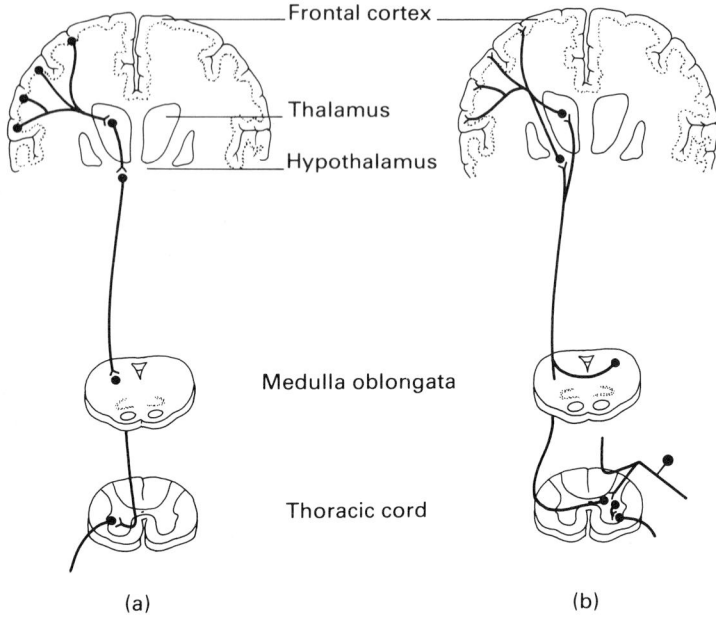

Frontal cortex

Thalamus

Hypothalamus

Medulla oblongata

Thoracic cord

(a)   (b)

Fig. 1.5 The sympathetic and parasympathetic nervous system.

lies a few centimetres from the vertebral column on each side of the spinal cord, running laterally from the level of the superior cervical ganglion downwards and thence to the pelvis. Postganglionic fibres arise from these ganglia and usually join spinal nerves; those to the head accompany the carotid artery.

Sympathetic fibres to the gut, however, do not relay in the sympathetic trunk, but in midline ganglia in front of the aorta (coeliac, superior and inferior mesenteric plexus).

THE PARASYMPATHETIC SYSTEM

This comprises a craniosacral outflow via the third, seventh, ninth and tenth cranial nerves and S2−S4. Postganglionic fibres are usually very short and may lie on the organ concerned. The functions of the parasympathetic system usually oppose those of sympathetic activity, although sweat glands contain sympathetic fibres only, which release acetylcholine and are blocked by atropine.

Central representation

Integration of autonomic and somatic activity maintains normal homeostasis, i.e. stable internal conditions despite a changing environment. This system is concerned with basic physiological functions such as cardiovascular control. CNS areas concerned with autonomic activity include nuclei in the hypothalamus around the third ventricle, a so-called vital centre which includes the supraoptic, paraventricular, dorsal and ventral medial hypothalamic, posterior hypothalamic and mamillary nuclei. The other vital centre lies within the medulla in the posterior fossa (see below). There is therefore close association with the frontal lobes and the posterior pituitary. The hippocampal circuit (hippocampus, fornix, mamillary body, anterior thalamic nuclei, cingulate gyrus, hippocampus) represents a continuous relationship between the cortex, thalamus and hippocampus, and is influenced by ascending pathways from the spinal cord and brainstem and by descending pathways from the cortex. This area is involved in emotional reactions which are often the result of somatic and emotional interactions (nausea, flushing) and with memory. The hypothalamus is also important in temperature regulation, the sleep/wake rhythm, endocrine and cardiovascular systems. Autonomic afferent fibres ascend through the cord and brainstem alongside somatosensory pathways to the hypothalamus, which acts as a relaying and redistribution centre, from which impulses are projected onwards to the thalamus and frontal cortex. Transmission of received information into action such as skeletal and cardiac muscle activation will not be considered.

Cranial nerves

These are situated on the base of the brain (Figs 1.6 and 1.7).

The *first cranial nerve*, the olfactory nerve, is a special visceral, afferent nerve, conveying impulses from the olfactory area of the nasal mucous membrane which traverses the cribriform plate of the ethmoid to the olfactory bulbs on the orbital surface of the frontal lobe.

The *second cranial nerve*, the optic nerve, is a special sensory afferent nerve carrying visual impulses from the retina back to the optic chiasma. An increase in cerebrospinal fluid (CSF) pressure will produce papilloedema within hours because this nerve is covered with a dural and arachnoid sheath, so that the subarachnoid space extends to the eyeball.

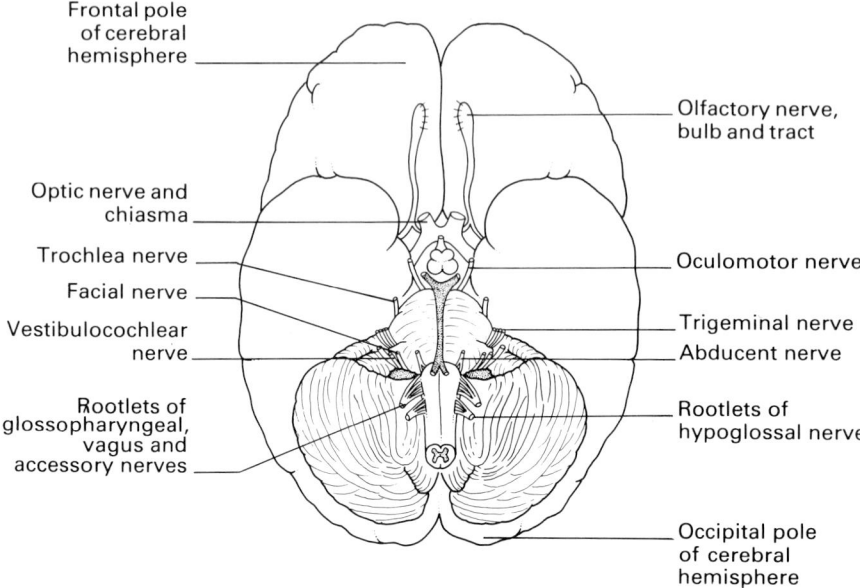

Fig. 1.6 Anatomical position of cranial nerves on the base of the brain.

Prolonged pressure on the optic nerve, for a period of weeks to months, produces optic atrophy. Vision may be tested by confrontation testing and the disc examined by fundoscopy.

The *third nerve*, the oculomotor, is a sensory afferent and efferent nerve and is the most important nerve concerned with the motor supply to the extrinsic and intrinsic eye muscles. Raised intracranial pressure (ICP) and tentorial herniation will dilate the pupil on the affected side.

The *fourth cranial nerve*, the trochlear, is a sensory afferent and efferent nerve and the only cranial nerve to arise from the dorsal aspect of the brainstem. It supplies the superior oblique muscle.

The *fifth nerve*, the trigeminal nerve, is a sensory afferent concerned with facial sensation, and a special visceral efferent nerve which supplies the muscles of mastication. Its cutaneous distribution is of great clinical importance for the localization of trigeminal neuralgia (Fig. 1.8). This nerve may be involved in a tumour such as an acoustic neuroma arising in the cerebellopontine angle along with involvement of the seventh and eighth cranial nerves.

The *sixth nerve*, the abducent, is a somatic afferent and efferent nerve supplying the lateral rectus muscle. It has the longest intracranial course

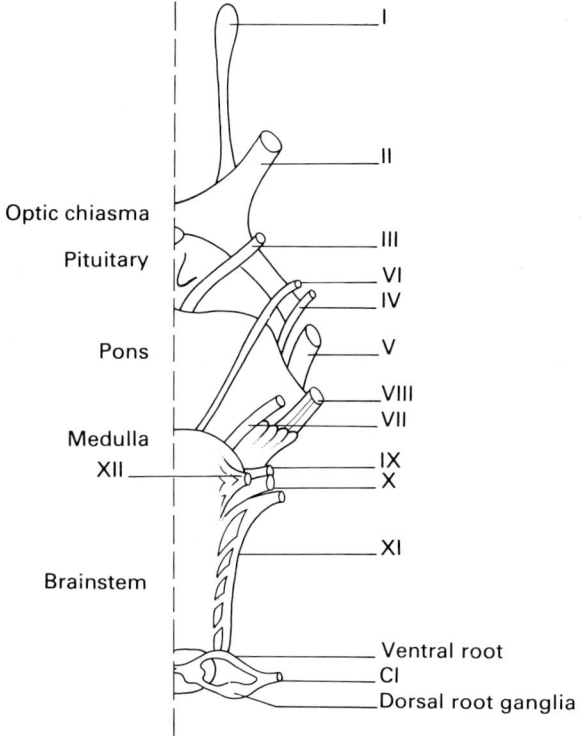

Optic chiasma

Pituitary

Pons

Medulla

XII

Brainstem

I

II

III

VI

IV

V

VIII

VII

IX

X

XI

Ventral root

CI

Dorsal root ganglia

Fig. 1.7 Relative position of cranial nerves.

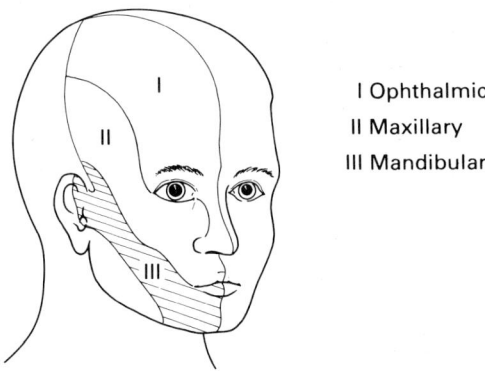

I Ophthalmic

II Maxillary

III Mandibular

Fig. 1.8 Cutaneous divisions of the fifth nerve.

and may be damaged in conditions producing a generalized rise in intracranial pressure, thereby creating a false localizing sign. The third, fourth and sixth nerves can be tested by comparing eye movements and examining for ptosis and diplopia.

The *seventh cranial nerve*, the facial, is a general and special visceral afferent and efferent nerve which forms the main motor supply to the face. Clinical testing involves requesting the patient to smile and raise the eyebrows, and testing for taste on the anterior two-thirds of the tongue.

The *eighth cranial nerve*, the auditory, is a special afferent nerve concerned with hearing and equilibrium, which may be tested by audiometry and caloric testing.

The *ninth cranial nerve*, the glossopharyngeal, is a general and special visceral afferent and efferent nerve which subserves one-third of taste and provides the motor supply to the pharynx.

The *tenth cranial nerve*, the vagus, supplies most motor and sensory modalities; it is the major motor nerve to the viscera, palate and vocal cords. Examination should include palatal movement, vocal and coughing ability.

The *eleventh cranial nerve*, the spinal accessory, is a general and special visceral efferent which supplies the sternomastoid and upper part of the trapezius muscle.

The *twelfth cranial nerve*, the hypoglossal, is a general somatic afferent and efferent nerve which is the motor nerve to the tongue. Examination should include inspection of the tongue for wasting, weakness and fasciculation.

Due to the close proximity of the last four cranial nerves, they may be involved together by pathology in the posterior fossa, producing a weak hoarse voice, nasal speech, difficulty in swallowing and regurgitation with production of an aspiration pneumonia. This constitutes a bulbar palsy and the airway should be protected.

Reports of cranial nerve dysfunction due to vascular compression are increasing (Janetta *et al*. 1984). Nerves most commonly involved are the fifth, seventh and eighth. Hypo- or hyperfunction of the affected nerve may result with classical tic doloreaux if the fifth nerve is affected.

Brainstem and midbrain function

The brainstem is that area of the brain which runs between the spinal cord and the midbrain. It is therefore infratentorial and limited inferiorly

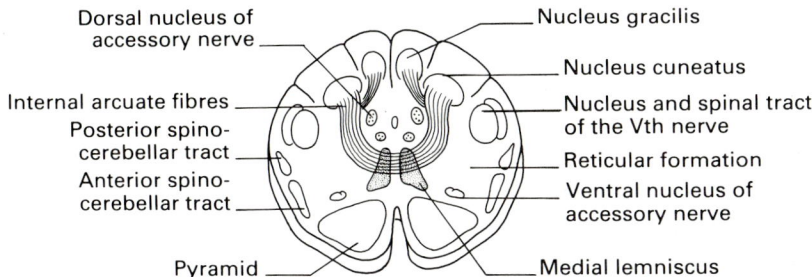

Dorsal nucleus of
accessory nerve

Internal arcuate fibres

Posterior spino-
cerebellar tract

Anterior spino-
cerebellar tract

Pyramid

Nucleus gracilis

Nucleus cuneatus

Nucleus and spinal tract
of the Vth nerve

Reticular formation

Ventral nucleus of
accessory nerve

Medial lemniscus

Fig. 1.9 Transverse section of the medulla at the level of the sensory decussation.

by the foramen magnum. The functions of the brainstem have been highlighted in recent years by the concept of brainstem death. An understanding of the functions requires some knowledge of the anatomy of the area. The medulla and the pons lie between the spinal cord and midbrain.

Medulla

1 Motor pathways are situated ventrally and comprise the corticospinal fibres. They traverse the internal capsule via the genu and are medially situated in the cerebral peduncle. Some cross the midline to supply the relevant cranial motor nerves of the opposite side. The remainder continue on the same side innervating the fifth and seventh cranial nerves. The motor nucleus of the fifth nerve, controlling the muscles of mastication, derives only half its innervation from the opposite hemisphere. The seventh nerve has similar innervation for the forehead muscles, but the muscles of the lower face are mainly innervated by crossed fibres. This has some clinical importance in that an upper motor neurone lesion of the facial nerve will cause total paralysis of the lower facial muscles but the upper facial muscles can still be moved owing to the bilateral innervation. Lower motor neurone lesions below the nucleus, on the other hand, cause complete paralysis of the muscles on one side.

Cranial nerve nuclei are situated in the dorsal area of the medulla.
2 Sensory pathways constitute the intermediate layer of the brainstem. The gracile and cuneate nuclei which arise from dorsal column sensory pathways are situated in the dorsal medulla. The spinothalamic tract is closely associated with descending sympathetic pathways.

The trigeminal sensory system is very complex. Information from one side of the face enters the brainstem in the fifth nerve at the level of the pons. Fibres concerned with the corneal reflex and touch decussate to run contralaterally. Pain and temperature fibres descend parallel to the descending nucleus of the fifth nerve, then relay to the opposite side in the lower medulla and become the secondary ascending tract of the fifth nerve adjacent to the medial lemniscus.

3 The brainstem contains cranial nerve nuclei of the third to the twelfth cranial nerves.

4 The brainstem controls respiration, heart rate and blood pressure. Within the medulla are the other so-called vital centres, which are groups of neurones in the floor of the fourth ventricle concerned with the automatic reflex control of the heart, lungs and circulation. This is further discussed in Chapter 9. Afferent fibres which originate in highly specialized visceral receptors, such as the carotid sinus and in receptor cells within the medulla itself, are responsive to changes in $Paco_2$. Swallowing, coughing and vomiting are also integrated in the medulla.

5 The fourth ventricle is situated within the brainstem in a dorsal position and connects with the third ventricle through the aqueduct of Sylvius.

Pons

The pons is situated above the medulla. A major feature of the pons is its peduncular connections. The medial lemniscus is the continuation upwards of the dorsal column sensory system.

Midbrain

This lies between the cerebrum and the pons, and contains the cerebral peduncles and the tectum. The aqueduct through the middle of the

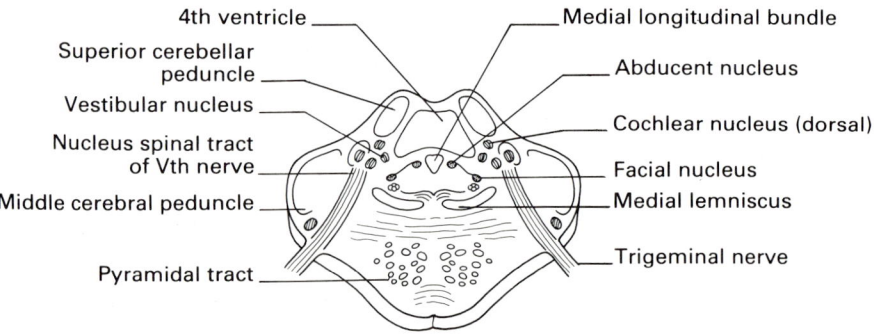

Fig. 1.10 Transverse section of the pons.

midbrain connects the third and fourth ventricles. The tectum contains the colliculi and receives some retinal fibres via the optic nerves, descending fibres from the optic cortex and ascending fibres from the cord.

The midbrain is responsible for coordination of input from the auditory areas of the temporal cortex and the cervical cord. The colliculi are also responsible for visual, auditory and vestibular reflexes.

The cerebral peduncles consist of a ventral aspect which becomes continuous with the internal capsule, the substantia nigra and a dorsal tegmentum. The corticonuclear, corticospinal and corticopontine fibres traverse the ventral aspect. The periaqueductal grey matter contains nuclei of the third and fourth cranial nerves and the mesencephalic nucleus of the fifth nerve. The red nucleus — which is an important relay station in pathways between cerebellum, corpus striatum and the spinal cord — is situated in the tegmentum.

The reticular formation

This constitutes the central core of the brainstem, projecting widely to the limbic system and cortex with many descending and ascending connections. Stimulation activates the cortex initiating an arousal reaction. This area is therefore responsible for generating the *capacity for consciousness*. This area is depressed in lesions of the pineal and somnolence results. Attention and circadian rhythms are also dependent upon the correct functioning of the reticular formation.

Common pathologies in the brainstem are vascular disturbances resulting in infarction, demyelination and tumour. The anatomical diagnosis of a brainstem lesion is not usually difficult, but frequently these lesions are untreatable.

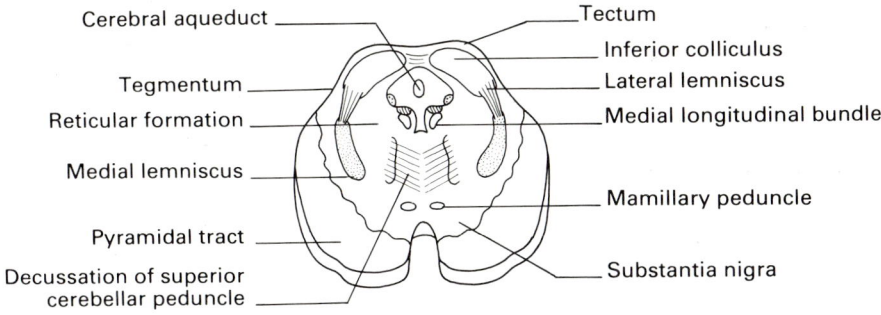

Fig. 1.11 Transverse section of the midbrain at the level of the inferior colliculi.

1 Bilateral medullary paramedial basal infarction results in a mute quadriplegic patient with impaired sensation over the whole body. This is the locked-in syndrome in which the patient is fully conscious but unable to communicate.

2 Intracranial haemorrhage into the pons produces unconsciousness, periodic respiration, pinpoint pupils, loss of reflex eye movement and a spastic quadriplegia which usually rapidly results in death, often accompanied by a rise in temperature to as much as 42°C.

Acute haemorrhage elsewhere in the brain, such as the cerebellum, may produce brainstem distortion.

The cerebral cortex

The surface anatomy of the cerebral cortex with its underlying functions is illustrated in Fig. 1.12.

The dominant hemisphere is that opposite the dominant hand for right-handed individuals, but is variable for left-handed ones. If the dominant hemisphere is destroyed early in life then the other can slowly but incompletely take over intellectual functions. The cerebral cortex is concerned with higher intellectual functions such as memory, learning and language. In the human there are three major association areas:

1 The frontal in front of the motor cortex.

2 The temporal between the superior temporal gyrus and limbic cortex.

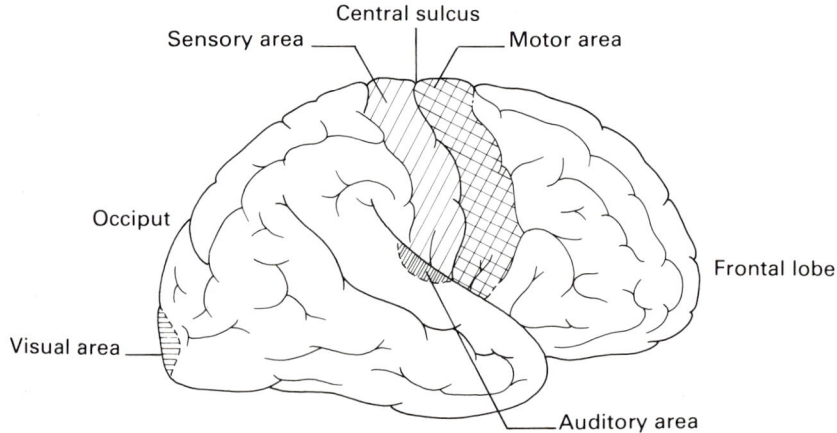

Fig. 1.12 Lateral aspect of the cerebral cortex.

3 The parieto-occipital between the sensory and visual cortex.
These areas have complex connections from the thalamus to each other
and the deeper cortex.

Language function

This involves understanding the written and spoken word and expression
of ideas, both written and oral. Abnormalities may occur with lesions
around the superior temporal sulcus and midfrontal regions. Those which
are not due to defects of vision, hearing or motor paralysis are called
dysphasias. Sensory or receptive dysphasia and motor or expressive
dysphasia are described. In a severe form of dysphasia the patient can
say only two or three words; often automatic words, such as days of the
week or swear-words.

A lesion in the parietal lobe area may lead to inability to recognize
the contralateral side of the body, the existence of which is often denied.
Astereognosis is inability to recognize an object by feel, and may occur
with lesions of either parietal lobe. Sensory loss or sensory inattention
may be associated with a hemianopia.

Ablation of the frontal lobes produces little change in intelligence but
clinical prefrontal leucotomy for severe obsessional delusions does relieve
tension by making the subject unconcerned. Unfortunately, lack of
concern tends to affect social integration and personal habits. There may
be striking memory impairment with dementia accompanied by fitting.
Bilateral hippocampal damage causes recent memory impairment. There
may be sudden attacks of altered behaviour. The temporal lobes contain
the central representation for taste and smell, and it is not uncommon
for temporal lobe epilepsy to be preceded by an aura which includes
taste or smell.

Lesions in the occipital lobes will produce a central abnormality of
vision. Extensive lesions in some areas of the cerebral cortex may produce
very little deficit, but a small lesion in the dominant hemisphere may
have a devastating effect on speech. Lesions such as tumours, in addition to
local signs and symptoms, may produce problems due to raised ICP,
cerebral oedema and displacement of the brain. However, non-specific
features are very common with impaired memory, lack of concentration,
irritability, loss of motor skills and inappropriate behaviour. In the elucidation of any defect, great care should be taken to distinguish between a
speech difficulty and simple confusion.

Cerebrospinal fluid (CSF)

CSF is formed by secretory cells of the choroid plexus with project into the lateral and third ventricles.

Fluid then traverses the third ventricle in the pons, passes through the aqueduct to the fourth ventricle to escape by two lateral foraminae of Luschka and the medial foramen of Magendie into the subarachnoid space around the brain and spinal cord. Large collections of CSF are called cisterns.

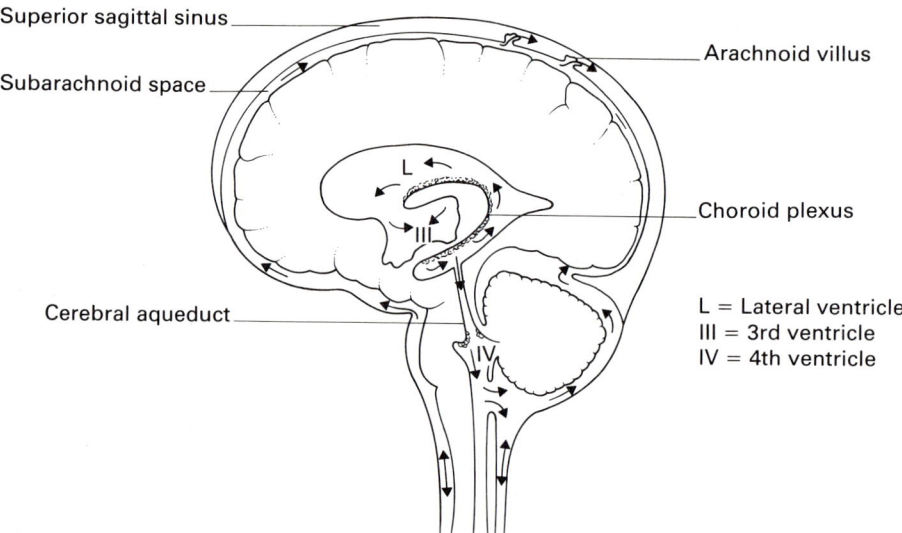

Fig. 1.13 The circulation of CSF.

Table 1.2 Comparison of plasma and cerebrospinal fluid

	Blood plasma (mmol l^{-1})	Cerebrospinal fluid (mmol l^{-1})
Urea	2.5−6.5	2.0−7.0
Glucose (fasting)	3.0−5.0	2.5−4.5
Sodium	136−148	144−152
Potassium	3.8−5.0	2.0−3.0
Calcium	2.2−2.6	1.1−1.3
Chloride	95−105	123−128
Bicarbonate	24−32	24−32
Protein	60−80 g l^{-1}	200−400 mg l^{-1}

CSF is produced at approximately $0.5\,\mathrm{ml\,min^{-1}}$. Its total volume is 150 ml. It is therefore exchanged once approximately every 4 h. Production must match absorption normally because there is no rise in pressure. Obstruction to the flow of CSF increases pressure with dilatation of the ventricles upstream from the obstruction.

Resorption is mainly into the venous system via arachnoid villi, which are areas where the arachnoid space invaginates into large venous sinuses. If the CSF pressure is less than venous pressure then the villi collapse. Some CSF is also probably absorbed around spinal nerves into spinal veins and through the ependymal lining of the ventricles.

CSF is a clear, colourless liquid of specific gravity 1005, with less than five lymphocytes per millilitre and pH 7.33.

CSF is probably produced from plasma by a combination of secretion and ultrafiltration. The high concentration of chloride occurs because carbon dioxide passes into glial cells where, by the action of carbonic anhydrase, it is hydrated to carbonic acid (H_2CO_3). Resulting bicarbonate ions (HCO_3^-) are then exchanged for chloride which passes into CSF against its concentration gradient. CSF is slightly hypertonic; sodium and magnesium ions are actively transported into it. Lipophilic substances readily pass from the blood to the brain but ionized hydrophilic substances pass only very slowly.

CSF acts as a cushion between the skull and the brain. It can accommodate a certain degree of change in brain volume by being displaced into the lumbar region. In conditions which produce cerebral atrophy there is an increase in CSF volume.

Solutes at higher concentration in the brain extracellular fluid diffuse into CSF and are carried into the blood at the arachnoid villi. Some substances are transported actively by cells of the choroid plexus from CSF into blood.

Electrophoresis of CSF proteins is now possible. CSF contains proteins which are partly derived by filtration of plasma, partly from brain interstitial fluid and brain cells and partly from cells of the CSF compartment itself. These proteins may reflect abnormalities of the filtration mechanism, of barrier function, brain metabolism and activities of the CSF. Electrophoresis has clinical application for investigation of certain neurological conditions such as multiple sclerosis, Guillain—Barré syndrome and neurosyphilis (Thompson & Johnson 1982).

The resting level of CSF pressure is $5-13\,\mathrm{mmHg}$ and represents the balance between production and resorption. Fluctuations in CSF pressure coincide with arterial pressure and respiration. Respiratory fluctuations follow changes in intrathoracic pressure and are probably due to transmission via the jugular and vertebral veins. Hydrocephalus results from obstruction of CSF pathways and is discussed in Chapter 13.

Cerebral circulation

The circle of Willis comprises an arterial circle at the base of the brain, supplied by two internal carotid and two vertebral arteries. In humans there is almost no anastomosis between internal and external carotid arteries but stenosis of one supplying vessel to the circle of Willis can be accommodated by an anastomotic collateral flow from other supplies. The branches of these four arteries communicate with each other over the surface of the cortex. Watershed areas between areas of major vessel supply are those most likely to be affected by hypoxia and ischaemia. Venous drainage is into sinuses which also receive CSF from arachnoid villi. Cerebral vessels have a prominent internal elastic lamina but less well-developed muscle coat. The white matter is less vascular than the grey.

Pain

Pain registered by stimulation of the skin has a pricking, itching quality and is well localized. The pain threshold may be increased by distracting

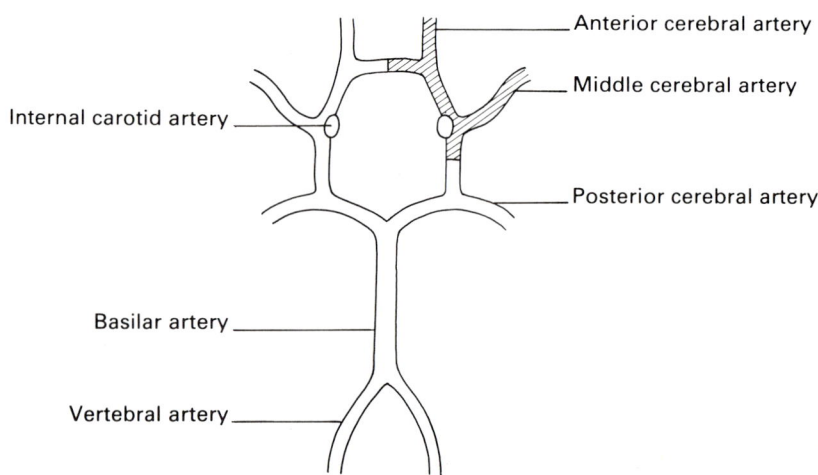

Fig. 1.14 The circle of Willis.

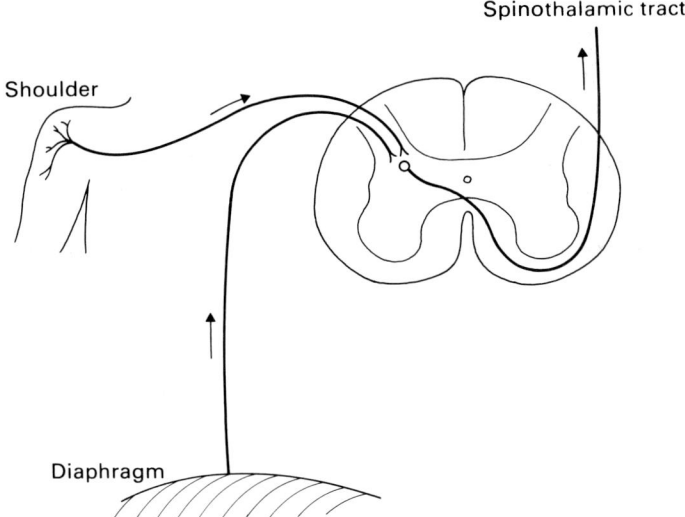

Fig. 1.15 Referred pain. Irritation of the diaphragm is felt in the shoulder tip. Nerves from these areas synapse with common neurones in the spinal cord.

the subject's attention and reduced by half in sunburnt skin. The first sensation of pain arises abruptly and is carried by moderately large fibres conducting impulses at $10 \, \text{m s}^{-1}$. The second sensation is slower and of a burning quality, probably being carried by unmyelinated fibres. Afferent

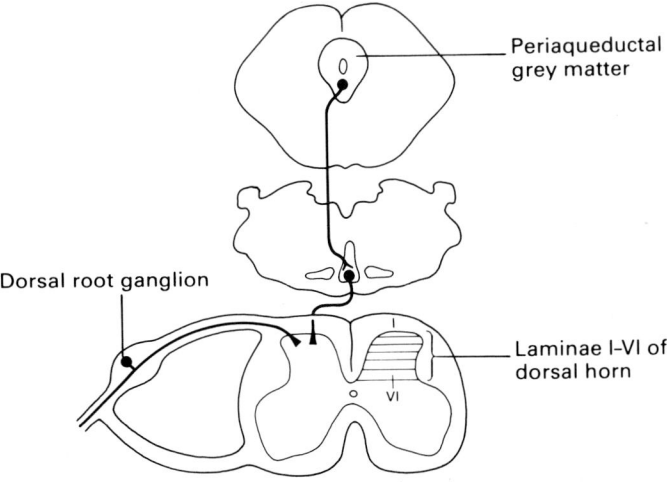

Fig. 1.16 Pain pathways.

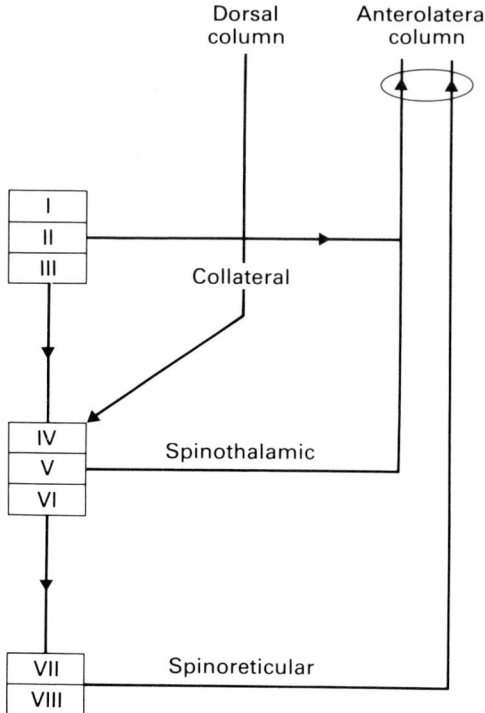

Fig. 1.17 Connections of the Rexed laminae.

sensations from viscera and vessels travel in autonomic nerves (see above) and are projected to a definitive position on the surface of the body; this is relevant when considering referred pain.

    Appreciation of noxious stimuli confers on the individual the ability to protect himself from adverse agents in the environment. Pain is a combination of severe discomfort, fear, autonomic changes, reflex activity and suffering. Nociceptors respond only to stimuli causing tissue damage which give rise to pain.

    Unmyelinated, peripheral, afferent fibres terminate in the substantia gelatinosa of the dorsal horn and smaller myelinated afferents (group 3) terminate in the nucleus proprius (which is lamina V of Rexed) and spinothalamic fibres at this level. Rexed, in 1952, showed that cells of the grey matter of the spinal cord are arranged in nine laminae, I–IX, from the dorsal to the ventral cord, the tenth lamina lying around the central zone.

Lamina I comprises the marginal zone, laminae II and III the substantia gelatinosa and laminae IV, V and VI the nucleus proprius. Small myelinated fibres activated by pinprick and hot and cold receptors terminate there. Lamina IX is the ventral horn and the output from this constitutes the ventral root. Transmission of information in the spinal cord is not one-for-one, but convergence and divergence occur at synapses and there is considerable anatomical variation in ascending tracts such that the response to surgical cordotomy is somewhat unpredicable.

References

Burdon J.G.W., Juniper E.F., Killian K.J., Hargreave F.E. & Campbell E.J.M. (1982) The perception of breathlessness in asthma. *American Review of Respiratory Diseases* **126**, 825−828.

Janetta P.J., Moller M.B. & Moller A.R. (1984) Disabling positional vertigo. *New England Journal of Medicine* **311**, 1053.

Rexed B. (1952) The cytoarchitectonic organisation of the spinal cord in the cat. *Journal of Comparative Neurology* **96**, 415.

Thompson E.J. & Johnson M.H. (1982) Electrophoresis of CSF proteins. *British Journal of Hospital Medicine* **28**, 600−608.

2
Neurophysiology

G. STUART INGRAM

Introduction

Whilst it is a truth universally acknowledged that the practice of rational anaesthesia requires a sound understanding of physiological principles, in neuroanaesthesia, although this maxim stills holds, it should be covered by at least two caveats. The enormous complexity of the brain warns that, important as the principles we currently understand may be, they are but small islands in a great sea of ignorance. In addition the neuro-anaesthetist is more often than not dealing with pathological situations in which the normal neurophysiological mechanisms are deranged. It is important, for instance, to understand the principle of autoregulation of the cerebral blood flow (CBF), but it is equally important to recognize that in many patients undergoing neurosurgery, either due to their pathology or the nature of the surgery, autoregulation has been lost.

Intracranial pressure (ICP)

In the adult the cranium forms an almost rigid container which is in direct communication with the vertebral canal. Normal ICP is 5–13 mmHg and shows small fluctuations related to arterial pulsations and respiration. The intracranial constituents and their relative volumes are shown in Table 2.1.

It is evident that any increase in volume of one constituent must result in either a similar reduction in volume of another or an increase in pressure. Thus a 'space-occupying lesion' within the skull such as a tumour or haematoma will initially be compensated for by the displacement of cerebrospinal fluid (CSF) into the spinal subarachnoid space, the reduction in intracranial blood volume due to the pressure exerted on the thin-walled cerebral veins and the increased reabsorption of CSF (Lofgren & Zwetnow 1973). When the volume increase takes place slowly the CSF changes are paramount, but if it is rapid then the changes

Table 2.1 Intracranial contents

	Volume (ml)	Percentage of total
Glia	700–900 ⎱	70–80
Neurones	500–700 ⎰	
CSF	130–150	10
Blood	100–150	5–10
ECF	<100	

in cerebral blood volume play the major role. As the main factors controlling the cerebral blood volume are similar to those controlling the CBF, during anaesthesia it is the anaesthetist's ability to manipulate the CBF that is crucial, even though, as can be seen in Table 2.1, cerebral blood volume represents a relatively small proportion of the total intra-cranial contents.

Figure 2.1 shows the relationship between cerebral volume and ICP, the initial compensatory phase in which there is increasing brain volume with little change in pressure is indicated by the long flat part of the curve (1–2). Although the ICP rises little in this phase there is a pro-gressive decrease in compliance. Should there be a brief rise in cerebral volume, as may occur with a cough, there will be a corresponding

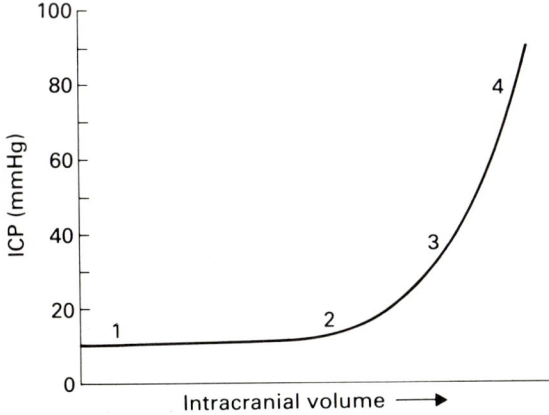

Fig. 2.1 Intracranial volume–pressure relationships: 1–2, compensation phase; 3–4, decompensation phase.

increase in pressure which would appear as a peak superimposed on the main curve. As intracranial compliance falls the magnitude of these peaks will become greater as the patient 'moves' to the right along the curve (Fig. 2.2). Finally with compliance low and the compensatory mechanism exhausted the ICP rises steeply with relatively small rise in volume, illustrated by the steep part of the curve 3–4 (Fig. 2.1).

In the clinical context it is well recognized that slowly developing lesions such as meningiomas are able to exploit the compensatory mechanisms to the full. The result is that they may develop to a very large size with a relatively small increase in ICP. With rapidly growing masses, however, much smaller lesions will cause marked increase in ICP, particularly if there is a significant amount of associated oedema. It is therefore not possible to assess the state of intracranial compliance and ICP merely by looking at the size of an intracranial lesion as shown on a computerized tomography (CT) or magnetic resonance imaging (MRI) scan.

In addition to increases in volume causing changes in ICP along a preset curve, changes in compliance may induce a shift in the curve

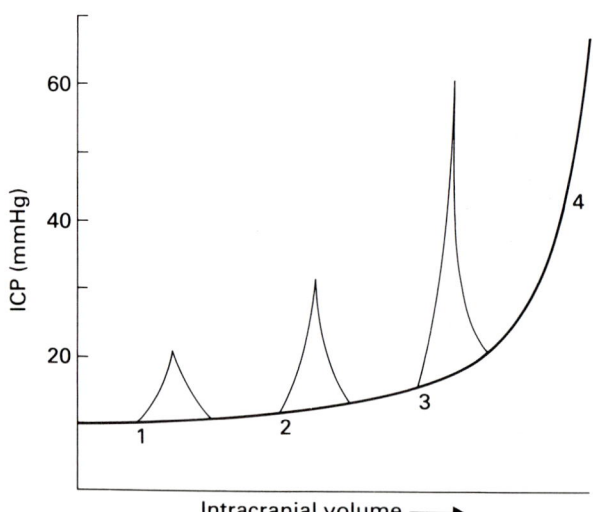

Fig. 2.2 Intracranial volume–pressure curve. As volume expands, compliance is reduced so each additional increment in volume causes a more marked rise in ICP. When ICP baseline is elevated (3) a small increase in intracranial volume will induce a marked surge in ICP.

itself. Thus it is recognized that brain oedema or an intracranial haemorrhage, for instance, will reduce the compliance of the brain as it becomes 'tighter' and move the volume–pressure curve to the left. By contrast steroids and mannitol lower the ICP, but by increasing the compliance of the brain they produce further benefit by moving the curve to the right (Miller & Leech 1975).

Testing compliance

In order to define the state of intracranial compliance and identify the relative position of an individual patient on the volume–pressure curve, volume–pressure response (VPR) testing has been developed. In a patient on ICP monitoring with a ventricular catheter, 1 ml of fluid is injected through the catheter and the increase in ICP noted. This increase in pressure can be used as an index of compliance. The VPR has been used to define the position of a patient on the volume–pressure curve and to predict impending decompensation. But although this and more complex tests have been of value experimentally, they have not as yet established themselves in clinical practice (Miller 1976).

The principal causes of increased ICP are listed below:

INCREASED BRAIN BULK

1 Space-occupying lesion:
   (i) cerebral tumour,
   (ii) intracranial haematoma,
   (iii) cerebral abscess.
2 Cerebral oedema.

INCREASED CSF VOLUME

1 Hydrocephalus.
2 Benign intracranial hypertension.

INCREASED BLOOD VOLUME

1 Increased cerebral blood flow — arterial blood volume:
   (i) hypoxia PaO_2 <60 mmHg
   (ii) hypercarbia $PaCO_2$ >45 mmHg
   (iii) halogenated anaesthetics.

2 Increased cerebral venous blood volume:
   (i) coughing, straining, increasing intrathoracic and intra-abdominal pressure,
   (ii) obstruction to free venous flow in the neck,
   (iii) head-down tilt.

Because the cerebral veins and dural venous sinuses within the cranium connect directly with the large veins in the neck, increases in intrathoracic pressure will therefore be transmitted through the venous system to the intracranial contents, raising ICP.

Coning

Unrelenting cerebral swelling from any cause, as well as raising ICP, will ultimately lead to brain displacement. This herniation typically takes place at the sites shown in Fig. 2.3.

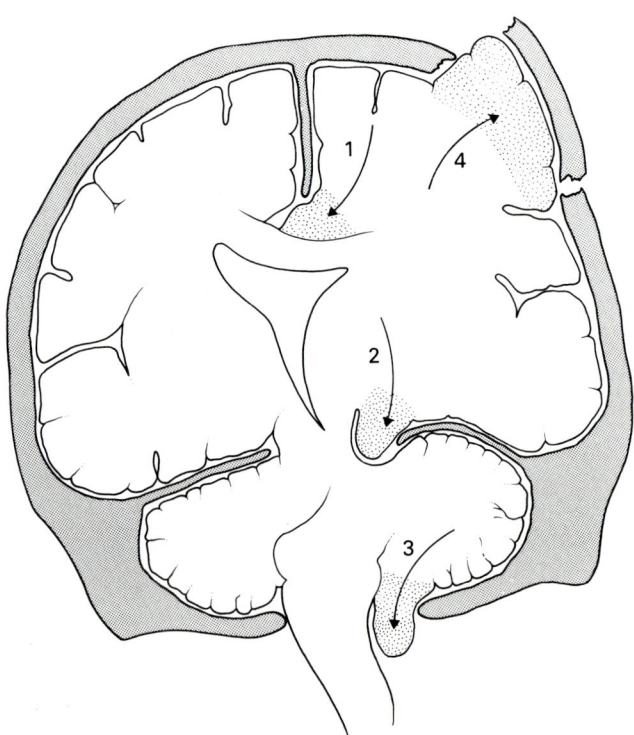

Fig. 2.3 Sites of brain herniation: (1) cingulate (subfalcine), (2) temporal (tentorial), (3) tonsillar or cerebellar (foraminal), (4) transcalvarial. After Fishman (1975).

CINGULATE (SUBFALCINE)

This is displacement of the medial surface of the hemisphere (cingulate gyrus) beneath the falx to the opposite side. Compression of the anterior cerebral artery may occur causing contralateral paralysis in the lower limb.

TEMPORAL (TENTORIAL)

The medial temporal lobe (the uncus) is displaced through the tentorial hiatus and compresses the midbrain, often referred to as temporal coning. The third nerve is compressed, causing pupillary dilatation on the same side. Pressure on the cerebral peduncle initially causes hemiparesis on the opposite side but with further pressure this may become bilateral. Direct pressure on the midbrain leads to fluctuation and deterioration of conscious level. The blood pressure rises and the pulse slows.

TONSILLAR OR CEREBELLAR (FORAMINAL)

This may occur as the final stage of progressive supratentorial swelling or result from a mass in the posterior fossa. If the herniation is limited to the cerebellar tonsils, neck stiffness and torticollis may be the only signs. The latter is a reflex attempt to relieve pressure on the medulla. However, further pressure forcing the cerebellum into the foramen magnum will result in medullary coning. Respiration changes, typically to Cheyne−Stokes or irregular breathing, and this may lead on to apnoea, which may be sudden.

TRANSCALVARIAL

Following a craniotomy or skull fracture herniation can occur through the skull.

The free flow of CSF ensures that normally, with allowance for gravity, pressure is the same throughout the cranium and spinal canal. But once swelling and herniation begin there will be blockage of CSF pathways and pressure gradients can develop. Pressure measurement at lumbar puncture in such situations will produce misleading information, and in addition the leakage of fluid may precipitate medullary coning. There is evidence that, with rapidly rising ICP, pressure differences may also be present transiently between intracranial compartments (Langfitt *et al.* 1964).

Intracranial pressure measurement

Continuous recording of ICP may be carried out in the ventricles, in the subdural space or in the extradural space. Each of these sites has advantages and disadvantages which need to be considered in relation to an individual patient (Dearden 1985).

VENTRICULAR MEASUREMENT

A catheter can be passed from a burr-hole through the brain into a lateral ventricle and a fluid-filled system set up for continuous measurement of ICP. Good-quality recordings can be obtained, and zeroing and calibration can be checked at any time. In addition the catheter makes it possible to withdraw CSF as a means of lowering ICP.

Disadvantages of this method include the risk of haemorrhage in passing the catheter, and of infection; generally a catheter is left in for only 2–3 days as otherwise the risk of infection becomes too great. If the ventricles are small, due to brain swelling, this technique may not be practical due to the difficulty of finding the ventricles, and at high ICP the tip of the catheter can be blocked by swollen brain.

EXTRADURAL MEASUREMENT

Having made a burr-hole, ICP can be measured by inserting a transducer or catheter into the extradural space. With the dura intact the risks posed by infection are greatly reduced, but against this the compliance of the dura may produce errors in measurement.

SUBDURAL MEASUREMENT

To overcome the problem of dural compliance the dura can be divided and a transducer or catheter can be passed into the subdural space; the quality of recording is improved but the risk of infection is once more increased.

When brain swelling is severe, subdural and extradural catheters may become blocked. If a fluid flush is used to clear the catheter this may then result in erroneously high pressures being recorded.

EQUIPMENT

Intraventricular catheters can be connected to pressure transducers via a fluid-filled system as with the measurement of intra-arterial pressure; the external transducer being mounted at the level of the external auditory meatus.

A similar system can also be used to measure extradural or subdural pressure via a 'Richmond' or 'Leeds' bolt. This and similar devices are screwed into a threaded burr-hole in the skull (Fig. 2.4); for subdural measurement the dura is incised when the burr-hole is made. The metal screws currently available may induce artefact on CT scanning and prevent the use of MRI.

A variety of transducers have been developed commercially for insertion through a burr-hole for ICP measurement. Once *in situ* zeroing and calibration cannot be checked and drift may lead to errors. Problems with some earlier designs resulted from the ease with which they were damaged in routine clinical use. The Camino transducer (Camino Laboratories, San Diego, USA) appears to have overcome these problems (Figs 2.5 and 2.6), this narrow fibreoptic catheter can be inserted through a small hole in the skull and pressure is measured from variation in the reflection of light from a diaphragm at its tip (Crutchfield *et al.* 1990).

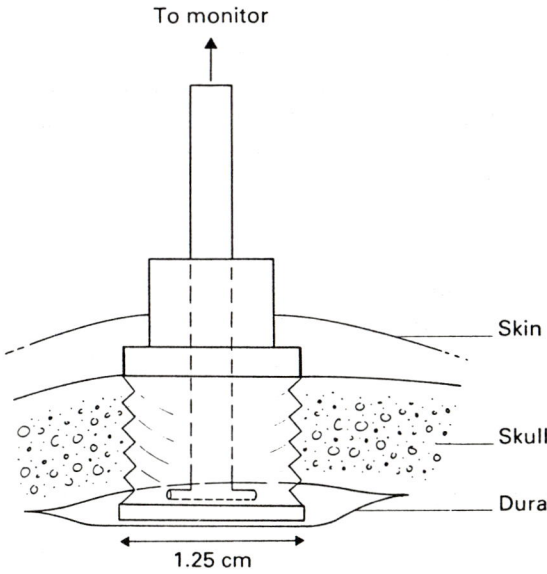

Fig. 2.4 The 'Richmond' bolt.

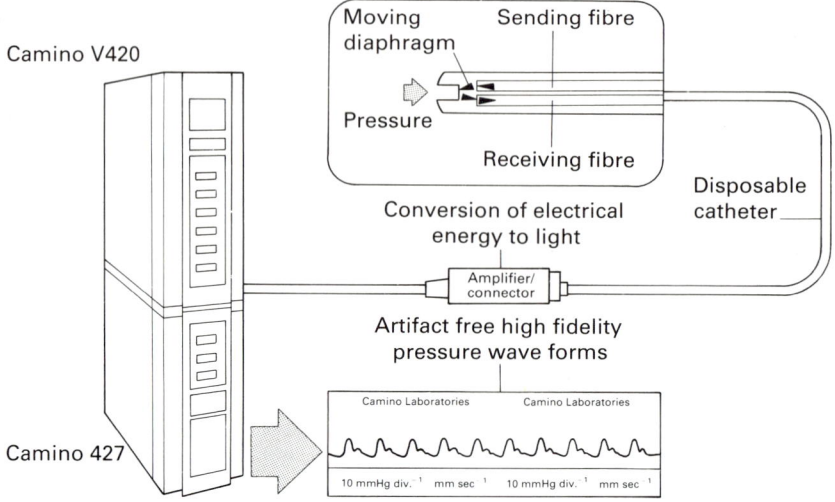

Fig. 2.5 Camino ICP monitor—a basic diagram of the fibreoptic, transducer-tipped, pressure monitoring catheter system.

Lundberg waves

In 1960 Lundberg identified three patterns of ICP fluctuation; they have become known as Lundberg waves (Fig. 2.7). Although descriptively helpful they are part of a spectrum of ICP variation in pathological states.

'A' WAVES

These are large plateau-like waves seen when the baseline ICP is already raised, recurring at intervals of 5−20 min, the ICP rising to 50−100 mmHg. They are generally seen in patients with raised ICP who have large space-occupying lesions. They are associated with transient neurological symptoms and the severity of the symptoms is related to the height of the pressure wave; each episode is followed by some degree of cerebral dysfunction. These waves can be ablated by lowering the baseline ICP, for instance with an infusion of mannitol.

'A' waves are related to intrinsic vasomotor control of the cerebral circulation: a specific event such as an increase in Pa_{CO_2}, a Valsalva manoeuvre or an epileptic fit may precipitate vasodilatation which increases cerebral blood volume and raises ICP in a patient with an already-reduced intracranial compliance. This is followed by a period of vasoconstriction during which ICP may fall below the original baseline.

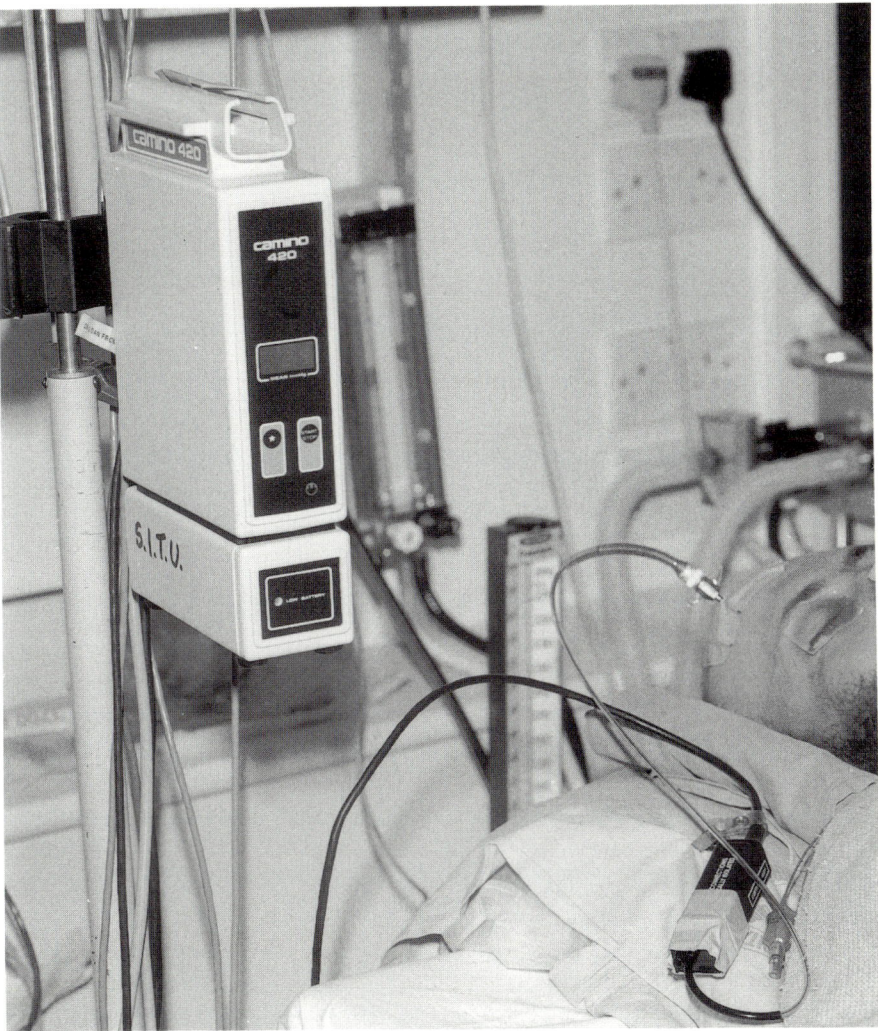

Fig. 2.6 Camino ICP monitor — ICP monitoring in the surgical intensive-care unit.

These waves are particularly sinister as they indicate that the normal compensatory mechanism is virtually exhausted.

'B' WAVES

These are smaller, sharper waves, usually occurring as rhythmic oscillations with a dominating frequency of about $1\,min^{-1}$, with ICP rising to

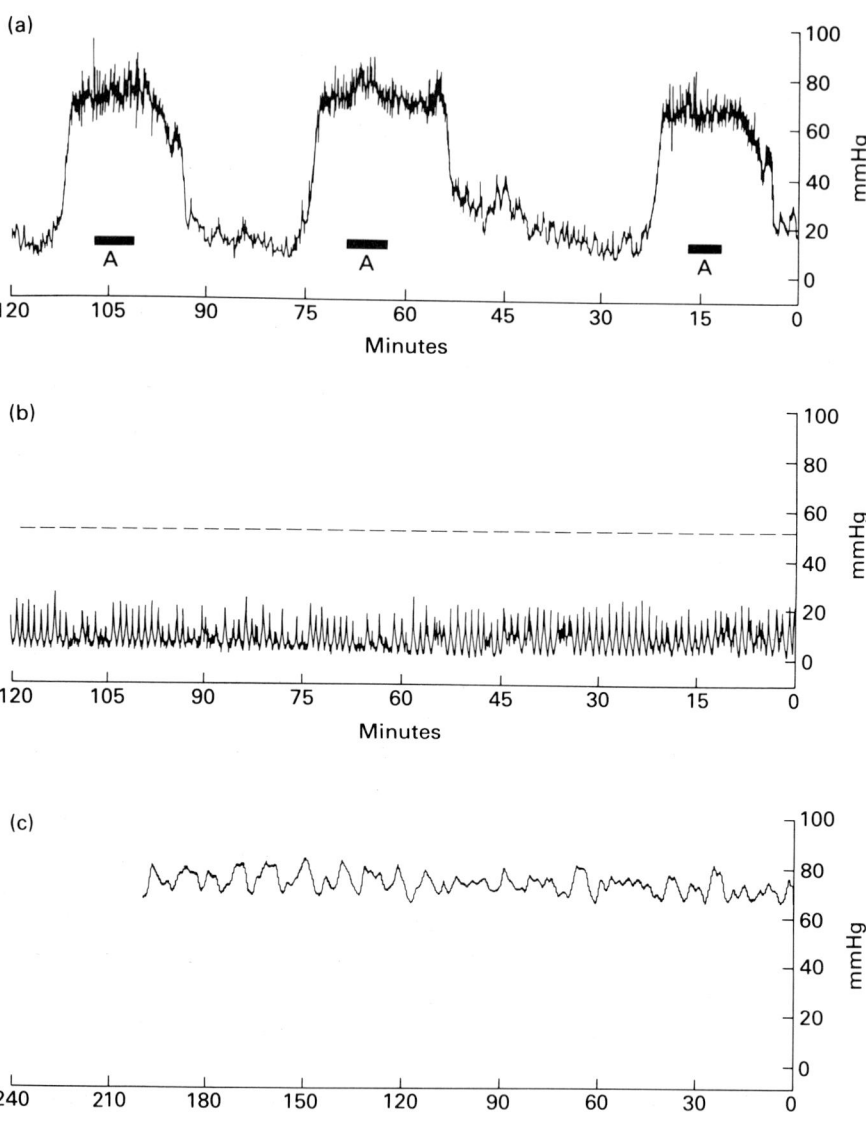

Fig. 2.7 (a) An 'A' wave where the intracranial pressure rises to more than 60 mmHg for 25 min. (b) A 'B' wave peaking at 20 mmHg in a patient with a cerebellar abscess. (c) A 'C' wave superimposed on a raised baseline ICP of 70 mmHg in a patient with a central glioma of the right cerebral hemisphere. The timescale in each example moves from the right-hand side, is in minutes in (a) and (b), and in seconds for (c). From Lundberg (1960).

50 mmHg. These fluctuations in ICP are related to periodic breathing and decreased wakefulness, becoming more marked as conscious level deteriorates. They are due to changes in blood pressure in the cerebral vascular bed and clinically they indicate the presence of functional disorders of the brainstem. Like 'A' waves they indicate failure of the compensatory mechanisms.

'C' WAVES

These are small rhythmic oscillations with a dominating frequency of about $6 \, min^{-1}$, the ICP rising up to 20 mmHg. 'C' waves may be seen superimposed on either the plateau of an 'A' wave or a raised baseline ICP. They are associated with cyclical changes in blood pressure, and although indicative of unstable control of CBF, they also occur in normal patients and are probably of little clinical significance.

Cerebral oedema

The mechanisms by which oedema may develop within the brain have been classified as vasogenic, cytotoxic and interstitial. Although useful particularly in relation to choice of therapy, in the clinical situation cerebral oedema is typically a combination of vasogenic and cytotoxic (Fishman 1975).

Vasogenic oedema This results from a failure of capillary permeability as occurs when the blood−brain barrier is disrupted. Plasma proteins leak into the brain parenchyma drawing water with them and producing a local increase in the extracellular fluid (ECF). ICP rises and further damage may follow. Hypertension, hypoxia and hypercarbia interfere with autoregulation and the integrity of the blood−brain barrier, and will therefore accentuate the development of vasogenic oedema (Reulen 1976).

Cytotoxic oedema Ischaemia or other factors which lead to a failure of the sodium−potassium pump in the cells of the brain, will result in the accumulation of sodium and water within these cells. The ECF may be reduced and, as fluid has shifted from one compartment to another, there may not be an overall increase in volume or rise in ICP (Klatzo 1985).

Interstitial oedema In hydrocephalus the pressure in the ventricles of the brain may cause CSF to leak into the ECF, increasing sodium and water in the white matter.

Blood−brain barrier (BBB)

The endothelial cells forming the walls of the cerebral capillaries are joined one to another by tight junctions around the entire periphery of each cell. They form the barrier between the blood and the brain, giving it the permeability characteristics of a cell membrane rather than the capillary endothelium in other parts of the circulation. The intact BBB restricts the passage of water-soluble molecules and proteins but is readily permeable to lipid-soluble substances. It acts as a semipermeable membrane and fluid movement is governed by factors controlling osmotic pressure. Total osmolality, defined by the activity of all particles in the blood and interstitium, becomes the overriding force, and the normal osmolality of about $285 \, \text{mosmol} \, \text{kg}^{-1}$ is determined almost entirely by small molecules. In the clinical setting this action of the BBB is important in the choice of intravenous fluids (see Chapter 7).

Cerebral blood flow (CBF)

Blood flow affects cerebral volume, oxygen delivery and removal of products of metabolism. In the adult the brain mass is approximately $1500 \, \text{g}$ and it receives a blood flow of $750 \, \text{ml} \, \text{min}^{-1}$, this represents 15−20% of the total cardiac output. Thus the normal CBF values can be given as follows:

Whole brain	$50 \, \text{ml} \, 100 \, \text{g}^{-1} \, \text{min}^{-1}$
Grey matter	$80 \, \text{ml} \, 100 \, \text{g}^{-1} \, \text{min}^{-1}$
White matter	$20 \, \text{ml} \, 100 \, \text{g}^{-1} \, \text{min}^{-1}$

In the newborn and elderly values are lower, but in young children they are significantly higher.

Measurement

The standard methods of measurement of CBF have been the inert gas clearance technique using arteriovenous content differences, and the indicator clearance method based on measurement of regional clearance. More recently positron emission tomography (PET) scanning has allowed both flow and metabolism within the brain to be studied simultaneously, but the need for positron-emitting radioisotopes with a short half-life has limited the technique to a few centres.

THE INERT GAS CLEARANCE TECHNIQUE

This relies on the Fick principle and involves delivering an inert indicator gas to the brain, while measuring its arterial and venous concentration. The Kety–Schmidt technique used nitrous oxide as the indicator, repeated samples being taken from an artery and the jugular venous bulb. More recently radioactive indicators, xenon-133 or krypton-85, have been employed. Mean flow can be calculated in an area determined by the venous drainage to the sampling site. The difficulties with the technique include obtaining a true jugular venous bulb specimen and the hazard involved in the cannulation. This technique is not used clinically today as the information is of limited use, being unable to detect small but significant changes in regional flow.

THE INDICATOR CLEARANCE TECHNIQUE

This relies on the principle that the rate at which an indicator is washed out of a tissue is proportional to the blood flow through it. Xenon-133, a radioactive inert gas, has been used, and is delivered to the brain following either arterial injection or inhalation. The washout is measured using a scintillation counter or gamma camera, depending on the indicator used. Using several detectors the size of the area studied can be varied, and by employing several transducers the blood flow in different regions can be recorded simultaneously. The chief advantage of the inhalational method is that it is non-invasive. There are two drawbacks: first the problem of recirculation, and secondly, the unwanted measurement of the clearance of the indicator from extracranial tissues.

Regulation of cerebral blood flow

The control of blood flow to the brain is primarily dictated by its metabolic needs and is mediated through chemical changes. Although disagreement exists as to the precise mechanism, it is simplest to regard this as being the result of changes in the pH of the brain ECF. If metabolism increases, carbon dioxide is produced and possibly lactic acid; the pH falls causing dilatation of the cerebral arterioles and this leads to a rise in CBF. Changes in arterial carbon dioxide which produce marked change in CBF can be regarded as exploiting the same mechanism. Neurogenic control through the sympathetic nervous system, although present, is of much less significance.

METABOLIC

In the normal brain there is a close 'coupling' between CBF and metabolism, if metabolism increases then CBF increases and if metabolism decreases then CBF decreases. On a global basis the highest levels of CBF will be seen in epileptic seizures when brain metabolism is maximal, and the lowest levels of CBF occur in coma (excluding hypothermic states). Similar changes can be demonstrated on a regional basis, an increase in blood flow can be shown experimentally in the contralateral cortex during voluntary muscle contraction, coincident with an increase in oxygen demand (Oleson 1971) (see Chapter 3). Similarly a painful stimulus will produce a direct increase in local blood flow even in an unconscious patient. This has clinical relevance in the management of a patient with multiple injuries which include a severe head injury. In the presence of raised ICP, inadequate analgesia in an unconscious patient who is paralysed and being ventilated may lead to intracranial decompensation because of an increase in CBF during a painful manoeuvre. It must be emphasized that the use of powerful analgesics in patients following head trauma is restricted to those who are being ventilated.

CARBON DIOXIDE

Changes in arterial carbon dioxide tension ($PaCO_2$) cause profound changes in CBF, in the range $22.5-75$ mmHg there is a linear relationship between $PaCO_2$ and CBF, each 7.5 mmHg change resulting in a rise or fall of $7-9$ ml $100 g^{-1} min^{-1}$ (Fig. 2.8). At 22.5 mmHg the CBF is reduced by about one-half and at 75 mmHg it is approximately doubled. Beyond these limits there is little further change, as can be seen in the flattening of the curve.

The way in which changes in $PaCO_2$ influence CBF is not fully understood, but it is thought that changes in $PaCO_2$ lead to changes in the pH of the CSF and as carbon dioxide crosses the BBB, freely, the pH of the brain ECF also changes, and this causes the constriction and dilatation of the cerebral arterioles. As bicarbonate ions do not cross the BBB, the acid–base balance of the ECF cannot easily be restored and the effect on the CBF therefore lasts for some hours (Jones 1981).

Hypocapnia reduces CBF and hence cerebral blood volume and ICP. Hypocapnia is used clinically in the short term to control intracranial hypertension with a response occurring within 20 min of the onset of hyperventilation. For reasons described above, the reduction in blood

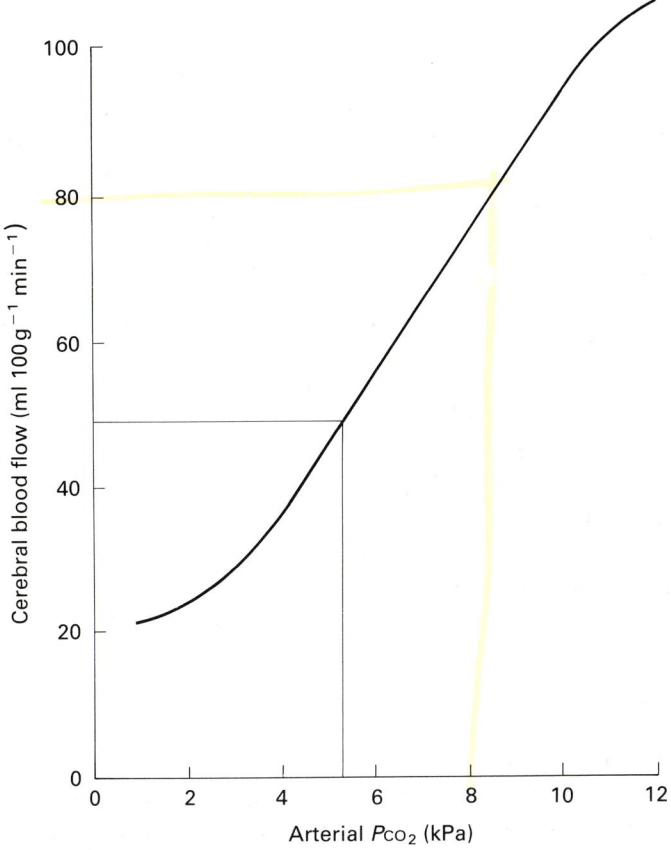

Fig. 2.8 Schematic representation of the relationship between cerebral blood flow and arterial carbon dioxide tension.

flow may only last for a few hours and is followed by an overshoot if $PaCO_2$ is returned rapidly to normal levels. When $PaCO_2$ is less than 22.6 mmHg vasoconstriction in the cerebral circulation can lead to demonstrable changes such as a decrease in reaction times, slow waves on the electroencephalogram (EEG) and an increase in cerebral lactate levels. In pathological states there is vasomotor paralysis which abolishes autoregulation and the normal carbon dioxide response. When a patient is hyperventilated it has been postulated that the healthy vessels constrict, thereby increasing the flow to the diseased areas. This phenomenon is known as '*inverse*' or '*counter steal*', but its clinical significance is less clear as recent work has cast doubt on this concept (see Chapter 4).

Hypercapnia causes brain swelling due to increase in CBF and cerebral blood volume. With pathological states the opposite to the situation described with hypocapnia will occur, the healthy vessels dilate producing a *'steal'* effect by increasing their flow at the expense of the pathological areas. Volatile anaesthetic agents also cause cerebral vasodilatation and raise CBF, thus they may also induce *'steal'*.

AUTOREGULATION

In normal humans CBF is held constant despite changes in arterial blood pressure. This autoregulation normally maintains the flow constant when mean arterial pressure is between 50 and 150 mmHg (Fig. 2.9). Below this minimum pressure there is a rapid fall-off in CBF and above the upper limit flow becomes pressure-dependent, the cerebral capillaries are then exposed to the high arterial pressure with the risk of break-through, leading to oedema and small haemorrhages (Strandgaard *et al.* 1973). When the blood pressure changes abruptly it takes about 1−2 min for autoregulation to act and restore the CBF. If the blood pressure falls the cerebral arterioles dilate, and if it rises they constrict. The mechanism involved may be a myogenic reflex, the vessels themselves sensing

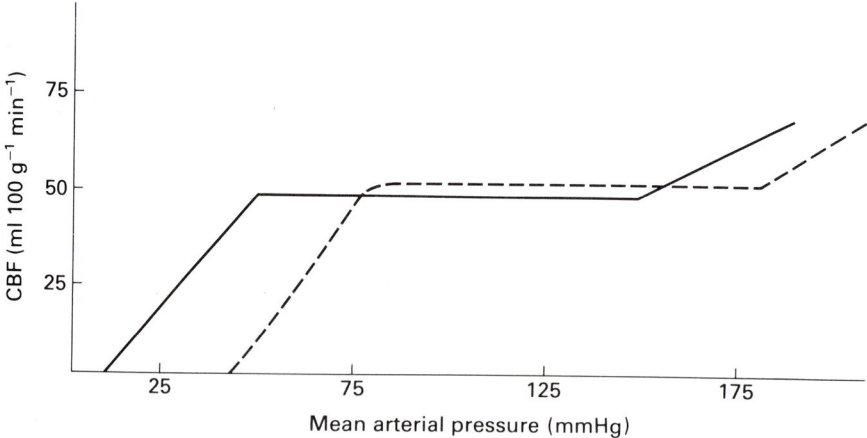

Fig. 2.9 Autoregulation of the cerebral blood flow with cerebral blood flow remaining constant over a mean arterial pressure range 50−150 mmHg. The curve is shifted to the right in patients with chronic hypertension (represented by the dotted line).

the change in pressure and responding, or metabolic changes may be involved.

In chronic hypertension the autoregulatory curve is shifted to the right (Fig. 2.9). This protects the small cerebral capillaries from the raised perfusion pressure; however, the lower limit for autoregulation is also raised. Therefore a blood pressure which may be adequate for a normal patient can lead to ischaemia in a hypertensive. In a treated hypertensive, as might be expected, the autoregulatory curve shifts back towards the left. In hypotension the situation is more complex. When the hypotension is induced by vasodilating drugs the lower end of the curve moves to the left, but when hypovolaemia is the cause, the generalized increase in sympathetic tone that occurs moves the curve to the right.

In the presence of brain tissue acidosis autoregulation is lost, the delicate cerebral vasculature is then vulnerable to a sudden increase in arterial pressure. If this occurs in a patient with critical ICP, the surge in CBF that follows will cause more oedema and capillary leakage. The result is ischaemia, a further increase in ICP and more brain tissue lactic acidosis, either local or global. Thus with trauma, haematoma, tumour, infection and subarachnoid haemorrhage when normal autoregulation is lost, this process of progressive deterioration can result.

OXYGEN

Changes in arterial oxygen tension (PaO_2) in general have little effect on CBF, but when the PaO_2 falls below 50 mmHg there is a rapid increase in blood flow (Fig. 2.10). Increasing PaO_2 causes a gradual decrease in flow until at 2 atm there is a 21% reduction.

NEUROGENIC

The cerebral vessels have a sympathetic nerve supply originating from the superior cervical ganglion and a parasymphathetic supply from the facial nerve. There appears to be little tonic autonomic control and maximum symphathetic stimulation will only produce a 5–10% decrease in CBF, but an increase in sympathetic tone can shift the autoregulatory curve to the right and this may help to protect against breakthrough at the upper end of the curve.

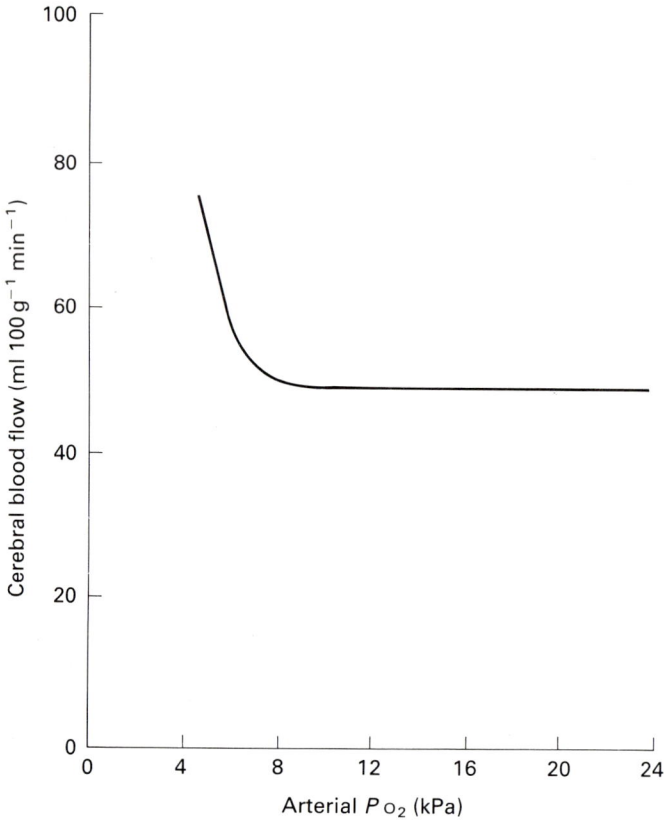

Fig. 2.10 Idealized curve of the relationship between cerebral blood flow and arterial oxygen tension.

OTHER FACTORS

Hypothermia Reduction in body temperature reduces cerebral metabolism and this will reduce CBF, metabolism falls by approximately 5% for each degree centigrade.

Blood viscosity Within the range 30−50% for the haemotocrit there is no effect on CBF, but outside this range the CBF will fall with increased viscosity and rise with decreased.

Cerebral perfusion pressure (CPP)

Physiological concept

Cerebral perfusion pressure (CPP) is the effective pressure which results in blood flow to the brain. The hydrostatic pressures which oppose perfusion are intracranial pressure (ICP) and venous pressure (VP). Therefore CPP is the difference between mean arterial pressure (MAP) and the sum of ICP and the pressure in the jugular venous bulb.

$$CPP = MAP - (ICP + VP)$$

As the venous pressure at the jugular bulb is usually zero or less, it can generally be ignored, and CPP related to MAP and ICP alone. With normal values of mean blood pressure (BP) of 100 mmHg and an ICP of 10 mmHg, the normal CPP will be about 90 mmHg.

Critical minimum values of CPP and CBF

Clearly if CPP falls to zero, CBF will cease and irreversible brain damage will soon follow. In determining critical levels for CPP and CBF which may result in irreversible damage, the time for which low levels are maintained has to considered, as does the state of the cerebral vessels; arteriosclerotic atheromatous arteries will not maintain flow as effectively as pristine blood vessels. Therefore any supposedly safe level of CPP will have to have a wide margin of safety. In Fig. 2.11 a comparison is made of the response of the brain's electrical activity to falling levels of CPP and CBF. If EEG changes are used as a criterion then in a lightly anaesthetized normothermic man slowing of the EEG occurs at a CBF of about 20 ml 100 g^{-1} min^{-1} and abolition at about 15 ml 100 g^{-1} min^{-1}. The latter can be related to a CPP of about 25−30 mmHg; in clinical practice these values would be regarded as being at the limits of safety. However, evoked potentials are not finally abolished until the CBF falls to 12 ml 100 g^{-1} min^{-1} and it is not until values below 10 ml 100 g^{-1} min^{-1} are reached that the efflux of potassium occurs indicating cellular failure. But even at these low levels there is potential for recovery if flow is restored, full recovery taking place following periods of ischaemic flow as long as 30−60 min (Branston 1987).

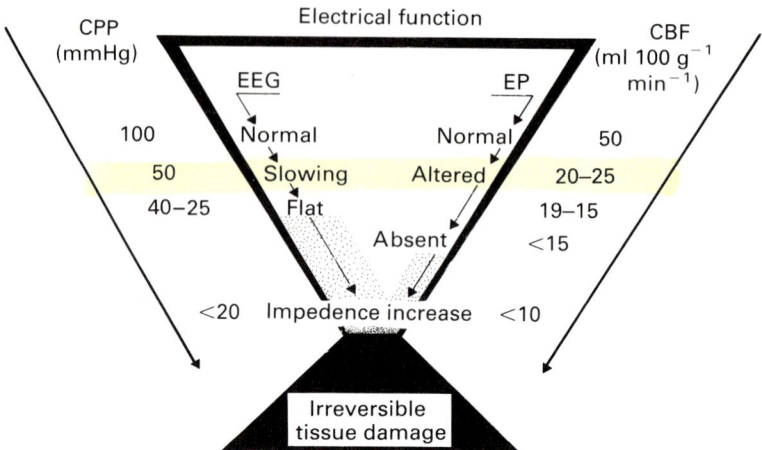

Fig. 2.11 Cerebral perfusion pressure and cerebral blood flow thresholds for changes in EEG and evoked potentials: EP, evoked potential; CPP, cerebral perfusion pressure. From Marsh *et al.* (1977).

Clinical implications

The complex interrelationship between CBF, CPP and ICP is best understood by considering different examples. Any fall in arterial pressure in a patient with raised ICP is potentially hazardous. Consider a patient after head trauma with a systolic arterial pressure of 120 mmHg. CPP can be calculated to give a value of 60 mmHg, assuming a mean arterial pressure of 100 mmHg and ICP of 40 mmHg. If the mean arterial pressure falls to 70 mmHg as a result of hypovolaemia from other injuries or the incautious administration of anaesthetic drugs, the CPP will fall to 30 mmHg and the patient's brain will be at great risk.

References

Branston N.M. (1987) Blood flow and electrophysiology: their relationships in normal and ischaemic brain. In: Jewkes D.A. (Ed.), *Clinical Anaesthesiology: Anaesthesia for Neurosurgery*, pp. 263–277. Baillière Tindall, London.

Crutchfield J.S., Narayan R.K., Robertson C.S. & Michael L.H. (1990) Evaluation of a fibreoptic intracranial monitor. *Journal of Neurosurgery* **72**, 482–487.

Dearden N.M. (1985) Intracranial pressure monitoring. *Care of the Critically Ill* **1**, 8–13.

Fishman R.A. (1975) Brain edema. *New England Journal of Medicine* **293**, 706−711.

Jones P.W. (1981) Hyperventilation in the management of cerebral oedema. *Intensive Care Medicine* **7**, 205−207.

Klatzo I. (1985) Brain oedema following brain ischaemia and the influences of therapy. *British Journal of Anaesthesia* **57**, 18−22.

Langfitt T.W., Weinstein J.D., Kassell N.F. & Simone F.A. (1964) Transmission of increased intracranial pressure. I: Within the cerebrospinal axis. *Journal of Neurosurgery* **21**, 989−997.

Lofgren J. & Zwetnow N.N. (1973) Cranial and spinal components of the cerebrospinal fluid pressure−volume curve. *Acta Neurologica Scandinavica* **49**, 575−585.

Lundberg N. (1960) Continuous recording and control of ventricular fluid pressure in neurosurgical practice. *Acta Psychiatrica et Neurologica Scandinavica* **36** (Suppl. 149), 1−193.

Marsh M.L., Marshall L.F. & Shapiro H.M. (1977) Neurosurgical intensive care. *Anesthesiology* **47**, 149−163.

Miller J.D. (1976) Intracranial pressure−volume relationships in pathological conditions. *Journal of Neurosurgical Science* **20**, 203−209.

Miller J.D. & Leech P.J. (1975) Assessing the effects of mannitol and steroid therapy on intra-cranial volume−pressure relationships. *Journal of Neurosurgery* **42**, 274−281.

Oleson J. (1971) Contralateral focal increase of cerebral blood flow in man during arm work. *Brain* **94**, 635−646.

Reulen H.J. (1976) Vasogenic brain oedema: new aspects in its formation, resolution and therapy. *British Journal of Anaesthesia* **48**, 741−752.

Strandgaard S., Olesen J., Skinhoj E. & Lassen N.A. (1973) Autoregulation of the brain circulation in severe arterial hypertension. *British Medical Journal* **1**, 507−510.

3
Cerebral metabolism

MIKE NEVIN

Introduction

Brain survival is totally dependent upon a continuous supply of adequate energy substrates, mainly oxygen and glucose, as well as the effective removal of the waste products of metabolism. Although regional metabolic requirements vary greatly, there exists within all brain tissue, under normal circumstances, a close relationship between oxygen supply and demand. Changes in metabolic requirements are mirrored by changes in cerebral blood flow (CBF) and hence in energy substrate supply. When cerebral function is depressed, such as during general anaesthesia or coma, energy requirements fall; resulting in parallel decreases in CBF, oxygen consumption and glucose utilization. In contrast, episodes of high substrate usage, such as hyperthermia or seizures, are associated with appropriate increases in supply. The mechanism of action of this *'flow—metabolism coupling'* remains unclear, although local metabolic factors, such as tissue pH, are likely to be prime contributors to the constancy of this relationship (Jones *et al.* 1985).

The metabolic requirements of the normal brain are considerable. Although only accounting for 2–3% of body weight, approximately 15% of the cardiac output is required to meet energy substrate demands. Under normal circumstances overall CBF is around $50 \, ml \, 100 \, g^{-1} \, min^{-1}$ (Lassen 1985) and cerebral metabolic rate for oxygen (CMRO$_2$), $3.8 \, ml \, 100 \, g^{-1} \, min^{-1}$ (Graham 1985). Whilst wide regional variations exist (Table 3.1), overall cerebral metabolism probably accounts for 20% of total body oxygen consumption; 60% of this energy is used to sustain synaptic function, as witnessed in the electroencephalogram (EEG), whilst the remaining 40% is devoted to the maintenance of cellular integrity. *Flow thresholds* describe the changes in functional brain activity that correlate with changes in CBF. Any reduction in energy substrate supply results in an immediate decrease in cerebral synaptic (EEG) activity; although once an isoelectric trace has been obtained further reductions in oxygen and glucose supply are likely to be associated

Table 3.1 Normal physiological parameters for the brain

Global CBF	$\approx 50\,\text{ml}\,100\,\text{g}^{-1}\,\text{min}^{-1}$
CBF (grey)	$\approx 80\,\text{ml}\,100\,\text{g}^{-1}\,\text{min}^{-1}$
CBF (white)	$\approx 20\,\text{ml}\,100\,\text{g}^{-1}\,\text{min}^{-1}$
CMR_{oxygen}	$\approx 3.5\,\text{ml}\,100\,\text{g}^{-1}\,\text{min}^{-1}$
$\text{CMR}_{glucose}$	$\approx 4.5\,\text{ml}\,100\,\text{g}^{-1}\,\text{min}^{-1}$
$\text{CBF}/\text{CMR}_{oxygen}$	≈ 15
Intracranial pressure	$5-12\,\text{mmHg}$
Venous P_{O_2}	$>35\,\text{mmHg}$

CBF, cerebral blood flow; CMR, cerebral metabolic rate.

with potentially irreparable cerebral cellular damage, unless immediate resuscitatory action is taken (Astrup *et al.* 1977, Prior 1985, Siesjo & Wieloch 1985) (Table 3.2).

Cerebral well-being under nonpathological conditions is safeguarded by the presence of an intact flow metabolism coupling system. There are occasions, however, when the efficiency of this linkage is severely disrupted, even in the 'normal' brain. It is important to understand clearly

Table 3.2 Pathophysiological changes associated with decreasing cerebral blood flow

CBF ($\text{ml}\,100\,\text{g}^{-1}\,\text{min}^{-1}$)	Index		
	Electrical	ECF ion activity	Metabolites
15–20	EEG silent SEP present but altered	—	—
15	EEG silent SEP absent	pH $\downarrow$	Lactate $\uparrow$ Creatine phosphate $\downarrow$
10–15	EEG silent	pH $\downarrow$ K_e $\uparrow$ Na_e $\downarrow$ Cl_e $\downarrow$	Lactate $\uparrow$ ATP and adenylate energy charge $\downarrow$
10	EEG silent	pH $\downarrow\downarrow$ K_e $\uparrow\uparrow$ Ca_e^{2+} $\downarrow$	Lactate $\uparrow\uparrow$ ATP and adenylate energy charge $\downarrow\downarrow$

ATP, adenosine triphosphate; EEG, electroencephalogram; SEP, somatosensory evoked potential; e, extracellular.

the significance of these factors under a variety of clinical and pathological circumstances.

Individual variations in $PaCO_2$, PaO_2 and cerebral perfusion pressure (CPP) are the factors which are likely to have the greatest effect on the preservation of cerebral defence mechanisms. Significant hypocapnia ($PaCO_2 < 30$ mmHg) is likely to be associated with a marked rise in cerebro-vascular resistance, even in the face of excessive metabolic requirements. Alternatively significant hypercapnia ($PaCO_2 > 60$ mmHg) will almost invariably produce maximum cerebral vasodilatation, a breakdown of flow−metabolism coupling and the production of a 'luxury-perfusion' state, as a result of the increases in CBF being in excess of cerebral metabolic requirements (Harper & Bell 1963). The supply of oxygen and glucose to the brain will also be dependent on the maintenance of an adequate CPP, defined as the difference between mean arterial pressure and either intracranial or cerebral venous pressure, whichever is the greatest. Although discussed in greater detail in Chapter 14, the adequacy of CPP and the presence or absence of 'cerebral autoregulation' play a major role in the aetiology of individual outcome following cerebral insult. Despite common belief that the maintenance of a CPP of greater than 50 mmHg ensures adequate substrate delivery (Stockard *et al.* 1974) this has not been proven. Indeed it seems likely that there will be no common lower autoregulatory limit: adequacy of perfusion in the individual being determined both by local cerebral activity and by the reactivity of the distributive microvasculature to changes in metabolic demands (Harper & Glass 1965).

The third physiological variable that has an effect on CBF is PaO_2 (McDowall 1966). Although these three factors are important in isolation, it is their interrelationship in the clinical setting that often has a major role to play in the preservation of cerebral well-being. Hypocapnia, whilst reducing CBF in reactive patients, is unlikely to result in global hypoperfusion because of the overriding effect of both global and focal reductions in PaO_2. In contrast hypercapnia not only increases intra-cerebral blood volume (and also intracellular pressure, ICP) as a result of maximal cerebral vasodilatation, but also reduces the capacity of the brain to respond to further stresses, whether they be hypoxaemic or hypotensive, as the cerebral vessels are already fully dilated (Harper & Glass 1965).

In summary the relationship between cerebral supply and demand is very closely controlled in 'normal' humans under 'normal' conditions. In many of the cases that present to the neurosurgical anaesthetist abnormal conditions prevail. This may be due to the presence of neo-plastic or inflammatory tissue, or it may be as a result of either traumatic or infective damage. Under any of the predisposing conditions it is dangerous to presume that the patient has either functional flow—meta-bolism coupling or cerebral autoregulatory capabilities. Any variations from normal energy substrate delivery, whether by hypoxia or hypoper-fusion, may expose the individual to ischaemic stresses to which he or she may be unable to respond.

Cerebral ischaemia

If the delivery of oxygen to the brain is less than metabolic requirements then cerebral ischaemia will occur. The reasons for this inadequacy of oxygen delivery may be either a reduction in supply as a consequence of a decrease in CBF, or secondary to an increase in cerebral oxygen requirements.

Decreases in substrate delivery may be due to either cerebral hypo-perfusion (as a result of either a fall in perfusion pressure or an increase in cerebrovascular resistance), to *arterial hypoxaemia* (acute respiratory failure, anaemia and decreased inspired oxygen concentration), or to *cytotoxic hypoxaemia* (failure to utilize available oxygen). Increased cer-ebral metabolic requirements occur during both excessive seizure activity and during periods of hyperpyrexia.

Classification of cerebral ischaemia

Cerebral ischaemia may be either global (affecting the whole brain) or focal (involving only specific regions); and is said to be either complete or incomplete depending on whether the blood flow is completely absent or merely reduced to levels below basal requirements (Fig. 3.1).

In *focal cerebral ischaemia*, for instance after regional arterial occlusion or embolization, compensatory flow via collateral vessels often limits the extent of the cerebral damage, which is therefore almost invariably incomplete. The overall degree of cerebral deficit correlates well with both the efficiency of the collateral circulation and with the duration of the insult. Although the maintenance of some cerebral flow throughout these episodes of hypoperfusion may seem a positive feature it is not always the case. The ischaemic areas continue to be supplied with not only oxygen but also glucose, which is then anaerobically converted to

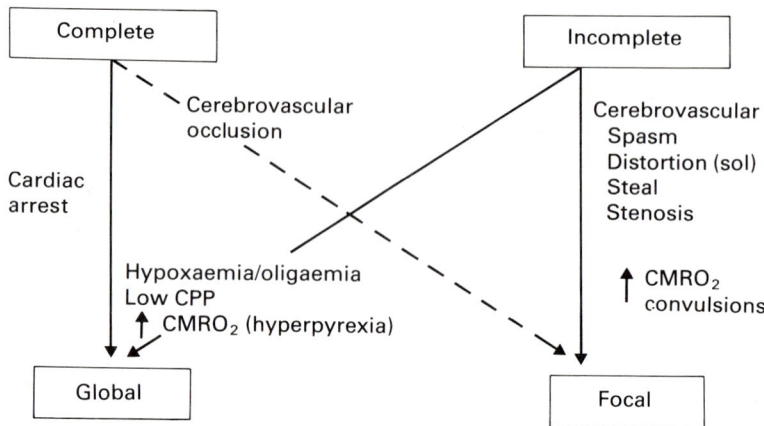

Fig. 3.1 Classification of cerebral ischaemia and its causes. CMRO$_2$, cerebral metabolic requirement for oxygen; CPP, cerebral perfusion pressure; sol, space occupying lesion.

lactate, increasing the degree of intracellular acidosis and possibly resulting in an extension of the original deficit (Kalimo *et al.* 1981, Heuser & Guggenberger 1985). Several mechanisms of injury by intracellular acidosis have been proposed. First, it results in an inhibition of mitochondrial phosphorylation and energy production; produces a denaturation of proteins and nucleic acid; whilst at the same time producing glial swelling, microcirculatory compromise and an increase in the production of free radicals. The significance of this 'lactate' pathway in determining eventual outcome is difficult to estimate, but it would seem reasonable to suggest that any management regimen for focal cerebral ischaemia should include the rapid restoration of 'normal' perfusion pressures, together with an absolute avoidance of intravenous dextrose solutions.

Flow thresholds in cerebral ischaemia

As CBF falls during a global ischaemic insult, flow thresholds have been identified which correlate well with cerebral electrical silence, ionic pump failure and lastly cellular membrane breakdown and death. An understanding of these thresholds and their metabolic consequences is vital if a logical response to any cerebral insult is to be made (Astrup *et al.* 1977).

CBF must fall by 60% before there are any changes in cerebral electrical activity suggestive of ischaemia. Around $20\,ml\,100\,g^{-1}\,min^{-1}$ changes in the distribution of electrical activity appear; often taking the form of a reduction in fast-wave activity (beta and alpha) and a generalized switch to slow-wave activity (theta and delta), often interspersed with transitory periods of burst suppression (Prior 1985).

Between 15 and $20\,ml\,100\,g^{-1}\,min^{-1}$ failure of electrical activity rapidly develops, EEG first followed later by evoked responses (Astrup *et al.* 1977). Cessation of synaptic function therefore serves as the first line of defence to the ensuing insult; allowing the conservation of all available energy for the maintenance of neuronal cellular integrity. As CBF falls even further the production of neurotransmitters ceases and the influx into cells of both water and sodium marks the onset of cerebral cytotoxic oedema. The effect of this oedema is to increase ICP, resulting in localized increases in vascular resistance which further reduce local CBF.

When CBF falls to around $10\,ml\,100\,g^{-1}\,min^{-1}$ there is a dramatic rise in glycolytic activity producing a marked lactic acidosis, the extent of which is often determined by the degree of continued supply of glucose (Siesjo & Wieloch 1985). Adenosine triphosphate (ATP) production fails almost immediately, with a resultant fall in adenylate energy charge and eventual ionic pump failure; resulting finally in the depolarization of the neuronal membrane following the efflux of potassium ions into the extracellular space.

A further fall of CBF to $6-10\,ml\,100\,g^{-1}\,min^{-1}$ is associated with the intracellular influx of calcium along voltage-gated channels. Detailed examination of this influx identifies two discrete events which both serve to extend the degree of the cerebral insult. First, the influx of calcium produces a rise in the release of excitatory neurotransmitters which then stimulate the voltage-gated channels so allowing a further influx of calcium ions, as well as the activation of a host of intracellular enzymes all of which result in a cascade of biochemical events all bent on the production of structural cellular damage. Lipase activation results in the formation of arachidonic acid, one of the precursors for the formation of both prostaglandins and leukotrienes, by the cyclo-oxygenase and lipoxygenase pathways respectively. Vasoconstriction, vasodilatation, leukotaxis and alterations in membrane permeability are only some of the effects of these substances. In addition free radicals (chemical species with an unpaired electron) formed as a result of this increase in cyclo-oxygenase and lipoxygenase activity add further to the degree of cellular structural damage (Kontos 1989, Schmidley 1990). The final event is the influx of calcium into the mitochondria; at which point neuronal death is inevitable (Fig. 3.2).

There is increasing evidence that the N-*methyl-*D-*aspartate* (NMDA) receptor is heavily involved in the production of cellular damage following periods of cerebral ischaemia. The hypothesis suggests that the pre-synaptic release of excitatory amino acids (glutamate and aspartate in particular) brings about an activation of the NMDA receptor resulting in a dramatic postsynaptic influx of calcium ions (Rothman & Olney 1986, Choi 1988, Siesjo 1988). Glutamate itself is not a neurotoxin; its role in the production of cellular damage hinges upon its ability to bring about the associated influx of sodium, chloride and hydrogen ions together with water into the cells. This rapidly results in neuronal swelling, dendritic osmolysis, intracellular acidosis and activation of the NMDA receptor, resulting in a sudden movement of calcium ions from the extracellular space into the cells (Siesjo 1988). Evidence in favour of this hypothesis is provided by the finding of glutamate throughout the CNS; a high concentration of excitatory amino acids following ischaemia and reperfusion; together with a high density of NMDA receptors in 'at-risk' areas of the brain such as the hippocampus. All of these findings are reinforced by the fact that selective blockade of these receptors may be

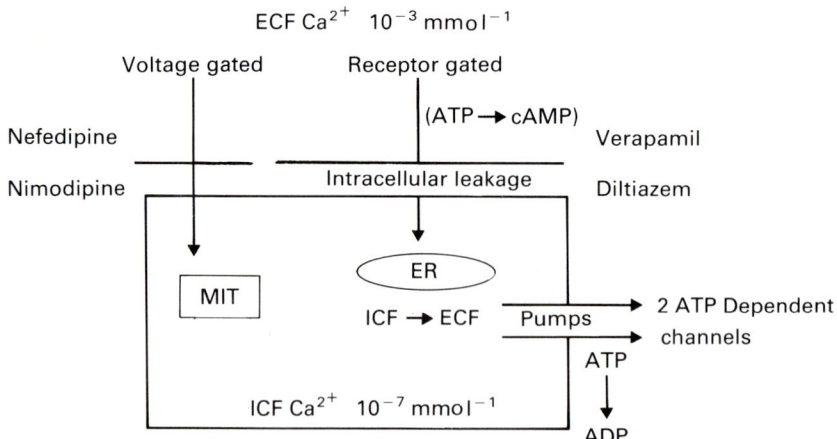

Fig. 3.2 Physiology of calcium fluxes between extracellular and intracellular compartments MIT, mitochondria; ER, endoplastic reticulum.

associated with significant improvements in deficit following ischaemic damage (Greenamyre *et al.* 1985, Church *et al.* 1988, Siesjo 1988).

Around all areas of neuronal infarction and cellular death there will be regions of brain in which structural destruction has not yet taken place, although CBF has fallen to levels ($6-10$ ml $100 \, g^{-1} min^{-1}$) that are barely sufficient to maintain cellular integrity. This region is often termed the ischaemic *'penumbra'*, and contains cells that, although electrically silent, remain potentially salvageable. The size of the eventual infarct will therefore be determined not only by the number of neurones suffering immediate infarction, but also by the peri-infarct management of the ischaemic penumbra and by the effect of reperfusion (itself associated with the production of vasogenic oedema and further structural damage), on this ischaemic tissue (Astrup *et al.* 1981a).

Global cerebral ischaemia differs from focal in that there is unlikely to be any significant collateral circulation. As a consequence of both this, and of the absence of any appreciable cerebral energy stores, complete cessation of cerebral flow on a global level will proceed to irreversible cellular damage within $4-5$ min unless flow is restored. If cerebral flow is restored then the severity of any permanent damage will be the product of both the duration of insult and the metabolic requirements of the brain during the period of ischaemia.

Incomplete global ischaemia, often arising as a result of inadequate oxygen supply secondary to a reduction in CPP, is normally concentrated on the areas of the brain most susceptible to marginal falls in CBF. These 'watershed regions' lie at the very extremes of territory of the three major cerebral arteries (Graham 1985). The occipitoparietal regions are perhaps one of the most sensitive areas to sudden falls in cerebral perfusion; a fact used to good effect by some workers who have used modified EEG monitoring (cerebral function analysing monitor), of these areas of the brain as a sensitive index of reduced cerebral perfusion (Maynard 1982, Nevin *et al.* 1989). Biochemical and electrical changes secondary to incomplete global ischaemia are identical to those for focal ischaemia.

Complete global ischaemia, such as that occurring following a cardiac arrest, produces biochemical and electrical changes that differ from those already mentioned. Following the cessation of CBF consciousness is lost within $10-15$ s, and all electrical activity stops within a further 10 s. Increasing acidosis ensues, producing an initial slow fall in pH, followed by a secondary rapid decrease and finally slowing down to produce an intracellular pH of around 6 after 5 min of ischaemia. High-energy phosphate stores are all empty within 3−4 min of cerebral standstill. ECF potassium levels initially rise slowly, but within 2 min of the commencement of ischaemia, and associated with cellular membrane depolarization, they rise rapidly to around 65 mmol l^{-1}. Over the following minutes if perfusion is not restored they rise even further, often to levels of 70−80 mmol l^{-1} immediately prior to cell death. Once cell depolarization commences it is associated with the opening of voltage-dependent gates producing a similar rapid influx of calcium ions and the activation of the catabolic cascade as described during focal ischaemia (Dearden 1990).

Cerebral protection

A clear differentiation must be made between 'cerebral protection' and 'cerebral resuscitation'. Cerebral protection involves either physiological or pharmacological interventions prior to the onset of any cerebral ischaemia, such prophylactic measures hopefully reducing the incidence of postoperative cerebral deficit a 'high-risk' population. In contrast cerebral resuscitation, whilst often utilizing similar clinical manipulations, is a response to a suspected or documented ischaemic insult; possibly representing, therefore, an exercise in damage limitation.

Principles of treatment

The ischaemic injury process has been shown clearly to be a cascade of biochemical events produced in response to cellular hypoxia. Any treatment regimen, whether designed for cerebral protection or cerebral resuscitatory purposes, should aim to limit both the severity of the initial energy imbalance whilst at the same time focusing on the individual components of the cascade (Fig. 3.3).

ENERGY FAILURE

Cerebral oxygen delivery must be at least as great as oxygen consumption if ischaemic damage is to be avoided. Possibilities for management therefore include measures both to decrease oxygen consumption, by reducing $CMRO_2$, as well as to increase oxygen delivery, either by increasing perfusion pressure or by selectively improving microcirculatory flow for any given CPP.

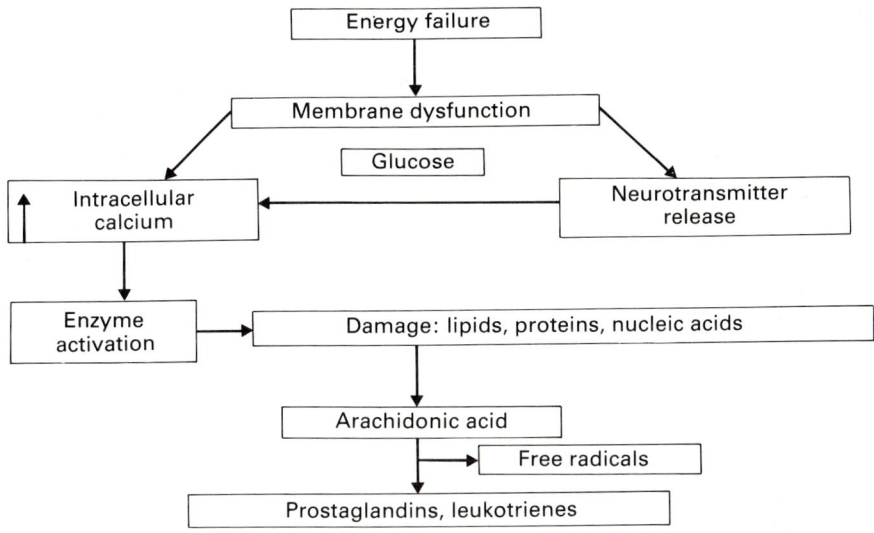

Fig. 3.3 The cascade of biochemical events initiated by cerebral ischaemia.

HYPOTHERMIA

$CMRO_2$ decreases by approximately 7% for every degree centigrade decrease in body temperature. As discussed above, energy usage by the brain is for both EEG activity (60%) and basal cellular integrity (40%). Hypothermia has the ability to reduce both of these components and, as a consequence may still have a role to play even in the presence of an isoelectric EEG. There is a considerable evidence that even mild hypothermia (2−4°C) can confer significant protective benefits (Busto *et al.* 1987, 1989a, Sano *et al.* 1992). Whilst the primary mode of protection is likely to be one of reduction in $CMRO_2$, recent animal studies have suggested that moderate hypothermia immediately post-ischaemia can provide protective benefits also (Boris-Moller *et al.* 1989, Busto *et al.* 1989a, Buchan & Pulsinelli 1990), thereby showing that other mechanisms may be involved. This hypothesis becomes more convincing after the discovery that hypothermia has a marked inhibitory effect on the release of neurotransmitters (Busto *et al.* 1989b). Deep levels of hypothermia necessitate the use of cardiopulmonary bypass equipment and dedicated technical assistance. In addition hypothermia at the end of a procedure is likely to be associated with hypertension and cardiac arrhythmias unless adequate time is allowed for rewarming. Because of these potential limitations deep hypothermia does not provide a realistic option for routine neurosurgical practice. On the other hand there would seem to be increasing evidence that the use of mild hypothermia has a major role to play in the routine management of high-risk cases; both peroperatively and also in an intensive-care setting. Hyperthermia should be avoided at all costs.

BARBITURATES

Thiopentone has been shown to reduce $CMRO_2$ in an approximately dose-related manner until an isoelectric EEG is produced (Steen & Michenfelder 1978). Barbiturates may also afford cerebral protection by a variety of other mechanisms, such as by the blackage of calcium channels, membrane stabilization and free-radical scavenging, as well as by reducing intracranial pressure (Warner *et al.* 1988, Milde 1990, Rockoff *et al.* 1979). At the present time available data do not support the use of barbiturates as a method of cerebral protection in the context of complete global ischaemia (Abramson *et al.* 1986). In cases of focal ischaemia the information available remains conflicting. There is anecdotal animal evidence that benefit may be obtained in complete focal cerebral ischaemia (Michenfelder 1974, Michenfelder *et al.* 1976, Selman *et al.* 1981, Nehls *et al.* 1987), but clinical studies have been unable to confirm these findings, and have often been limited by the cardiovascular side-effects of these drugs (Shapiro 1985). Barbiturates may have a role to play in instances of temporary focal ischaemia, such as following cerebral embolization during cardiac surgery, where a significant reduction in stroke rate has been shown following the routine use of thiopentone, titrated to produce an isoelectric EEG, during periods of cardiopulmonary bypass (Nussmeier *et al.* 1986, Michenfelder 1986). There is no evidence to suggest that thiopentone, or any other barbiturate, has a place in the protective management of the acute head trauma patient. This is discussed further in Chapter 14.

ISOFLURANE

Isoflurane is capable of producing a reduction in $CMRO_2$ as well as an increase in CBF. It remains unique among all the volatile agents in that it is capable of bringing about an isoelectric EEG trace at 2.0 minimal alveolar concentration (MAC). Despite these potential advantages there is no evidence to suggest that a reduction in post-ischaemic cerebral deficit can be affected using this agent. Studies comparing isoflurane with halothane have produced no evidence of significant protective differences between the two (Ruta *et al.* 1991). Isoflurane (2.0 MAC) compared with nitrous oxide/fentanyl control group again showed no differences in cerebral deficit between the groups (Nehls *et al.* 1987). Finally, in an attempt to put in true perspective the relative value of isoflurane as a protective agent, Sano *et al.* (1992) compared isoflurane (1.3 MAC) at normothermia with halothane (1.3 MAC) at normothermia, and also at 33°C, on a model of temporary forebrain ischaemia. Isoflurane (normothermia) showed no cerebral protective benefit over halothane (normothermia), whereas mild hypothermia significantly reduced ischaemic brain injury in the 1.3 MAC halothane group. This lack of benefit on the part of isoflurane can perhaps be explained on the basis of its ability to vasodilate non-ischaemic areas, so producing an intra-cerebral steal, as well as the potential for raising ICP as a result of an increase in CBF.

OTHER ANAESTHETIC AGENTS

Etomidate has been shown to reduce $CMRO_2$ and CBF in a similar fashion to barbiturates. Both potentiate gamma-aminobutyric acid-ergic (GABAergic) activity at the GABA-A—benzodiazepine receptor complex, and the available data suggest that they do so by activity at the same modulator site. The cardiovascular stability of etomidate has earned it possibly a higher ranking as a protective agent than thiopentone in some neurosurgical centres. Despite this enthusiasm neuroprotective studies in animals remain inconclusive (Venables *et al.* 1986, Smith *et al.* 1989) and future usage is likely to be limited by the detrimental effects of this drug on the adrenal function of critically ill patients; even after a single intravenous dose (Ledingham & Watt 1983).

Benzodiazepines reduce CBF and $CMRO_2$, but again there is minimal evidence that they have a role in cerebral protection. Narcotic agents, by removing pain as well as reducing conscious awareness, reduce $CMRO_2$. While their cardiovascular stability and easy reversibility make their usage in neurosurgical anaesthesia very popular, there is no evidence to suggest that they have intrinsic cerebral protective capabilities. Further investigation into the protective properties of opiate receptor agonists acting selectively at the kappa receptor subtype is ongoing.

Lignocaine reduces $CMRO_2$ and at higher doses (160 mg kg^{-1}) is capable of abolishing EEG activity. As with hypothermia it is capable of reducing $CMRO_2$ even after the production of an isoelectric EEG. Cerebral protection in these instances may involve the blockade of neuronal Na^+ channels by abolishing synaptic electrical activity as well as by reducing the amount of energy required to maintain ionic gradients by impending Na^+/K^+ exchange (Astrup *et al.* 1981b). Routine usage is likely to be limited by the epileptogenicity and cardiotoxicity of the drug at higher dosage levels. Lignocaine has also been used at lower doses to obtund rises in ICP secondary to stimuli such as physiotherapy (Evans & Kobrine 1987).

The role of propofol will be examined in greater detail in the section on free-radical scavenging agents later in this chapter.

Osmotic diuretics such as mannitol and dismethylsulphoxide (DMSO) are effective in cytoxic brain oedema (Gisvold & Steen 1985) while vasogenic oedema can be treated by promoting diuresis and reducing CSF production with agents such as frusemide and acetazolamide (Klatzo 1985).

Hyperexcitability following cerebral ischaemia is extremely likely, and should be treated immediately the diagnosis is made. The routine use of devices such as the cerebral function analysing monitor (CFAM) is likely to make early diagnosis possible. Phenytoin not only reduces $CMRO_2$ but, in addition, has a stabilizing effect on cell membranes, delaying the dissipative ion fluxes associated with cerebral ischaemia (Artru & Michenfelder 1981).

HAEMODYNAMIC MANAGEMENT

When considering appropriate cerebral protective policies much emphasis is placed on pharmacological methods of treatment. Other simple treatment modalities should not be forgotten. The maintenance of an appropriate cerebral perfusion pressure is one that is often underplayed in review articles on this subject. After an episode of cerebral ischaemia, with the restoration of an adequate CPP, cerebral blood flow normally increases to hyperaemic levels for about 15 min. This is routinely followed by a decrease in CBF to less than normal levels, despite the maintenance of a normal CPP (phase of delayed hypoperfusion) (Sundt & Waltz 1971). There is extensive evidence available, both in human and animal models, to suggest that the brain in exquisitely sensitive to these episodes of cerebral hypoperfusion (Bouma *et al.* 1991); perhaps as a result of impaired autoregulatory capabilities following the initial ischaemic insult. This vulnerability is especially recognizable in patients who have sustained a head injury, in those suffering subarachnoid haemorrhage and in those suffering acute episodes of acute focal ischaemia (Araki *et al.* 1990, Giannotta *et al.* 1991). Increasing systemic perfusion pressure in the immediate post-ischaemic period is thought to bring about an opening of collateral vessels, thereby improving blood flow to the ischaemic areas (Symon *et al.* 1976). Hypertensive management utilizing vasoactive compounds such as methoxamine or noradrenaline have been shown to be associated with consistently decreased cerebral deficit in the rat model of middle cerebral artery ischaemia (Drummond *et al.* 1989). Worries remain in the minds of many clinicians regarding the incidence of iatrogenic cerebral oedema or rebleeding following the use of such techniques. This has resulted in an underuse of the technique in routine clinical practice even though evidence is accumulating that its use in patients with vasospastic ischaemia may be beneficial (Awad *et al.* 1987). There is a clear need for urgent investigation in this area.

MICROCIRCULATORY IMPROVEMENT

During the phase of delayed hypoperfusion following cerebral ischaemia, capillary blood flow may be detrimentally affected by both platelet activation and increased red cell stiffness (Gisvold & Steen 1985), as well as by oedema and astrocytic swelling in the perivascular space (Siesjo & Wieloch 1985). Flow in the microcirculation can be improved by manipulating the haematocrit by the administration of either albumin or low molecular weight dextrans; such interventions, if conducted immediately following the ischaemic insult, have been associated with an improved outcome (Hoff 1986). In addition a combination of heparin, indomethacin and prostacyclin administered after an ischaemic insult has been shown to improve post-ischaemia CBF (Hallenbeck & Furlow 1979). The use of oxygen-carrying perfluorochemicals, such as fluosol-DA, has been extensively investigated in animal models of focal ischaemia. Whilst fluosol-DA has a lower viscosity than blood, does not increase its viscosity at low flow rates and results in an improved outcome following acute ischaemia (Faithfull 1987), its use in clinical practice is extremely limited due to the long-term inhibitory effects this group of chemicals have both on the reticuloendothelial system and on leucocyte function (Kahn *et al.* 1985). At present investigations are focused on the use of haemodilution with an artificial haemoglobin and macromolecules which have the ability to seal a leaky blood–brain barrier after an acute ischaemic event (Schell *et al.* 1991). The use of anticoagulants following cerebral ischaemia is based on the ability of such drugs to limit thrombus formation. Thrombus formation may be either the cause or effect of acute cerebral ischaemia. Improvement in microcirculatory flow has been shown to be associated with the use of systemic anticoagulation immediately following a focal ischaemic episode. Limitations to the routine application of anticoagulation therapy lie mainly in the reservation of individual clinicians; some are unwilling to expose the individual patient to the risk of further intracerebral bleeding.

CALCIUM ENTRY BLOCKERS

Any increase in intracellular and mitochondrial Ca^{2+} following cerebral ischaemia leads to activation of phospholipases, membrane disruption and the production of other mechanisms of cellular injury. The idea that it might be possible to interrupt this cascade of events as a result of pharmacologically limiting the intracellular influx of Ca^{2+} seemed extremely appealing; especially as many of the likely candidates also possessed vasodilatory properties, with the added possibility of increasing CBF to damaged neurones. Despite great enthusiasm, some of the early calcium antagonists proved disappointing in this respect; perhaps mainly due to their poor blood−brain barrier transmission. More recently three newer agents—nimodipine, lidoflazine and flunarizine—have been investigated extensively, and initial results are proving to be promising. They are not, however, without side-effects. Nimodipine obtunds cerebral autoregulation as well as reducing CPP, secondary to both a decrease in mean arterial pressure (MAP) as well as an increase in ICP. It also increases the potential for intracerebral steal as a result of a reduction in carbon dioxide reactivity, and raises the CBF thresholds at which structural neuronal damage is likely. In addition there is little evidence to suggest that in clinically acceptable doses it has any effect on the influx of Ca^{2+} ions into the cell following ischaemia (Symon 1985). Despite these findings, the use of nimodipine in experimental ischaemia results in a significant improvement in post-ischaemic flow associated with both an increase in cerebral oxygen delivery and a reduction in oxygen debt. Drugs such as nimodipine may be providing benefit either as a result of their effect on cerebral vascular endothelium or by their effects on platelet activation and blood viscosity, rather than by reducing the intracellular influx of calcium ions (Church *et al.* 1988).

Calcium antagonists have been shown to be of cerebral protective benefit under a variety of circumstances. Evidence related to their use in focal ischaemia would suggest that an improvement in outcome (i.e. a reduction in the extent of the initial neurological deficit) is achieved only if they are given prior to the ischaemic event occurring (Myers & Yamaguchi 1977, Mohamed *et al.* 1985), although improved recovery is likely to be associated with a reduction in post-ischaemia hypoperfusion, a feature achieved with these agents even when they are given immediately after the period of cerebral ischaemia (Milde *et al.* 1986). They may yet have a role to play in the immediate management of patients suffering cardiac arrests. A recent prospective, double-blind trial of nimodipine given within 24 h of the onset of an acute stroke demonstrated significant improvements in the severity of ischaemic deficit as well as a reduction in mortality (Gelmers *et al.* 1988). Initial results from controlled, double-blind studies in patients suffering subarachnoid haemorrhage (SAH), reported a reduction in the incidence of neurological deficits associated with arterial spasm but no reduction in the occurrence of vasospasm or improvement in outcome when compared with controls. Further, more encouraging, evidence is emerging that nimodipine 60 mg 4-hourly orally (given for 21 days and commenced within 96 h of SAH confirmed by CT scan) reduces significantly the number and size of infarcts, based on CT and postmortem data, and improves significantly 3-month outcome (Pickard *et al.* 1989). Calcium antagonists therefore probably do have a place in cerebral protection as well as in cerebral resuscitation; although the mode of action seems likely to be by improvement in microcirculatory flow rather than by any action on intracellular calcium flux.

NMDA RECEPTOR ANTAGONISM

The discovery of excitatory amino acid (EAA) receptors, in close proximity to calcium ion channels, in areas of the brain that are especially sensitive to ischaemia has raised much interest in identifying their role in the ischaemic process. To date four different groups of EAA receptors have been identified: one NMDA and three non-NMDA types (Cotman & Iversen 1987). A suggested hypothesis is that during any period of ischaemia an increase in cytosolic calcium concentration in susceptible neurones triggers the release of extracellular EAAs (e.g. glutamate and aspartate) which then bind to membrane-associated NMDA receptors with the resultant opening of voltage-gated Ca^{2+} channels (Rothman & Olney 1986, Siesjo & Smith 1991) (Fig. 3.4). The concentration of EAA in the extracellular space may increase by 200-fold in a 30-min period if ischaemia is persistent, their uptake being obtunded by the concomitant presence of arachidonic acid. Both competitive (D-AP5) and non-competitive NMDA receptor antagonists have been identified, although many are too toxic for clinical use. Of those that may have some clinical application, ketamine and MK-801, two phencyclidine receptor agonists, appear the most promising. Both cross the blood–brain barrier and act as non-competitive NMDA receptor antagonists. The use of ketamine is likely to be limited as it increases cerebral metabolism and ICP, but results from experimental studies using MK-801 are extremely encouraging; especially as benefit appears to result whether the agent is given before or even after the ischaemic insult (Kemp *et al.* 1987, Gill & Woodruff 1990, Van Rijen *et al.* 1991). Dextromethorphan, an antitussive agent with non-competitive NMDA receptor antagonistic properties, and kyenuric acid, a broad-spectrum EAA antagonist with both competitive and non-competitive NMDA receptor activity, are two other agents whose use has been associated with attenuation of ischaemic injury in exper-

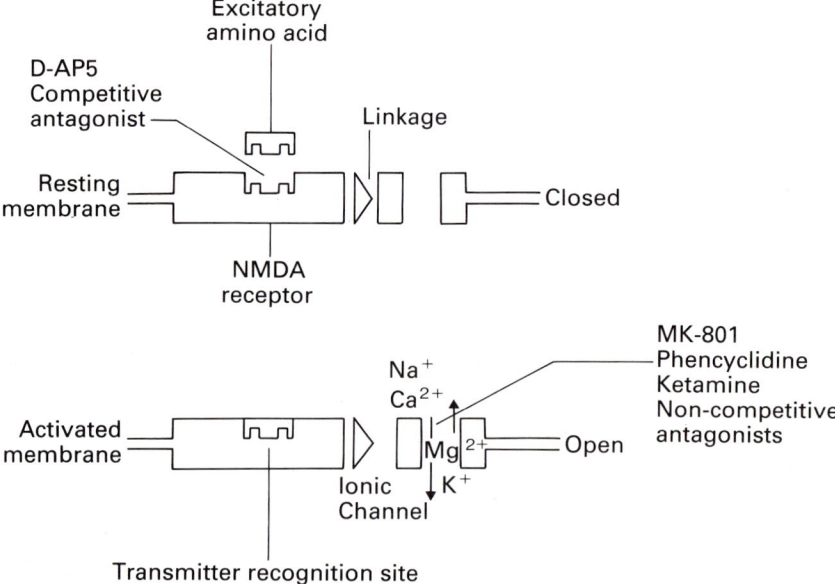

Fig. 3.4 Control of ionic channel calcium influx by adjacent NMDA receptors; site of action of NMDA receptor antagonists.

imental models. Further investigation into the role of NMDA receptor antagonists in the clinical management of cerebral ischaemia is eagerly awaited.

INHIBITORS OF ARACHIDONIC ACID METABOLISM

One of the final common pathways after the ischaemic activation of intracellular lipases and proteases, the forerunners of neuronal death, is the generation of free fatty acids, including arachidonic acid. Numerous investigations into the possible protective use of drugs which limit the metabolism of arachidonic acid have therefore been conducted. Aspirin, indomethacin, prostacyclin and eicosapentaenoic acid all appear to have little effect on outcome following focal or global cerebral ischaemia. However, a relatively new thromboxane synthetase inhibitor, trapidil, may be of some benefit in patients suffering SAH (Tani *et al.* 1984), although the effects of this drug on the incidence of rebleeding, due to its inherent ability to reduce platelet aggregation, are raising some concerns and need further investigation.

FREE-RADICAL SCAVENGERS

The reperfusion of ischaemic areas of the brain is associated with the generation of free radicals from abnormal mitochondrial electron transfer. Free radicals increase lipid peroxidation, prostaglandin synthesis and membrane damage (White *et al.* 1985). As well as the release of free radicals, the presence of oxygen in previously ischaemic areas is associated with the release of pro-oxidant iron, which is then able to act as a catalyst in free-radical reactions, so increasing the degree of cerebral damage. Although free radicals represent extremely destructive compounds the brain does, under normal circumstances, possess natural free-radical scavenging agents. Two of these scavenging agents, catalase and mitochondrial superoxide dismutase, are lost early in the ischaemic process, while glutathione peroxidase is absent from some of the most ischaemically vulnerable areas of the brain. Attention has therefore been focused on the use of drugs with free-radical scavenging properties as means of providing protection against reperfusion injury. Results following the use of mannitol, thiopentone, chlorpromazine, allopurinol and vitamins C and E remain inconclusive (Halliwell & Gutteridge 1985, Symon 1985) although there is new evidence to suggest that the anaesthetic agent propofol (2,6-diisopropylphenol) is an extremely efficient free-radical scavenger. The phenolic structure within propofol allows it to scavenge free radicals in a similar way to vitamin E and other phenol-based antioxidants. The addition of propofol to plasma increases the total radical antioxidant potential. Liver homogenates of rats anaesthetized with clinical doses of propofol show a delayed fall in PaO_2 after the addition of a free-radical generator compared with liver homogenates from control rats (Murphy *et al.* 1992). While further clinical investigation is still needed, the *in vitro*, free-radical scavenging ability of propofol does not seem in doubt. Giving substances such as superoxide dismutase and catalase are not feasible ways of boosting the bodily defences in the event of ischaemia and reperfusion. In addition it takes up to 6 weeks to charge up the intracellular content of vitamin E. The interest in propofol is not just that it may be effective, but also that its action may be immediate.

References

Abramson N.S., Safar P. & Detre K.M. (1986) Randomized clinical study of thiopental loading in comatose survivors of cardiac arrest. *New England Journal of Medicine* **314**, 397−403.

Araki T., Kato H. & Kogure K. (1990) Neuronal damage and calcium accumulation following repeated brief cerebral ischemia in the gerbil. *Brain Research* **528**, 114−122.

Artru A.A. & Michenfelder J.D. (1981) Anoxic cerebral potassium accumulation reduced by phenytoin: mechanism of cerebral protection? *Anesthesia and Analgesia* **60**, 41−45.

Astrup J., Siesjo B.J. & Symon L.S. (1981a) Thresholds in cerebral ischaemia — The ischemic penumbra. *Stroke* **12**, 723−725.

Astrup J., Skovsted P., Gjerris F. & Sorensen H.R. (1981b) Increase in extracellular potassium in the brain during circulatory arrest: effects of hypothermia, lidocaine, and thiopental. *Anesthesiology* **55**, 256−262.

Astrup J., Symon L., Branston N.M. & Lassen N.A. (1977) Cortical evoked potential and extracellular K^+ and H^+ at critical levels of brain ischemia. *Stroke* **8**, 51−57.

Awad I.A., Carter L.P., Spetzler R.F., Medina M. & Williams J.F.G. (1987) Clinical vasospasm after subarachnoid hemorrhage: response to hypervolemic hemodilution and arterial hypertension. *Stroke* **18**, 365−372.

Boris-Moller F., Smith M. & Siesjo B.K. (1989) Effects of hypothermia on ischemic brain damage: a comparison between pre-ischemic and post-ischemic cooling. *Neuroscience Research Committee* **5**, 87−93.

Bouma G.J., Muizelaar J.P., Choi S.C., Newlon P.G. & Young H.F. (1991)

Cerebral circulation and metabolism after severe traumatic brain injury: the elusive role of ischemia. *Journal of Neurosurgery* **75**, 685−693.

Buchan A. & Pulsinelli W.A. (1990) Hypothermia but not the N-methyl-D-aspartate antagonist MK-801, attenuates neuronal damage in gerbils subjected to global ischemia. *Journal of Neuroscience* **10**, 311−316.

Busto R., Dietrich W.D., Globus M.Y-T., Valdes I., Scheinberg P. & Ginsberg M.D. (1987) Small differences in intraischaemic brain temperature critically determine the extent of ischaemic neuronal injury. *Journal of Cerebral Blood Flow and Metabolism* **7**, 729−738.

Busto R., Globus M.Y-T., Dietrich W.D., Martinez E., Valdes I. & Ginsberg M.D. (1989a) Effect of mild hypothermia on ischaemia-induced release of neurotransmitters and free fatty acids in rat brain. *Stroke* **20**, 904−910.

Busto R., Dietrich W.D., Globus M.Y-T. & Ginsberg M.D. (1989b) Post-ischemic moderate hypothermia inhibits CA1 hippocampal neuronal ischemic injury. *Neuroscience Letters* **101**, 299−304.

Choi D.W. (1988) Glutamate neurotoxicity and diseases of the central nervous system. *Neuron* **1**, 623−634.

Church J., Zeman S. & Lodge D. (1988) The neuroprotective action of ketamine and MK-801 after transient cerebral ischaemia in rats. *Anesthesiology* **69**, 702−709.

Cotman C.W. & Iversen L.L. (1987) Excitatory amino acids in the brain. Focus on NMDA receptors. *Trends in Neuroscience* **10**, 263−265.

Dearden N.M. (1990) The management of the post-ischaemic brain. *Current Anaesthesia and Critical Care* **1**, 105−114.

Drummond J.C., Oh Y-S., Cole D.J. & Shapiro H.M. (1989) Phenylephrine induced hypertension reduces ischemia following middle cerebral artery occlusion in rats. *Stroke* **20**, 1538−1544.

Evans D.E. & Kobrine A.I. (1987) Reduction of experimental intracranial hypertension by lidocaine. *Neurosurgery* **20**, 542−547.

Faithfull N.S. (1987) Fluorocarbons: current status and future applications. *Anaesthesia* **42**, 234−242.

Gelmers H.J., Gorter K., DeWeerdt C.J. & Wiezer H.J.A. (1988) A controlled trial of nimodipine in acute ischemic stroke. *New England Journal of Medicine* **318**, 203−207.

Giannotta S.L., Oppenheimer J.H., Levy M.L. & Zelman V. (1991) Management of intraoperative rupture of aneurysm without hypotension. *Neurosurgery* **28**, 531−536.

Gill R. & Woodruff G.N. (1990) The neuroprotective actions of kynurenic acid and MK-801 in gerbils are synergistic and not related to hypothermia. *European Journal of Pharmacology* **176**, 143−149.

Gisvold S.E. & Steen P.A. (1985) Drug therapy in brain ischaemia. *British Journal of Anaesthesia* **57**, 96−109.

Graham D.I. (1985) The pathology of brain ischaemia and possibilities for therapeutic intervention. *British Journal of Anaesthesia* **57**, 3–17.

Greenamyre J.T., Olson J.M.M., Penney J.B. & Young A.B. (1985) Autoradiographic characterisation of N-methyl-D-aspartate-quisqualate- and kainate-sensitive glutamate binding sites. *Journal of Pharmacology and Experimental Therapeutics* **233**, 254–263.

Hallenbeck J.M. & Furlow T.W. (1979) Prostaglandin I_2 and indomethacin prevent impairment of post-ischemia brain perfusion in the dog. *Stroke* **10**, 629–637.

Halliwell B. & Gutteridge J.M.C. (1985) Review: oxygen radicals and the nervous system. *Trends in Neuroscience* **8**, 22–26.

Harper A.M. & Bell R.A. (1963) The effect of metabolic acidosis and alkalosis on the blood flow through the cerebral cortex. *Journal of Neurology, Neurosurgery and Psychiatry* **26**, 341–344.

Harper A.M. & Glass H.I. (1965) Effects of alterations in the arterial carbon dioxide tension on the blood flow through the cerebral cortex at normal and low arterial blood pressures. *Journal of Neurology, Neurosurgery and Psychiatry* **28**, 449–452.

Heuser D. & Guggenberger H. (1985) Ionic changes in brain ischaemia and alterations produced by drugs. *British Journal of Anaesthesia* **57**, 23–33.

Hoff J.T. (1986) Cerebral protection. *Journal of Neurosurgery* **65**, 579–591.

Jones J.G., Heneghan C.P.H. & Thornton C. (1985) Functional assessment of the normal brain during general anaesthesia. In: Kaufman L (Ed.), *Anaesthesia Review 3*, pp. 83–98. Churchill Livingstone, Edinburgh.

Kahn R.A., Allen R.W. & Baldassare J. (1985) Alternate sources and substitutes for therapeutic blood components. *Blood* **66**, 1–12.

Kalimo H., Rehncrona S., Soderfeldt B., Olsson Y. & Siesjo B.K. (1981) Brain lactic acidosis and ischaemic cell damage. 2 Histopathology. *Journal of Cerebral Blood Flow and Metabolism* **1**, 313–327.

Kemp J.A., Foster A.C. & Wong E.H.F. (1987) Non-competitive antagonists of the excitatory amino acid receptors. *Trends in Neuroscience* **10**, 294–298.

Klatzo I. (1985) Brain oedema following brain ischaemia and the influence of therapy. *British Journal of Anaesthesia* **57**, 18–22.

Kontos H.A. (1989) Oxygen radicals in CNS damage. *Chemical–Biological Interactions* **72**, 229–255.

Lassen N.A. (1985) Normal average value of cerebral blood flow in younger adults is 50 ml/100 g/min. *Journal of Cerebral Blood Flow and Metabolism* **5**, 347–349.

Ledingham I.McA. & Watt I. (1983) Influence of sedation in critically ill multiple trauma patients. *Lancet* **i**, 1270.

Maynard D.E. (1982) Cerebral function analysing monitor (CFAM): detection of cerebral ischaemia. *Electroencephalography and Clinical Neurophysiology* **54**, 20–25.

McDowall D.G. (1966) Inter-relationships between oxygen tensions and cerebral blood flows. In: Payne J.P. & Hill D.W. (Eds), *Oxygen Measurements in Blood and Tissues*, pp. 205−214. J. & A. Churchill, London.

Milde L.N. (1990) Cerebral protection. In: Cucchiara RF & Michenfelder JD (Eds), *Clinical Neuroanesthesia*, p. 171. Churchill Livingstone, New York.

Milde L.N., Milde J.H. & Michenfelder J.D. (1986) Delayed treatment with nimodipine improves cerebral blood flow after complete cerebral ischemia in the dog. *Journal of Cerebral Blood Flow and Metabolism* **6**, 332−337.

Michenfelder J.D. (1974) The interdependency of cerebral function and metabolic effects following massive doses of thiopental in dog. *Anesthesiology* **41**, 231−236.

Michenfelder J.D. (1986) A valid demonstration of barbiturate-induced brain protection in man − at last. *Anesthesiology* **64**, 140−142.

Michenfelder J.D., Milde L.N. & Sundt T.M. (1976) Cerebral protection by barbiturate anesthesia: Use after middle cerebral artery occlusion in Java monkeys. *Archives of Neurology* **33**, 345−350.

Mohamed A.A., Gotoh O. & Graham D.I. *et al.* (1985) Effect of pretreatment with the calcium antagonist nimodipine on local cerebral blood flow and histopathology after middle cerebral artery occlusion. *Annals of Neurology* **18**, 705−711.

Murphy P.G., Myers D.S., Davies M.J., Webster N.R. & Jones J.G. (1992) The antioxidant potential of propofol (2,6-diisopropylphenol). *British Journal of Anaesthesia* **68**, 613−618.

Myers R.E. & Yamaguchi S. (1977) Nervous system effects of cardiac arrest in monkeys: preservation of vision. *Archives of Neurology* **34**, 65−74.

Nehls D.G., Todd M.M., Spetzler R.F., Drummond J.C., Thompson R.A. & Johnson P.C. (1987) A comparison of the cerebral protective effects of isoflurane and barbiturates during temporary focal ischemia in primates. *Anesthesiology* **66**, 453−464.

Nevin M., Colchester A.C.F., Adams S. & Pepper J.R. (1989) Prediction of neurological damage after cardiopulmonary bypass surgery: use of the cerebral function analysing monitor. *Anaesthesia* **44**, 725−729.

Nussmeier N.A., Ralund C. & Slogoff S. (1986) Neuropsychiatric complications after cardiopulmonary bypass: cerebral protection by a barbiturate. *Anesthesiology* **64**, 165−170.

Pickard J.D., Murray G.D., Illingworth R. *et al.* (1989) Effect of oral nimodipine on cerebral infarction and outcome after subarachnoid haemorrhage: British aneurysm nimodipine trial. *British Medical Journal* **298**, 636−642.

Prior P.F. (1985) EEG monitoring and evoked potentials in brain ischaemia. *British Journal of Anaesthesia* **57**, 63−81.

Rockoff M.A., Marshall L.F. & Shapiro H.M. (1979) High-dose barbiturate therapy in humans: a clinical review of 60 patients. *Annals of Neurology* **6**, 194−199.

Rothman S.M. & Olney J.W. (1986) Glutamate and the pathophysiology of hypoxic—ischaemic brain damage. *Annals of Neurology* **19**, 105—111.

Ruta T.S., Drummond J.C. & Cole D.J. (1991) A comparison of the area of histochemical dysfunction after focal cerebral ischaemia during anaesthesia with isoflurane and halothane in the rat. *Canadian Journal of Anaesthesia* **38**, 129—135.

Sano T., Drummond J.C., Patel P.M., Grafe M.R., Watson J.C. & Cole D.J. (1992) A comparison of the cerebral protective effects of isoflurane and mild hypothermia in a model of incomplete forebrain ischemia in the rat. *Anesthesiology* **76**, 221—228.

Schell R.M., Cole D.J. & Osborne T.N. (1991) Pentastarch decreases blood—brain barrier permeability following temporary cerebral ischemia in rats. *Anesthesia and Analgesia* **72** (Suppl.), S235.

Schmidley J.W. (1990) Free radicals in central nervous system ischaemia. *Stroke* **21**, 1086—1090.

Selman W.R., Spetzler R.F. & Roski R.A. (1981) Barbiturate resuscitation from focal cerebral ischemia—a review. *Resuscitation* **9**, 189—196.

Shapiro H.M. (1985) Barbiturates in brain ischaemia. *British Journal of Anaesthesia* **57**, 82—95.

Siesjo B.K. (1988) Acidosis and ischaemic brain damage. *Neurochemistry and Pathology* **9**, 31—88.

Siesjo B.K. & Smith M.L. (1991) The biochemical basis of ischemic brain lesions. *Arzneimittelforschung/Drug Research* **41**, 288—292.

Siesjo B.K. & Wieloch T. (1985) Cerebral metabolism in ischaemia: neurochemical basis for therapy. *British Journal of Anaesthesia* **57**, 47—62.

Smith D.S., Keykhah M.M. & O'Neill J.J. (1989) The effect of etomidate pretreatment on cerebral high energy metabolites, lactate, and glucose during severe hypoxia in the rat. *Anesthesiology* **71**, 438—443.

Steen P.A. & Michenfelder J.D. (1978) Cerebral protection with barbiturates: relation to anaesthetic effect. *Stroke* **9**, 140—142.

Stockard J.J., Bickford R.G., Myers R.R. & Aung M.H. (1974) Hypotension induced changes in cerebral function during cardiac surgery. *Stroke* **5**, 730—738.

Sundt T.M. & Waltz A.G. (1971) Cerebral ischemia and reactive hyperemia. Studies of cortical blood flow and microcirculation before, during and after temporary occlusion of middle cerebral artery of sqirrel monkeys. *Circulation Research* **28**, 34—43.

Symon L. (1985) Flow thresholds in brain ischaemia and the effects of drugs. British Journal of Anaesthesia 57, 34—43.

Symon L., Branston N.M. & Strong A.J. (1976) Autoregulation in acute focal ischaemia. *Stroke* **7**, 547—554.

Tani E., Maeda Y., Fukurmori T. *et al.* (1984) Effect of selective inhibitor thromboxane A_2 synthetase on cerebral vasospasm after early surgery. *Journal of Neurosurgery* **61**, 24—29.

Van Rijen P.C., Verheul H.B., van Echteld C.J.A. *et al.* (1991) Effects of dextro-methorphan on rat brain during ischemia and reperfusion assessed by magnetic resonance spectroscopy. *Stroke* **22**, 343—350.

Venables G.S., Strong A.J., Miller S.A., Gibson G. & Hardy J.A. (1986) The effects of etomidate in the cat middle cerebral artery occlusion model of brain ischemia. *Neurology Research* **8**, 209—213.

Warner D.S., Godersky J.C. & Smith M.L. (1988) Failure of pre-ischemic lido-caine administration to ameliorate global ischemic brain damage in the rat. *Anesthesiology* **68**, 73—78.

White B.C., Krause G.S., Aust S.D. & Eyster G.E. (1985) Postischemic tissue injury by iron-mediated free radical lipid peroxidation. *Annals of Emergency Medicine* **14**, 804—809.

4
Neuropharmacology

EDWARD MOSS

Introduction

The rational management of anaesthesia and intensive care for patients with intracranial pathology requires knowledge of the effects of drugs on cerebral matabolism, cerebral blood flow (CBF), intracranial pressure (ICP) and cerebral perfusion pressure (CPP). In addition, any effects of these drugs on the physiology of normal and pathological brain must be clearly understood.

Physiology

Drugs used during anaesthesia are unlikely to affect the volume of the brain tissue but, by causing hypertension in the presence of defective autoregulation, may cause an increase in brain extracellular fluid volume. Many drugs are cerebral vasodilators, either having a direct effect on the blood vessels or acting indirectly by depressing respiration and causing an increase in arterial carbon dioxide concentration. Cerebral vasodilatation increases CBF causing an increase in cerebral blood volume (CBV) (Smith *et al.* 1971) which in turn causes an increase in ICP. This effect will be small in patients with normal brain but, when intracranial compliance is reduced due to a space-occupying lesion or diffuse cerebral oedema, the increase in ICP will be greater. Thus, in the presence of intracranial hypertension, ICP changes will tend to parallel those in CBF. The increase in ICP causes a reduction in CPP which causes further vasodilatation and increase in ICP. In the absence of a compensatory increase in arterial pressure this will ultimately cause a reduction in CBF but, because the increase in ICP is caused by increasing CBF, the extent of intracranial hypertension is self-limiting. Any associated reduction in arterial pressure will also limit the increase in ICP, but it will be associated with a marked fall in perfusion pressure to inadequate levels.

Cerebral vasodilators will modify the normal autoregulatory process, making CBF dependent on the arterial pressure. When there is a reduction in arterial pressure there may be either no change or an increase in CBF initially, and CBF is maintained to pressures below the lower limit of autoregulation, but as the arterial pressure is reduced further CBF will start to decrease. Therefore, the change in blood flow is the result of the complex interrelationships between the direct effect of the agent on the vessels, autoregulation and CPP. If arterial pressure is reduced by an agent which does not cause cerebral vasodilatation CBF is maintained until the lower limit of autoregulation is reached; as the arterial pressure is reduced further flow decreases passively.

Cerebrovascular disease may lead to areas of incomplete ischaemia because of arterial narrowing which may be fixed due to atherosclerotic disease or reversible as in vasospasm. Other cerebral lesions may cause cerebral vasoparalysis due to local loss of autoregulation and carbon dioxide reactivity. In either of these situations cerebral vasodilators, by dilating vessels which can respond, will cause cerebral steal and exacerbation of regional ischaemia. On the other hand, drugs which produce vasoconstriction should induce inverse steal, altering the distribution of blood flow to improve oxygenation of pathological areas of the brain. In the presence of cerebral vasospasm cerebral vasodilatation will improve the situation only if the pathological narrowing of the vessel is reversed. Recent evidence has cast doubt on the concept of intracerebral steal by showing that vasodilators such as carbon dioxide, papaverine or nimodipine decrease the resistance of vessels supplying ischaemic tissue and increase flow in the ischaemic areas (Scremin 1991).

Drugs may influence ICP by altering the rate of production or the resistance to reabsorption of cerebrospinal fluid (CSF). CSF pressure represents an equilibrium between the rates of production and reabsorption of CSF. If the rate of production is increased and/or the resistance to reabsorption through the arachnoid villi is increased CSF pressure will increase until a new equilibrium is reached. CSF is produced at the rate of approximately $0.5 \, \text{ml} \, \text{min}^{-1}$ (Rubin *et al.* 1966, Cutler *et al.* 1968), so any change in ICP by this mechanism will occur slowly.

An increase in ICP will cause a reduction in CPP which may cause cerebral ischaemia and internal pressure gradients which may produce brain shift (Fig. 4.1). The brain may herniate through the foramen magnum with distortion of the brainstem, through the tentorium cerebelli, underneath the falx and, if the dura is open, through the craniotomy defect. Differential pressures occur in the brain because the vessels in normal and diseased brain tissue respond differently to vasodilators and

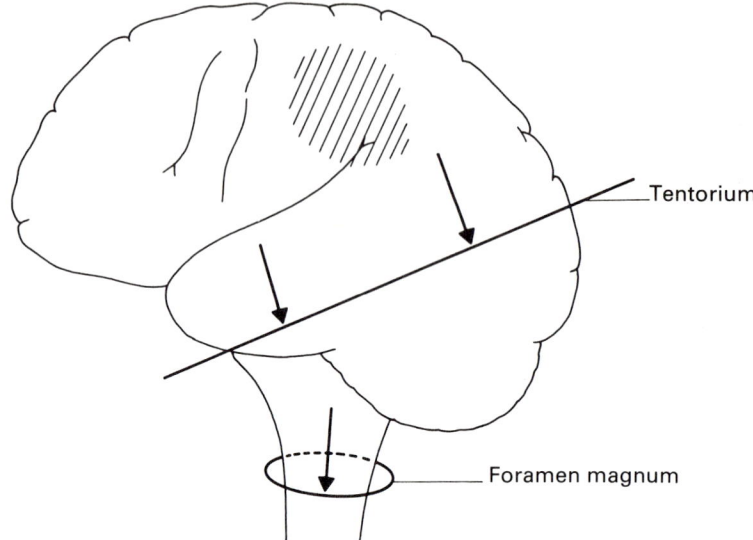

Fig. 4.1 Schematic drawing of intracranial pressure gradients indicating brain shift which can develop in the presence of a space-occupying lesion indicated in the parietal region.

the compliance of diseased brain is altered, so the various intracranial compartments will have different changes in volume and pressure. When the dura is incised ICP falls to zero, but if ventricular CSF volume or brain bulk is increased the brain will appear tight, surgical access will be hampered and the brain may herniate through the skull defect. Lesser increases in brain bulk will result in increased retraction pressures on the brain which may cause cerebral ischaemia (Rosenorn & Diemer 1982).

Cerebral metabolic rate and CBF usually increase or decrease in parallel, thus matching the oxygen supply to demand. Under normal circumstances global CBF does not alter significantly and blood is diverted from less active to more active areas, so that regional flow changes but global flow remains constant. Drugs which reduce cerebral metabolic rate usually reduce CBF and ICP, but volatile anaesthetics are the exception to this rule, reducing cerebral metabolic rate whilst increasing CBF.

Nitrous oxide can increase ICP by a unique mechanism. It diffuses into air spaces at approximately 30 times the rate that nitrogen diffuses out. Therefore, if there is a pocket of air inside the cranium following air encephalography (Campkin & Turner 1972) or posterior fossa surgery

(MacGillivray 1982) it will increase in size rapidly, causing an increase in ICP.

Cerebral autoregulation and the carbon dioxide reactivity of the cerebral vessels are important homeostatic mechanisms. Therefore, it is desirable for anaesthetic agents to have little or no effect on cerebral autoregulation or carbon dioxide reactivity.

The effects of drugs on cerebral metabolic rate, CBF and ICP have been studied in animals and humans, both with and without intracranial pathology. Some results are conflicting, possibly due to different animal species and experimental design involving different arterial carbon dioxide tensions and cerebral perfusion pressures. In interpreting the results of these studies it must be remembered that an increase in global CBF may mask regional steal effects and significant cerebral ischaemia. The effects of the individual drugs are discussed below and summarized in Table 4.1 (see pp. 80–82).

Volatile anaesthetic agents

All volatile anaesthetic agents increase CBF and ICP and reduce cerebral metabolic rate for oxygen ($CMRO_2$). This represents an uncoupling of the usual relationship between cerebral metabolism and CBF, and indicates a direct vasodilating effect on the cerebral vessels (Jensen *et al.* 1992). These changes in ICP are greater in patients with increased ICP (Jennett *et al.* 1969, Gordon 1970) because as the volume of a space-occupying lesion increases, the intracranial compliance is reduced and the same degree of cerebral vasodilatation will cause a greater increase in ICP (Fitch & McDowall 1971) (Fig. 4.2). Volatile anaesthetics increase ICP and decrease mean arterial pressure (MAP) so CPP is reduced. Halothane causes the greatest increase in CBF and ICP and isoflurane the least (Eger 1981) (see Fig. 4.3). Cerebrovascular autoregulation is gradually abolished as the dose of volatile anaesthetic is increased, with CBF becoming more pressure-dependent (Fig. 4.4). Carbon dioxide reactivity is increased during halothane (Alexander *et al.* 1964, Young *et al.* 1991) and isoflurane anaesthesia (Young *et al.* 1971, Drummond & Todd 1985). Thus the CBF–carbon dioxide response curve is shifted to the left (Fig. 4.5) so that hypocapnia will still reduce flow but any rise in $PaCO_2$ will cause an exaggerated increase in CBF. There is no significant difference in the slope of the CBF–carbon dioxide response curves for equal maximal allowable concentration (MAC) multiples of isoflurane, halothane and

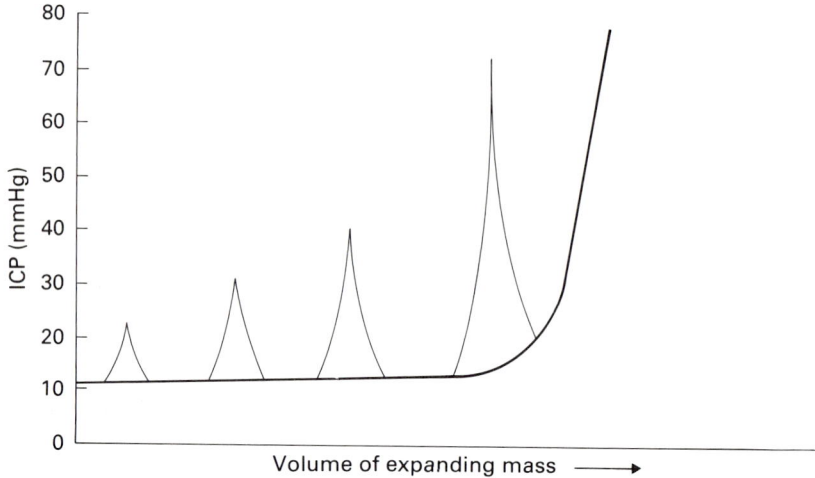

Fig. 4.2 The pressure–volume curve of the cranial contents. As the volume of an expanding intracranial mass increases ICP rises only slightly until the compensatory mechanisms are overcome. This point is reached at the elbow of the curve when further expansion of the mass causes a steep increase in ICP. Administration of a cerebral vasodilator such as halothane causes a small increase in ICP at the left-hand end of the curve (with a return to the previous value due to compensatory mechanisms), but will cause larger increases as the volume of the mass increases and intracranial compliance is reduced (Fitch & McDowall 1971).

methoxyflurane in dogs (Smith & Wollman 1972) (Fig. 4.6). There is experimental evidence that, in the presence of cerebral oedema, volatile anaesthetics cause significant further increases in oedema and ICP (Scheller *et al.* 1987) whereas pentobarbitone or nitrous oxide, fentanyl and droperidol anaesthesia do not (Smith & Marque 1976).

HALOTHANE

Halothane causes an increase in ICP (Jennett *et al.* 1969) and CBF (Christensen *et al.* 1967), an effect which is most marked in the neocortex (Hansen *et al.* 1988). It reduces $CMRO_2$ but does not appear to provide cerebral protection, and high concentrations may induce cerebral acidosis (Michenfelder & Theye 1975). If ICP is elevated hyperventilation for at least 10 min before halothane is introduced can prevent large increases in ICP (Adams *et al.* 1972), but when ICP is markedly elevated this may not be effective (Jennett *et al.* 1969, Gordon 1970) and halothane is best

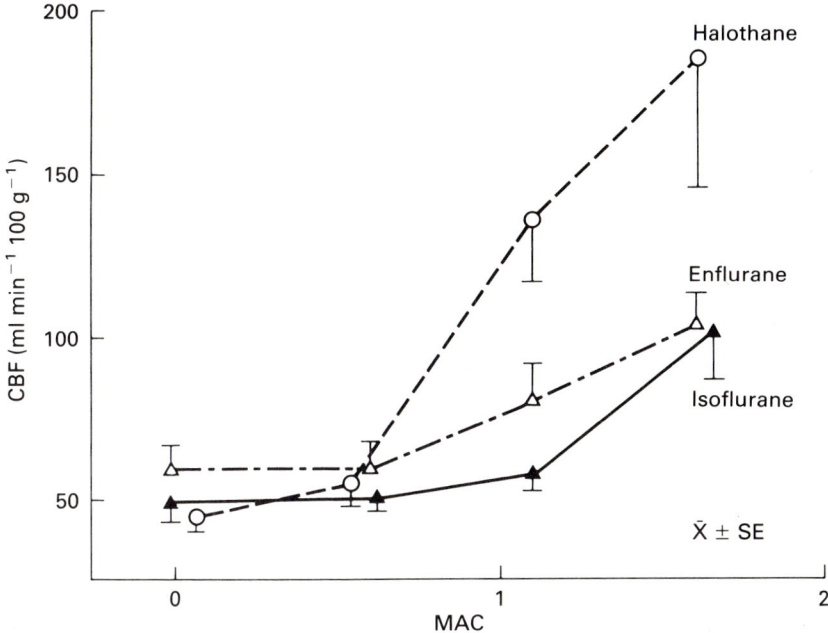

Fig. 4.3 CBF measured in normocapnic volunteers awake and anaesthetized with nitrous oxide and different volatile agents. Systemic pressure was maintained at normal levels by infusion of phenylephrine. From Eger (1981).

avoided until the dura has been incised and the patient is hypocapnic. The rate of CSF production is unaltered by halothane but the resistance to absorption is increased (Artru 1984). Autoregulation is disturbed by halothane 1% inspired concentration and abolished by halothane 2% (Morita *et al.* 1977) and may not return to normal for 2 h after discontinuation of the halothane. Halothane does not cause seizure activity on the electroencephalogram (EEG) (Kaven *et al.* 1974).

ENFLURANE

The majority of studies show that enflurane has less effect on CBF and ICP than halothane, and the largest reported increases in ICP with enflurane are significantly smaller than those reported with halothane (Moss *et al.* 1983). Enflurane (1 MAC) has little effect on CBF and ICP even in patients with intracranial space-occupying lesions, but MAP is reduced, which decreases CPP and may mask any cerebral vasodilatation

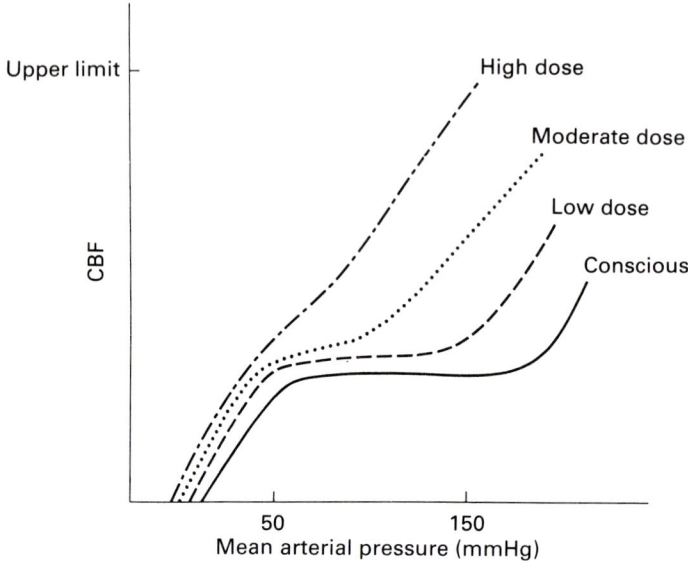

Fig. 4.4 Idealized curves of the effect of a progressively increased dose of a volatile anaesthetic agent on CBF autoregulation.

(Moss *et al.* 1983). Like halothane, enflurane reduces $CMRO_2$ (De Rood *et al.* 1980). The EEG shows high-voltage slow waves and hypersynchrony in concentrations up to 1.5 MAC (Kaven *et al.* 1974), but greater concentrations cause high-amplitude spikes or spike-and-wave complexes, particularly during hypocapnia and auditory stimulation (Neigh *et al.* 1971). This epileptiform activity will increase $CMRO_2$ and CBF. However, enflurane is no more likely than isoflurane to cause convulsions after intracranial surgery when inspired concentrations of 2% or less are used (Christys *et al.* 1989). The rate of production and resistance to reabsorption of CSF are increased by enflurane, which contributes to the increase in ICP associated with its administration (Artru 1984).

ISOFLURANE

CBF and CBV are not affected by inspired concentrations of 0.6–1.1 MAC of isoflurane, but 1.6 MAC isoflurane doubles CBF (Eger 1981). ICP is similarly unaffected by less than 1 MAC isoflurane (Adams *et al.* 1981, Campkin 1984), but higher concentrations increase ICP (Gomez-Sainz *et al.* 1988). The rate of CSF production or reabsorption is not affected by isoflurane (Artru 1984). The carbon dioxide reactivity of the cerebral

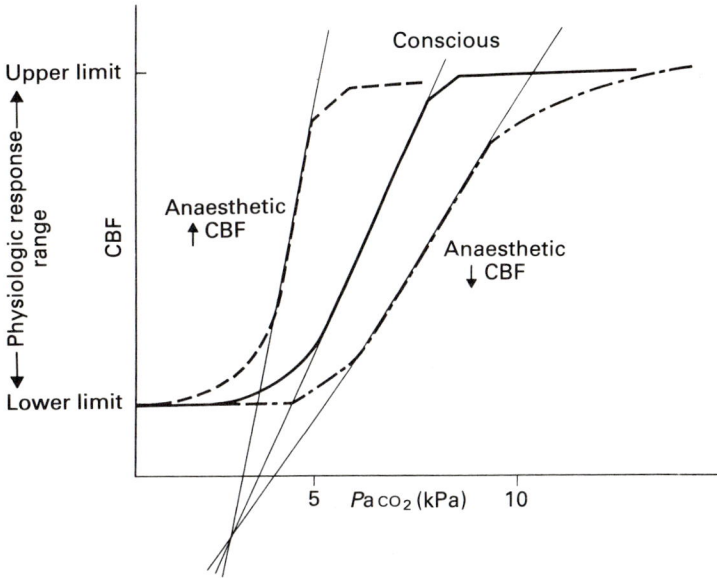

Fig. 4.5 Effects of anaesthetic agents on the CBF–carbon dioxide response curve. Idealized curves indicating the effects of carbon dioxide and volatile agents. The slope of the thin line indicates that CBF–carbon dioxide sensitivity is increased with agents which increase cerebral blood flow, such as volatile agents.

vessels is increased (Drummond & Todd 1985) and maintained even when high concentrations are given (McPherson *et al.* 1989). Isoflurane causes less impairment of cerebrovascular autoregulation than halothane (Mutch *et al.* 1990), and autoregulation is significantly impaired only by concentrations greater than 1 MAC (Alad *et al.* 1991). The depression of CMRO$_2$ is greater with isoflurane than halothane (Algotsson *et al.* 1988) and progressive metabolic depression occurs with concentrations greater than 1 MAC until, at approximately 2.5 MAC, the EEG becomes isoelectric (Newberg *et al.* 1983). The concentrations necessary to abolish cortical activity have no direct toxic effect on cerebral metabolic pathways. If has been suggested that isoflurane has a cerebral protective effect against ischaemia in animals (Newberg *et al.* 1984) and in humans (Michenfelder *et al.* 1987), but a study in primates showed that during profound hypotension isoflurane gave no more cerebral protection than halothane and sodium nitroprusside combined (Gelb *et al.* 1989). In concentrations up to 1.5 MAC isoflurane has similar effects on the EEG to enflurane, causing high-voltage slow waves and hypersynchrony (Kaven *et al.*

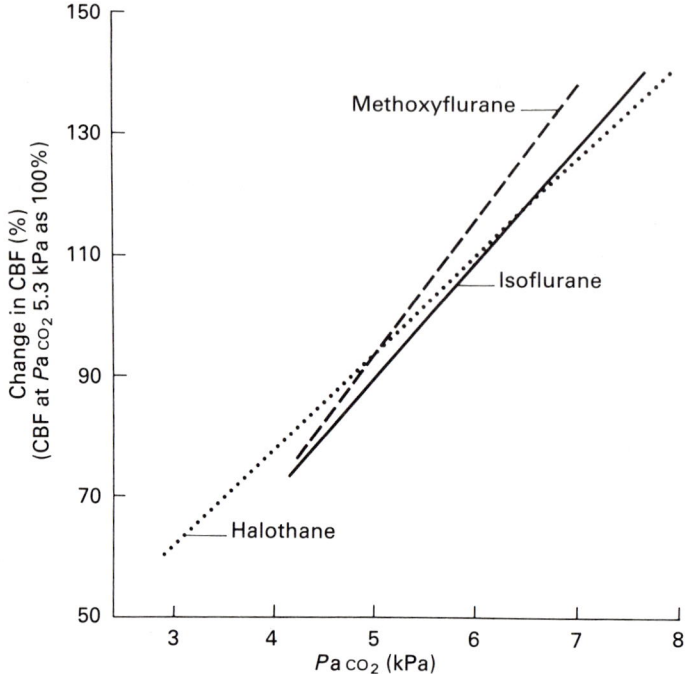

Fig. 4.6 CBF—carbon dioxide response curves with isoflurane, halothane and methoxyflurane in dogs. From Smith & Wollman (1972).

1974), but the EEG becomes isoelectric at higher concentrations (Newberg *et al.* 1983). However, convulsions have been reported during or following anaesthesia in patients who had no history of epilepsy (Hymes 1985, Poulton & Ellingson 1984).

SEVOFLURANE

Present evidence indicates that sevoflurane has a minimal effect on CBF and increases ICP very slightly (Scheller *et al.* 1988). Its effects on the EEG are similar to those of isoflurane. It causes dose-related cardiovascular depression (Kazama & Ikeda 1985) so CPP will be reduced. This agent is available for clinical use in Japan but not in the UK.

DESFLURANE

In dogs desflurane causes a dose-related reduction in cerebral vascular resistance and 1.5 MAC desflurane increases CBF by 25% (Lutz *et al.*

1990). The reduction in CMRO$_2$ is comparable to other volatile anaesthetics. CBF and CMRO$_2$ are both reduced during hypotension induced with desflurane, and there is no decrease in high-energy phosphates even with profound hypotension (Milde & Milde 1991). The cardiovascular effects are similar to those of isoflurane so there will be a reduction in CPP (Weiskopf *et al.* 1991). Equipotent concentrations of desflurane have similar effects on the EEG to isoflurane with progressive depression of the EEG (Rampil *et al.* 1988, Lutz *et al.* 1990), but the effects of higher concentrations on EEG activity may decrease with time. This agent is at present undergoing clinical trials but is not yet available for clinical use.

Anaesthetic gases

NITROUS OXIDE

Nitrous oxide increases CMRO$_2$ and CBF in dogs (McDowall & Harper 1965, Theye & Michenfelder, 1972) but reports in humans are conflicting (Wollman *et al.* 1965, Sakabe *et al.* 1976, Algotsson *et al.* 1992). There is no doubt that nitrous oxide increases ICP during established anaesthesia with hypocapnia in patients with cerebral tumours (Misfeldt *et al.* 1974) and in hypocapnic patients with head injury (Moss & McDowall 1979). The increase in ICP must be caused by cerebral vasodilatation, which suggests that the conflicting results regarding CBF are methodological. CBF measurements can be made only intermittently, and the experimental error is fairly large, thus a change in CBF can be missed. If hypocapnia is established for 10 min before the administration of nitrous oxide its effects on ICP are reduced (Misfeldt *et al.* 1974, Jorgensen & Henriksen 1973). Therefore, in patients with raised ICP, nitrous oxide should be avoided until after intubation and hyperventilation with 100% oxygen is established (Henriksen & Jorgensen 1973). Nitrous oxide does not affect cerebral autoregulation or carbon dioxide reactivity (Wollman *et al.* 1965). The depression of CMRO$_2$ caused by 0.5 and 1 MAC isoflurane is reversed by nitrous oxide possibly attenuating any cerebral protection against ischaemia which may be offered by isoflurane (Baughman *et al.* 1989). However, most published work suggests that nitrous oxide has a minimal effect on cerebral metabolism (Baughman *et al.* 1990, Algotsson *et al.* 1992). In rats the addition of 0.5 MAC nitrous oxide to 0.5 MAC halothane causes similar increases in CBF to the addition of a further 0.5 MAC halothane, and adding 0.5 MAC nitrous oxide to 0.5 MAC

Table 4.1 Summary of the effects on the cranial contents of agents used during anaesthesia

Agent	CMRO$_2$	CBF	ICP	CO$_2$ reactivity	Cerebral autoregulation	CSF production	Resistance to reabsorption CSF
Volatile anaesthetics							
Halothane	–	+	+	+	–	0	+
Enflurane	–	+	+	+	–	+	+
Isoflurane	–	+	+	+	–	0	–
Sevoflurane	–	+	+	?	?	?	?
Desflurane	–	+	?+	?	?	?	?
Anaesthetic gases							
Nitrous oxide	+	+	+	0	0	0	0
Cyclopropane	?	+	+	+	?	?	?
Intravenous anaesthetics							
Thiopentone	–	–	–	0	0	0–*	0–*
Methohexitone	–	–	–	0	0	?	?
Etomidate	–	–	–	0	0	0–*	0–*
Propofol	–	–	–	0	0	?	?
Ketamine	?+	+	+	0	0	0	+
Benzodiazepines							
Diazepam	–	–	0	0	?	?	?
Lorazepam	–	–	?	?	?	?	?
Midazolam	–	–	0	?	?	0–*	0+*
Flumazenil	0	0	0	?	?	?	?

Analgesics							
Morphine	0	0	0	?	0	?	?
Pethidine	–	–	?	?	?	?	?
Phenoperidine	0	?+	?+	?	?	?	?
Fentanyl	0	0	0	+	0	0	?
Alfentanil	0	+	+	?	?	0	–
Sufentanil	?–	+	+	?	?	?	?
Tramadol	?	?	?	?	?	?	?
Muscle relaxants							
Suxamethonium	0	+	+	?	?	?	
Non-depolarizing	0	0	0	?	?	?	
Other agents							
Droperidol	0	–	0	?	?	?	
Lignocaine	–	–a	–	?	?	?	
Naloxone	0	0	0	?	?	?	
Alpha$_2$ agonists	0	–	?–	?	?	?	
Diuretics							
Mannitol	0	0b	–b	0	0	0	–
Frusemide	0	0	–	0	0	0	–

Continued on p. 82

Table 4.1 (*Continued*)

Agent	CMRO$_2$	CBF	ICP	CO$_2$ reactivity	Cerebral autoregulation	CSF production	Resistance to reabsorption CSF
Hypotensive agents							
Sodium nitroprusside	0	+	+	0	1		
Glyceryl trinitrate	0	?+	+	0	?		
Trimetaphan	0	0	0c	0	0		
Labetalol	0	0	0	0	0		
Hydralazine	0	+	+	0	?		
Captopril	0	0	0	+	0		
Adenosine	?	+	+	?	?		
Urapidil	?	?	0	?	?		
Prostaglandin E$_1$	0	0	0	0	0		
Calcium antagonists							
Nimodipine	0	+	?+	–	0		
Nicardipine	?	?+	?	0	?		

0, no change; +, increase; –, decrease; ?, unknown; ?+, possible increase; ?–, possible decrease; a, very large doses; b, increases initially; c, may increase if intracranial compliance reduced; 1, impaired.
* Dependent on dose.

isoflurane produces CBF values significantly greater than those caused by 1 MAC isoflurane alone (Hansen *et al.* 1989). This indicates that 0.5 MAC nitrous oxide causes similar increases in CBF to 0.5 MAC halothane. Similar findings have been reported in dogs (Roald *et al.* 1991). The background anaesthetic may alter the response to nitrous oxide; for example, the effect of nitrous oxide on CBF is less if an opioid is used (Drummond *et al.* 1987).

Intravenous anaesthetic agents

Provided that there is no respiratory depression, the intravenous anaesthetic agents reduce cerebral metabolic rate, CBF and ICP, and through their effects on arterial pressure CPP is reduced. The exception is ketamine, which has a different mode of action. The reduction in ICP is greater in patients with higher ICP values (Turner *et al.* 1973) and, in these patients, the reduction in ICP may be greater than the reduction in MAP, resulting in an increase in CPP. Propanidid and Althesin are no longer available for clinical use, but the steroid anaesthetic, pregnanolone, is undergoing clinical trials and might be expected to have similar effects on CBF, $CMRO_2$ and ICP to Althesin. Midazolam and thiopentone may increase the resistance to reabsorption of CSF whereas etomidate has no effect (Artru 1988), but these results are unlikely to be clinically relevant because the response to different doses of these agents was variable.

Barbiturates

Thiopentone and methohexitone are the barbiturates commonly used to induce anaesthesia. Pentobarbitone is used in the management of severe head injuries and Reyes syndrome, but is not available for clinical use in the UK. However, significant cardiovascular depression is easily induced causing a reduction in CPP, so barbiturates should be used only with careful monitoring in these situations. Barbiturates do not reduce $CMRO_2$, CBF or ICP until consciousness is lost, after which there is rapid dose-dependent depression of metabolism until the EEG becomes isoelectric, whereupon additional increases in barbiturate tissue levels do not reduce $CMRO_2$ further (Steen *et al.* 1983). There is a significant correlation between $CMRO_2$ and CBF in dogs treated with thiopentone (Kassell *et al.* 1980) and this decrease in metabolic rate and the rate of production of acid metabolites is the most likely cause of barbiturate-induced vasoconstriction.

Barbiturates may induce inverse steal by inducing vasoconstriction in normal vessels and preferentially directing flow to areas where there is vasomotor paralysis and hypoperfusion. They can reduce ICP by controlling epileptic fits and oedema formation. Epileptiform activity is often associated with head injury and hypoxia, and leads to a marked increase in cerebral metabolism, resulting in lactic acidosis and an increase in CBF and ICP. Thus the barbiturates are able to break the vicious cycle of hypoxia, convulsions, intracranial hypertension and further fits. Barbiturates, by inducing arteriolar constriction, may also protect damaged capillaries and reduce oedema formation (Smith & Marque 1976).

THIOPENTONE

Thiopentone reduces $CMRO_2$ and CBF (Pierce *et al.* 1962, Cote *et al.* 1979), causing a reduction in ICP (Horsley 1937, Sondergard 1961, Shapiro *et al.* 1973) and an increase in intracranial compliance (Artru 1989). The carbon dioxide reactivity of the cerebral vessels is not affected (Pierce *et al.* 1962). It has been used by infusion to maintain anaesthesia during neurosurgery (Hunter 1972a) and in the management of severe head injury, but cumulation due to slow metabolism limits its use in these situations.

METHOHEXITONE

Methohexitone reduces CBF (Herrschaft & Schmidt 1974) and ICP (Takasaki *et al.* 1973, Cunitz *et al.* 1978) and has also been used by infusion to maintain anaesthesia during neurosurgery (Hunter 1972b). However, it can produce epileptiform activity on the EEG and is used during surgery for temporal lobe epilepsy to stimulate epileptiform activity and help identify the focus by electrocorticography (Paul & Harris 1970; Musella *et al.* 1971).

ETOMIDATE

Etomidate reduces $CMRO_2$, CBF (Van Aken & Rolly 1976; Renou *et al.* 1978) and ICP (Moss *et al.* 1979) and increases intracranial compliance (Artru 1989). CPP is usually well maintained (Moss *et al.* 1979) and cerebrovascular carbon dioxide reactivity is preserved (Cold *et al.* 1985).

As the brain concentration of etomidate increases EEG activity is depressed (Cold *et al.* 1986). The drug has anticonvulsant properties (Wauquier 1983) but convulsions have occurred after a short general anaesthetic in which only etomidate was used (Hansen & Drenck 1988). Etomidate has been used by infusion to maintain anaesthesia during neurosurgery, but many neuroanaesthetists formed the clinical impression that this increased the incidence of vomiting after craniotomy. It is now known that etomidate causes adrenocortical suppression due to inhibition of 11 beta-hydroxylation, 17 alpha-hydroxylation and other intramitochondrial hydroxylation reactions, thus depressing 17 alpha-hydroxyprogesterone, aldosterone and corticosterone production (Moore *et al.* 1985). This caused an increase in mortality in multiple-trauma patients sedated by etomidate infusion on an intensive therapy unit (Watt & Ledingham 1984). Etomidate is no longer recommended for use by continuous infusion but, if used, steroids must be administered and continued for at least 24 h after the cessation of the infusion. However, it has been used to prevent the increase in ICP associated with intubation while maintaining a normal CPP by infusion to the point of burst suppression on the EEG (Modica & Tempelhoff 1992).

PROPOFOL

Propofol reduces $CMRO_2$, CBF (Stephan *et al.* 1987, Vandesteene *et al.* 1988) and ICP (Mazzarella *et al.* 1987, Van Hemelrijck *et al.* 1989) but CPP may be reduced due to a marked reduction in MAP (Mazzarella *et al.* 1987, Van Hemelrijck *et al.* 1989). Propofol also reduces the pressure under the brain retractor during intracranial surgery, but significant reduction in CPP may occur (Moss & Price 1990). The carbon dioxide reactivity and autoregulation of the cerebral vessels is well maintained during propofol anaesthesia (Stephan *et al.* 1987, Van Hemelrijck *et al.* 1990). EEG activity is depressed by propofol (Stephan *et al.* 1987) but spikes and slow waves have been demonstrated on electrocorticography in patients undergoing temporal lobectomy (Hodkinson *et al.* 1987), and a grand-mal convulsion has been reported following anaesthesia with propofol in a patient with no previous history of epilepsy (Victory & Magee 1988). In experimental animals anaesthetic doses of propofol have an anticonvulsant effect (Lowson *et al.* 1990) and the duration of convulsions during eletroconvulsive therapy is reduced (Simpson *et al.* 1988). It appears that propofol does not have proconvulsant properties but, during recovery from anaesthesia, the blood level falls quickly, causing rapid termination of the anticonvulsant activity which may allow convulsions to occur in susceptible patients.

Infusion of propofol with or without nitrous oxide has proved very satisfactory for maintenance of anaesthesia during craniotomy (Freedman & Levy 1988, Merckx *et al.* 1988). Its pharmacokinetic properties allow infusion for several hours without significant cumulation (Shafer *et al.* 1988). Propofol reduces but does not abolish the hypertensive response to intubation (Coates *et al.* 1987, Roberts *et al.* 1988). It does not suppress adrenocortical function significantly, having a similar effect to thiopentone on adrenal steroidogenesis (Lambert *et al.* 1985, Fragen *et al.* 1987). Propofol has free-radical scavenging properties (Murphy *et al.* 1992), which may explain the improved neurological outcome following incomplete ischaemia in experimental animals when propofol is used (Kochs *et al.* 1992).

KETAMINE

Ketamine is a phenyl cyclohexamine which induces dissociative anaesthesia. In contrast to the other anaesthetic agents it stimulates the cardiovascular system and causes minimal respiratory depression, but produces significant emergence sequelae. Ketamine increases CBF (Takeshita *et al.* 1972), the power of the EEG, cerebral blood flow velocity (Kochs *et al.* 1991), ICP (Gardner *et al.* 1972, Gibbs 1972) and the resistance to reabsorption of CSF (Mann *et al.* 1980), but increases in $CMRO_2$ have been described only in animals (Dawson *et al.* 1971). The increases in ICP are exacerbated in patients with intracranial space-occupying lesions (Shapiro *et al.* 1972). The reactivity of the cerebral circulation to carbon dioxide is not altered by ketamine (Sari *et al.* 1972a). It has a similar potency to methohexitone as an anticonvulsant (Wardley-Smith *et al.* 1988). Ketamine has been used by infusion during intracranial surgery in combination with drugs such as benzodiazepines or lignocaine, which obtund its effects on cerebral metabolism and CBF. Its action as a non-competitive antagonist at NMDA receptors may offer protection from the adverse effects of cerebral ischaemia.

Benzodiazepines

Benzodiazepines may be given orally as anxiolytics before operation or parenterally for sedation on the intensive care unit (ICU) and for induction and maintenance of anaesthesia. They reduce CBF and $CMRO_2$; therefore their use is safe in patients with intracranial decompensation. However, they are of little therapeutic value in the treatment of intracranial hypertension. As with all sedatives, they should be used with caution and careful monitoring in patients who are breathing spontaneously because of the potential for respiratory depression.

DIAZEPAM

Diazepam reduces $CMRO_2$ and CBF without affecting the carbon dioxide reactivity of the cerebral vessels (Cotev & Shalit 1975) but has no effect on ICP in dogs (Campan & Lazorthes 1976) or neurosurgical patients (Tateishi *et al.* 1981). If the arterial pressure is reduced CPP will decrease. The effects of diazepam on CBF and $CMRO_2$ are potentiated by nitrous oxide (Carlsson *et al.* 1976). It has little effect on the cardiovascular system but does cause slight respiratory depression.

LORAZEPAM

Lorazepam reduces $CMRO_2$ and increases cerebral vascular resistance, thereby reducing CBF in primates (Rockoff *et al.* 1980). The absence of cerebral metabolic changes indicative of ischaemia in Rockoff's study suggests that the reduction in $CMRO_2$ is proportional to or exceeds the decrease in CBF.

MIDAZOLAM MALEATE

Midazolam is a water-soluble benzodiazepine with an elimination half-life of 2 h, which is noticeably shorter than that of diazepam. It can be used intravenously to induce anaesthesia and has minimal cardiovascular effects. Midazolam increases cerebral vascular resistance (Forster *et al.* 1982, 1987) but did not reduce ICP in patients with brain tumours or abolish increases in ICP associated with laryngoscopy and intubation (Griffin *et al.* 1984). An associated small reduction in arterial pressure may reduce CPP, but CPP is better maintained with midazolam than with thiopentone. Large doses of midazolam reduced $CMRO_2$ in dogs, and brain biopsies after midazolam administration revealed a normal energy state (Nugent *et al.* 1982). Midazolam provided greater protection against hypoxia than diazepam, but less than thiopentone. Infusion of midazolam and alfentanil does not suppress adrenocortical function significantly (Nilsson *et al.* 1988). Midazolam can be used by infusion for maintenance of anaesthesia, but it causes quite prolonged sedation postoperatively (Nilsson & Persson 1988). This would be a disadvantage in neurosurgery because neurological assessment is required as soon as possible after surgery.

FLUMAZENIL

Flumazenil is a specific benzodiazepine antagonist which reverses the effects of benzodiazepines on CBF, but has no effect on CBF when administered alone (Forster *et al.* 1987). Other workers have failed to demonstrate a change in CBF when midazolam was reversed with flumazenil (Knudsen *et al.* 1991) but because of the intermittent nature of CBF measurements a change may have been missed. If flumazenil is used to rouse midazolam-sedated patients with pathological intracranial compliance, it should be titrated very carefully to avoid dangerous increases in CBF and ICP (Schulte am Esch & Kochs 1990) and the precipitation of a convulsion in an epileptic.

Neuroleptics

DROPERIDOL

Droperidol reduces CBF in dogs but has no effect on $CMRO_2$ (Michenfelder & Theye 1971). It appears to have little effect on ICP in humans (Misfeldt *et al.* 1976), although when combined with fentanyl it has been shown to reduce ICP in patients with intracranial space-occupying lesions (Fitch *et al.* 1969). Animal work suggests that oedema formation following trauma may be reduced when neuroleptic drugs are used rather than halothane (Smith & Marque 1976).

Analgesics

The narcotic analgesics have little effect on CBF and ICP if respiratory depression with a consequent increase in $PaCO_2$ is avoided. Thus morphine has no effect on CBF (Moyer *et al.* 1957, Jobes *et al.* 1977) or ICP (Keats & Mithoefer 1955) if $PaCO_2$ remains constant. Pethidine causes slight reductions in CBF and $CMRO_2$ in dogs (Messick & Theye 1969). Cerebrovascular autoregulation is not affected by fentanyl or morphine (Farrar *et al.* 1981, Jobes *et al.* 1975). The effects of the individual agents are discussed below, but in general, provided the patient is being ventilated, these drugs are both safe and useful in neurosurgical patients undergoing surgery or being treated in the ICU. Their analgesic properties attenuate the increase in CBF associated with painful stimulation. The shorter-acting agents are preferable to longer-acting agents because their respiratory depressant effects are less likely to continue into the postoperative period.

PHENOPERIDINE

When given with droperidol at constant $PaCO_2$, phenoperidine causes small changes in CSF pressure which can be in either direction (Fitch *et al.* 1969) and CBF is unaltered (Wilkinson & Browne 1970). Phenoperidine has been widely used for sedation of patients with head injury during mechanical ventilation, but increases in ICP, possibly by causing vasodilatation which triggered A waves (Grummitt & Goat 1984), and reduction in CPP have been reported (Bingham & Hinds 1987).

FENTANYL

Fentanyl has little effect on ICP (Moss *et al.* 1978b) and decreases the resistance to absorption of CSF (Artru 1984). When given in large doses it tends to reduce CPP (Cuillerier *et al.* 1990). $CMRO_2$ and CBF are reduced in dogs anaesthetized with nitrous oxide in oxygen (Michenfelder & Theye 1971) but, when given with droperidol in humans, fentanyl does not affect $CMRO_2$ or CBF (Sari *et al.* 1972b, Vernhiet *et al.* 1977). Fentanyl increases cerebral vascular reactivity to carbon dioxide (Vernhiet *et al.* 1977) and has no effect on cerebrovascular autoregulation (Farrar *et al.* 1981).

Grand-mal convulsions have occurred following the administration of fentanyl (Rao *et al.* 1982, Safat & Daniel 1983) and it is generally accepted that they are most likely to occur with large doses, but in one report only 100 µg of fentanyl had been given (Hoien 1984). The respiratory depressant effects of fentanyl are of short duration because of its short half-life. This is an advantage in intracranial surgery because postoperative respiratory depression will induce cerebral vasodilatation which will increase ICP and the formation of cerebral oedema. However, respiratory depression will occur if the dose is not carefully controlled, and reversal with naloxone may be required.

ALFENTANIL

The literature regarding the effects of alfentanil on CBF and ICP is conflicting. There is little doubt that bolus doses of alfentanil can cause increases in ICP which are greater if intracranial compliance is reduced (Jung *et al.* 1990, Moss 1992) and, in rats, it can be demonstrated that alfentanil induced rigidity causes an increase in ICP by increasing CVP (Benthuysen *et al.* 1988). Cerebrovascular autoregulation and carbon dioxide reactivity is not affected by large doses of alfentanil (McPherson *et al.* 1985). There is no doubt that bolus doses of alfentanil reduce CPP in patients with intracranial lesions (Cuillerier *et al.* 1990, Moss 1992) and, although it reduces the haemodynamic response to intubation, it should not be given as a bolus for this purpose unless administered cautiously. It is commonly given by infusion to sedate patients who are mechanically ventilated after severe head injury, and does not appear to increase ICP. Slow infusions produce stable cardiovascular parameters (Stuart-Taylor & Sleigh 1987) and, by avoiding sudden changes in arterial pressure, have no effect on ICP and can be safely employed in these circumstances. Spindle activity is prominent on the EEG following the administration of alfentanil, which causes an increase in delta-activity, a reduction in the higher-frequency components and less synchronization of the EEG than do fentanyl or sufentanil (Bovill *et al.* 1983). Alfentanil has the shortest half-life of the opioids available for clinical use in the UK, and would be expected to cause less postoperative respiratory depression than fentanyl. However, it is cumulative and infusion should be discontinued at least 30 min before the end of surgery.

SUFENTANIL

Sufentanil is an opioid analgesic structurally related to fentanyl and alfentanil, and is not available in the UK. Although some authors have been unable to demonstrate any effect on CBF (Mayer *et al.* 1990, Werner *et al.* 1991) there are reports that it is a cerebral vasodilator causing increases in CBF (Vernhiet *et al.* 1977, Milde & Milde 1989) and ICP and a reduction in CPP (Marx *et al.* 1988, Cuillerier *et al.* 1990). It has been shown to reduce $CMRO_2$ in dogs (Milde *et al.* 1990). The increase in ICP and the reduction in CPP associated with its use make it less appropriate than other available analgesics for use during intracranial surgery.

PENTAZOCINE

Pentazocine causes small decreases in ICP in patients undergoing intra-cranial surgery when ventilation is controlled to maintain a constant $PaCO_2$ but, when given to patients with cerebral trauma who are breathing spontaneously, $PaCO_2$ and ICP increase (Barker *et al.* 1972).

TRAMADOL

Tramadol is an opioid which has very little depressant effect on respiration (Vickers *et al.* 1992) and may prove useful for postoperative analgesia following intracranial surgery. At the time of writing it is being assessed in clinical trials in the UK and is not available for general use.

Neuromuscular blocking drugs

With the exception of d-tubocurarine, the non-depolarizing muscle relaxants have no direct effect on CBF (Alexander *et al.* 1964, Wollman *et al.* 1964, 1965) or ICP in humans, but the depolarizing relaxants cause muscle fasciculations and increase ICP. In patients who are mechan-ically ventilated, muscle relaxants may reduce ICP by reducing inflation pressures and CVP.

SUXAMETHONIUM

Suxamethonium increases lumbar CSF pressure (Halldin & Wahlin 1959) and ICP (Marsch *et al.* 1980). This is probably caused by muscle fascicu-lations which increase intra-abdominal, intrathoracic and central venous pressures. The increase in CVP is transmitted to the valveless epidural veins increasing the epidural blood volume which squeezes the dura mater increasing CSF pressure and ICP. Lanier and colleagues (1986) demon-strated an increase in CBF following the administration of suxamethonium to dogs lightly anaesthetized with halothane, which they attributed to afferent muscle spindle activity and a secondary rise in $PaCO_2$ consequent upon muscle fasciculations. This increase in CBF may be responsible for part of the increase in CSF pressure with suxamethonium. When suxamethonium is given to patients already paralysed with a non-depolarizing muscle relaxant ICP is not affected, so pretreatment with a small dose of non-depolarizing relaxant may prevent the increase in ICP by reducing the fasciculations (Minton *et al.* 1986). Unfortunately, this manoeuvre can make the intubating conditions less satisfactory. It is generally accepted that the effect of suxamethonium on ICP is moderate (approximately 5—10 mmHg) and short-lived (Marsh *et al.* 1980, Minton *et al.* 1986), therefore, if suxamethonium is indicated, as in the head injury patient with a full stomach, it should be used, and measures to reduce ICP should be employed as soon as the patient is safely intubated.

D-TUBOCURARINE

The literature regarding the effects of d-tubocurarine on ICP is conflicting. Sondergard (1961) found that there was no effect on ICP provided that the $PaCO_2$ was not allowed to increase, and others have failed to demonstrate any increase in ICP when bolus doses of 45 mg were given (Moss *et al.* 1978a). However, Tarkkanen and colleagues (1974) showed an increase in ICP following d-tubocurarine 0.6 mg kg^{-1} which they attributed partly to histamine release causing cerebral vasodilatation. Other factors including an increase in $PaCO_2$ and increased arousal may have contributed to the increase in ICP in this study. d-Tubocurarine is a useful agent for neurosurgery when induced hypotension is planned because its ganglion-blocking properties help in the control of arterial pressure, but if used at induction of anaesthesia with thiopentone a marked fall in arterial pressure and CPP may occur (Moss *et al.* 1978a).

PANCURONIUM

Pancuronium does not affect ICP during induction of anaesthesia (McLeskey *et al.* 1974) and has no effect on $CMRO_2$, CBF or the EEG in dogs (Lanier *et al.* 1985). It may cause arterial hypertension (Kelman & Kennedy 1971), which can cause problems during some intracranial procedures.

ALCURONIUM AND ATRACURIUM

These have no effect on ICP (Greenbaum *et al.* 1975, Unni *et al.* 1986) and atracurium does not affect $CMRO_2$ or CBF in dogs (Lanier *et al.* 1985).

VECURONIUM

Vecuronium has been shown to cause a small reduction in ICP and MAP without significant changes in CPP, probably due to muscle relaxation causing a decrease in CVP (Rosa *et al.* 1986, Stirt *et al.* 1987).

Other agents

LIGNOCAINE

Lignocaine $1.5 \, mg \, kg^{-1}$ prevents increases in ICP associated with tracheal intubation in patients with cerebral tumours (Bedford *et al.* 1980) and is commonly used during induction of anaesthesia for intracranial surgery. A similar dose reduces ICP in patients with head injury (Donegan & Bedford 1980). In animals $CMRO_2$ is reduced by a dose of $3 \, mg \, kg^{-1}$, but much larger doses are needed to reduce CBF (Sakabe *et al.* 1974). In addition to its suppressant effect on synaptic transmission lignocaine has a specific membrane-stabilizing effect by blocking sodium channels and restricting sodium−potassium leak fluxes. The load on the ion pump is reduced and metabolism decreased. Thus further metabolic depression (15−20%) can be achieved after the EEG has become isoelectric (Astrup *et al.* 1981).

NALOXONE

Reversal of opioid analgesia with naloxone increases heart rate, cardiac output and arterial pressure (Desmonts *et al.* 1978) due to an action on specific receptors near the cardiovascular control centre (Artru *et al.* 1980). Therefore, when it is used to reverse the residual effects of opioids after intracranial surgery, it should be carefully titrated to effect. The administration of naloxone has been associated with an improvement in neurological status in some patients with acute stroke (Jabaily & Davis 1984).

DOXAPRAM

Doxapram has some stimulant effects on the brain, so it would be expected to stimulate cerebral metabolism and cause increases in CBF and ICP. Therefore, it would be wise to avoid this agent after intracranial surgery despite a report of its use to stimulate respiration in a brain-damaged infant without any increase in ICP (Fisher & Rodarte 1987).

ALPHA₂ AGONISTS

In dogs dexmedetomidine, an alpha₂-adrenergic agonist, reduces cardiac output and CBF without influencing $CMRO_2$ (Karlsson *et al.* 1990, Zornow *et al.* 1990). There is a loss of high-frequency activity on the EEG similar to that seen with 1.9% isoflurane, and these EEG effects can be reversed by the alpha₂ antagonist idazoxan. This agent may prove useful as a supplementary agent during neuroanaesthesia by allowing a reduction in the doses of other agents.

Dehydrating agents

OSMOTIC DIURETICS

The role of hypertonic agents to reduce brain water was first described by Javid in 1958 with the use of urea. Urea is no longer used because the small molecule penetrates the blood–brain barrier easily, causing a rebound increase in ICP, significant tubular reabsorption occurs and it is irritant, so that accidental leakage into the tissues causes local tissue damage. Osmotic diuretics are freely filtrable at the glomerulus, undergo limited reabsorption by the tubule and are pharmacologically inert. In order to reduce brain water these agents require an intact blood–brain barrier so that they can draw water out of normal brain into the vascular space from where it is excreted by the kidney. If the blood–brain barrier is damaged, osmotic diuretics will pass freely into the brain extracellular fluid, increasing brain osmolality and causing a rebound increase in ICP. The ideal osmotic gradient for the treatment of cerebral oedema is $10-15\,\text{mosmol}\,\text{kg}^{-1}$ between CSF and blood (Marshall *et al.* 1978). The normal plasma osmolality is $285 \pm 6\,\text{mosmol}\,\text{kg}^{-1}$ so this does not need to be increased to more than $305\,\text{mosmol}\,\text{kg}^{-1}$. A satisfactory effect can be achieved with 20% mannitol $0.25-0.5\,\text{g}\,\text{kg}^{-1}$ infused over a period of 10 min, although larger doses may be indicated in an emergency (Marshall *et al.* 1978, Smith *et al.* 1986). However, these larger doses may increase the requirements for further doses of mannitol. Rapid infusion of mannitol causes an initial increase in circulating blood volume and arterial pressure, which can be reduced if a loop diuretic is administered first. However, the combination of frusemide and mannitol is more effective if mannitol is given first (see below). The reduction in blood viscosity increases CBF and cerebral blood volume, which may cause a transient increase in ICP (Cottrell *et al.* 1977, Ravussin *et al.* 1985) before an autoregulatory response causes a compensatory vaso-constriction which leads to a fall in ICP (Muizelaar *et al.* 1983). This cerebrovascular response to mannitol occurs only if autoregulation is intact (Muizelaar *et al.* 1984). The more prolonged reduction in ICP following mannitol is due to its osmotic effects withdrawing water from normal rather than oedematous tissue (Pappius & Dayes 1965). Therefore, osmotic diuretics reduce ICP rather than treating the cause of raised ICP. Mannitol also increases intracranial compliance, as shown by a reduction in the response of ICP to injection of 1 ml of saline into a lateral ventricle (Miller & Leech 1975). Mannitol causes increased excretion of sodium and potassium in the urine and may cause hyponatraemia and hypo-kalaemia following repeated administration, or in patients with a chronic deficit. Sodium and potassium excretion is greater when mannitol is given in combination with frusemide (Schettini *et al.* 1982), a combination often used to reduce brain bulk during neurosurgery because the effect is greater and its duration is 5 h as opposed to 3 h when mannitol alone is used (Pollay *et al.* 1983). The combination is more effective in reducing ICP if mannitol is given 15 min before rather than after the frusemide (Roberts *et al.* 1987). There is some evidence that mannitol may offer some cerebral protection against ischaemia following occlusion of cerebral vessels (Brown *et al.* 1978, Little 1978). Hypertonic glucose and glycerol have been used to reduce ICP, but are not widely used. Glycerol can be given orally, but has a tendency to cause gastric irritation and, if given intravenously in effective concentrations, intravascular haemolysis and haemoglobinuria can occur (Hagnevik *et al.* 1974).

When large and frequent doses of mannitol are infused it is important to monitor serum osmolality because when serum osmolality exceeds $320\,mosmol\,kg^{-1}$ renal failure and severe metabolic acidosis occur (Becker & Vries 1971). It is also wise to measure ICP in order to assess the effectiveness of the dosage used, because widespread passage of mannitol across the blood—brain barrier can occur, making further administration of this agent ineffective (Stuart *et al.* 1970, Becker & Vries 1971).

There are some situations in which osmotic diuretics are contraindi-cated or should be used with extreme care. The initial increase in cerebral blood volume may be critical if intracranial compliance is low, and osmotic diuretics should be used cautiously in this situation. However, they are sometimes used in this situation to produce a temporary reduction in ICP and gain time immediately before surgery. They are contraindicated when neurogenic pulmonary oedema is present, and it is also wise to avoid them in patients with head injury who show marked sympathetic overactivity even when there is no pulmonary oedema (Clifton *et al.* 1983). Hypertonic solutions are contraindicated in patients with renal disease, and should be used with caution if myocardial function is compromised because a sudden increase in circulating blood volume can precipitate left ventricular failure. Patients who are receiving these agents should have a urinary catheter inserted to prevent discomfort and measure urinary excretion of water and electrolytes.

OTHER DIURETICS

The rate of CSF production is reduced by frusemide, ethacrynic acid, triamterene and thiazide diuretics, but is significantly increased by spironolactone (Domer 1969).

Frusemide reduces ICP mainly by reducing the circulating and cerebral blood volumes, but also decreases CSF production by suppressing sodium transport (Melby *et al.* 1982, Pollay *et al.* 1983). Loop diuretics offer certain advantages over osmotic diuretics in that they do not expand the circulating blood volume, they do not cause an initial increase in ICP, they lower ICP from peak diuresis and they produce smaller losses of sodium and potassium and smaller changes in serum osmolality than osmotic agents (Cottrell *et al.* 1977). These authors recommended frusemide $1 \, mg \, kg^{-1}$ instead of mannitol when a diuresis is required in patients with raised ICP, cardiac disease or electrolyte abnormalities.

Vasoconstrictor drugs

Adrenaline in moderate doses has little action on CBF or $CMRO_2$ provided that autoregulation and the blood—brain barrier remain intact (Olesen 1972, Abdul Rahman *et al.* 1979). Larger doses will increase $CMRO_2$ and CBF, probably secondary to arousal and an increase in arterial pressure which allows translocation of adrenaline into the cerebral extracellular fluid (King *et al.* 1952, Dahlgren *et al.* 1980).

Noradrenaline and *metaraminol* produce minimal cerebral vasoconstriction with little effect on CBF (Greenfield & Tindall 1968, Olesen 1972), and *phenylephrine* restores peripheral vascular tone without affecting cerebrovascular resistance or cerebral metabolism (Schleien *et al.* 1989, Sokrab & Johansson 1989). *Ephedrine* dilates the cerebral vessels and increases flow. *Angiotensin* has no effect on cerebral vessels and is used to raise the arterial pressure and test the integrity of autoregulation (Greenfield & Tindall 1968, Olesen 1972). *Isoprenaline* may increase CBF, and different authors have demonstrated increases and decreases in CBF with *dopamine* (Edvinsson & MacKenzie 1976). Investigations in cats indicate that dopamine may reduce the beneficial effects of barbiturate therapy on cerebral metabolism (Sato *et al.* 1991).

Cerebral vasoconstrictors will decrease overall CBF and include the hypnotics, as discussed above, and xanthine derivatives such as aminophylline (Bowton *et al.* 1988).

Vasodilator drugs

The alpha sympathomimetic blocking drugs, phenoxybenzamine and phentolamine, have no direct influence on CBF, but may cause a small increase in flow due to their effects on sympathetic tone. Papaverine, histamine, sodium nitroprusside, glyceryl trinitrate, hydrallazine, adenosine and those calcium antagonists which are highly lipid-soluble and readily penetrate the blood–brain barrier, nimodipine and nicardipine, induce cerebral vasodilatation. In healthy brain they will increase flow but, in the presence of vasomotor paralysis, have the potential to induce inverse steal.

Hypotensive agents

SODIUM NITROPRUSSIDE

Sodium nitroprusside (SNP), sodium nitroferricyanide, is a powerful vasodilator affecting both resistance and capacitance vessels. It is unstable in solution and is reconstituted from a freeze-dried powder with 5% glucose and diluted to form a 0.01% solution. Alternatively, 0.9% saline can be used for dilution, thus avoiding the infusion of glucose during periods of potential cerebral ischaemia. The solution should be wrapped in the silver foil provided, because it rapidly decomposes in light and should be discarded after 4 h. The solution is pale brown and should be discarded if there is any tendency to blue or green coloration caused by a change from ferric to ferrous iron. Hypotension occurs within 60–90 s of administration and recovery occurs equally quickly on cessation of the infusion, so direct monitoring of arterial pressure is essential.

SNP breaks down in the plasma with the release of cyanide ions which combine with thiosulphate to form thiocyanate, a reaction which is catalysed by the enzyme rhodanase in the liver. In excess there is accumulation of cyanide which inhibits the cytochrome oxidase system and blocks intracellular respiration, causing histotoxic hypoxia and rapidly increasing metabolic acidosis (Creiss *et al*. 1976, Michenfelder & Tinker 1977, Bryson 1977). The use of SNP is contraindicated in patients with vitamin B_{12} deficiency, tobacco amblyopia, Leber's optic atrophy, severe renal disease, impaired liver function and hypothyroidism, because cyanide interferes with vitamin B_{12} metabolism (Creiss *et al*. 1976). The use of hydroxocobalamin, which absorbs free cyanide radicals, has been suggested to reduce the possibility of toxicity, but it is expensive and not generally available. SNP crosses the placenta and is not recommended for use during pregnancy, but has been used during aneurysm surgery with no adverse effect on the fetus (Donchin *et al*. 1978).

The total dose of SNP given over a short period should not exceed $1.5\,mg\,kg^{-1}$ (Vesey *et al*. 1976) and the infusion rate should not be more than $10\,\mu g\,kg^{-1}\,min^{-1}$. If a prolonged infusion is required the maximum safe sustained dose is about $4\,\mu g\,kg^{-1}\,min^{-1}$ with a total dose of $70\,mg\,kg^{-1}$ in patients with adequate renal function (Vesey & Cole 1985).

Poisoning should be treated with sodium thiosulphate (Michenfelder & Tinker 1977) in 300 mg increments intravenously up to a total of $150\,mg\,kg^{-1}$ over 10 min to provide more substrate for the synthesis of thiocyanate. Sodium nitrite ($5\,mg\,kg^{-1}$ intravenously over 3 min) oxidizes haemoglobin to methaemoglobin, which competes preferentially with cytochrome for the cyanide radical to form cyanmethaemoglobin releasing free cytochrome a_3. However, nitrites cause hypotension and may induce hypoxia if too much metahaemoglobin is formed. Cobalt edetate (Kelocyanor), a chelating agent, can be given slowly intravenously in increments of 300 mg (Bryson 1977) up to a total dose of 900 mg. Side-effects of cobalt edetate include hypotension, transient tachycardia and anaphylactoid reactions.

SNP is a potent vasodilator which produces a significant fall in cerebrovascular resistance (Griffiths *et al*. 1974) and abolishes cerebrovascular autoregulation, which is not restored for at least 1 h after SNP is stopped. The autoregulatory response to hypertension returns more rapidly (15–25 min) than the response to hypotension (Stange *et al*. 1991). The cerebral vasodilatation allows the maintenance of normal cerebral blood flow at arterial pressures below the lower limit of autoregulation (Henriksen *et al*. 1983, Keaney *et al*. 1973). However, when regional as opposed to global CBF was studied in goats there was a marked reduction in flow to white matter and the thalamus during profound hypotension with SNP (Miletich *et al.* 1980).

The cerebral vasodilatation caused by SNP, particularly its effect on the capacitance vessels (Michenfelder & Milde 1988), leads to an increase in cerebral blood volume and ICP with the potential for aggravating transtentorial pressure gradients (Morris *et al.* 1982a). The increase in ICP can be attenuated by hypocapnia and, when the mean arterial pressure is reduced to 70% of the control level, ICP returns to the initial value (Turner *et al.* 1977). However, cerebral perfusion pressures as low as 45 mmHg were recorded.

After termination of the SNP infusion rebound hypertension frequently occurs. This is thought to be due to reduced baroreceptor activity during hypotension leading to increased secretion of renin from the juxtaglomerular apparatus of the kidney, and overactivity of the renin—angiotensin system (Khambatta *et al.* 1979, Fahmy *et al.* 1979). This rebound hypertension is a significant complication, as the cerebral capillaries are unprotected because of the absence of autoregulation. Propranolol reduces renin release (Pettinger 1978) and has proved effective in reducing rebound hypertension (Khambatta *et al.* 1981).

In animal studies profound hypotension with SNP produced a smaller reduction in CBF than did a similar reduction in arterial pressure induced by trimetaphan (Morris *et al.* 1982a). There was a smaller reduction in cortical pH and a smaller increase in cortical potassium concentrations with SNP. In a similar model cortical blood flow, PO_2 and EEG activity was better preserved during profound hypotension (mean arterial pressure 30—40 mmHg) induced by SNP when compared with trimetaphan hypotension (Maekawa *et al.* 1979, Ishikawa & McDowall 1981). Thus SNP hypotension causes less disturbance of brain function than trimetaphan.

In summary, SNP is a useful drug for rapid control of arterial pressure during neurosurgery but, because it increases ICP, it should be avoided in patients with intracranial hypertension until after the dura has been incised and the brain decompressed. Combination with other drugs such as trimetaphan or beta-blockers will reduce the dose required, and lessen the risk of toxicity and rebound hypertension.

GLYCERYL TRINITRATE

The nitrates are some of the oldest and most potent drugs used to induce smooth muscle relaxation and vasodilatation. The predominant effect of the drug is on the capacitance vessels reducing venous return, but some direct arteriolar dilatation does occur. The drug is diluted to a 0.01% solution in glass or polyethylene containers, and infused through poly-ethylene tubing because it is rapidly absorbed by polyvinyl chloride. Rarely an excessive dose will lead to methaemoglobinaemia.

Initial reports suggested that arterial pressure was easily controlled, starting to fall within 2−3 min and returning to control values after approximately 10 min following the termination of the infusion (Fahmy 1978). However, others have found it unreliable in reducing arterial pressure during intracranial surgery, and that very high doses are required in those patients who respond (Guggiara *et al.* 1985).

Glyceryl trinitrate (GTN) increases ICP, causing a significant reduction in perfusion pressure (Gagnon *et al.* 1979, Morris *et al.* 1982b). When the arterial pressure is reduced by more than 25% of control, a small reduction in ICP is observed, but cerebral perfusion pressure is markedly reduced (Cottrell *et al.* 1980). It was believed that the increase in ICP was due to an increase in CBF, but animal work has shown that the increase in ICP is not associated with an increase in CBF. It is possible that dilatation of the cerebral veins with an associated increase in CBV is the cause of the increase in ICP when compliance is low (Cottrell *et al.* 1980).

Rebound hypertension has not been reported following the use of GTN. As with SNP the net effect of GTN on the cerebral dynamics is the result of changes in ICP, perfusion pressure and effects on the cerebral vasculature. It may be of benefit in patients with coronary artery disease, but is of limited value in neuroanaesthesia. Like SNP it should be avoided until the dura has been incised in patients with intracranial mass lesions.

TRIMETAPHAN

Trimetaphan is a bisquaternary ammonium compound which is used to induce arterial hypotension by infusion of a 0.1% solution in saline. It is a short-acting ganglion-blocking drug producing both arterial and venous dilatation. The arterial pressure starts to fall within 3−4 min, and on discontinuation of the infusion the pressure usually returns to normal within 10−15 min but hypotension may persist for up to 30 min. Although histamine release occurs it does not play an important role in the haemodynamic effects of the drug in humans (Fahmy & Soter 1985).

Trimetaphan (TMP) has a minimal effect on ICP in most patients, but when intracranial compliance is markedly reduced it may increase ICP (Turner *et al.* 1977). Autoregulation is preserved (Fitch *et al.* 1976) so the brain is protected against hypertension in the early postoperative period. However, CBF is reduced to a greater extent and ischaemia is more severe during profound hypotension with TMP compared with SNP.

A 10 : 1 mixture of TMP with SNP is chemically stable and gives rapid control of arterial pressure. The drugs have a synergistic effect which allows reduced dosage of each agent to induce the required level of hypotension (Macrae *et al.* 1981). There is no information available on the effects of this combination on cerebral dynamics. Rebound hypertension does not appear to be a problem when TMP is stopped either when used alone or as a mixture. As it is a ganglion-blocker it will cause pupillary dilatation and thus complicate the interpretation of clinical signs postoperatively.

If the ICP is raised, TMP appears to be safer than SNP or GTN for induction of moderate hypotension before the skull is opened. If profound hypotension is required an alternative drug would be preferred to maintain adequate cerebral perfusion.

LABETALOL

Labetalol has alpha- and non-cardioselective beta-adrenergic blocking actions. The beta-blocking effects are stronger and more prolonged than the alpha effects. It has a plasma half-life of about 5 h. It has no effect on ICP in dogs with normal or raised ICP (Van Aken *et al.* 1982) and does not alter CBF or cerebrovascular carbon dioxide reactivity in human volunteers (Schroeder *et al.* 1991).

Labetalol acts synergistically with halothane and enflurane, and is commonly used in conjunction with either of these volatile agents to induce hypotension (Scott *et al.* 1972). The initial dose is 10−15 mg intravenously, and it is most effective in the presence of tachycardia. The hypotension can be readily reversed by discontinuation of the volatile agent and the administration of atropine.

HYDRALAZINE

Hydralazine acts centrally and peripherally, producing relaxation of vascular smooth muscle and reducing arteriolar tone. The arterioles are dilated more than the capacitance vessels. The effect of hydralazine starts 15 min after an intravenous bolus of 5−10 mg and the plasma half-life is about 3 h. It causes cerebral vasodilatation (Overgaard &

Skinhoj 1975) and increases ICP when used in combination with enflurane to induce hypotension in patients with cerebral tumours (James & Bedford 1982).

ANGIOTENSIN CONVERTING ENZYME INHIBITORS

Pretreatment with captopril 1 mg kg^{-1} causes a reduction in CBF during anaesthesia (Jensen *et al.* 1989). However, in human volunteers captopril caused no change in CBF and CMRO$_2$ and carbon dioxide reactivity was increased (Schmidt *et al.* 1990). Induced hypotension with captopril and SNP to an MAP of 46 mmHg did not affect CBF and CMRO$_2$ with the exception of one patient who developed a critically low CBF (Thomsen *et al.* 1989).

ADENOSINE

Adenosine triphosphate and adenosine have been used as hypotensive agents. Adenosine triphosphate is converted rapidly to adenosine by 5-nucleotidase so that the major effect is caused by adenosine. Adenosine is a potent vasodilator with rapid onset and recovery. It does not exhibit tachyphylaxis or rebound hypertension following termination of the infusion, and there is no increase in plasma renin activity (Lagerkrauser *et al.* 1985). Bradycardia occurs when the arterial pressure falls. An infusion rate of 0.2−0.6 mg kg^{-1} min^{-1} has been used clinically to reduce the mean arterial pressure to approximately 60 mmHg. Adenosine triphosphate is effective in attenuating the hypertensive response to laryngoscopy and tracheal intubation (Mikawa *et al.* 1991).

An infusion of 1 mg kg^{-1} min^{-1} increased ICP and reduced intracranial compliance in dogs with normal and raised ICP (Van Aken *et al.* 1984). Adenosine reduces the arterial to jugular venous oxygen content difference without signs of lactate formation, indicating an increase in CBF (Sollevi *et al.* 1984). Therefore, this drug can be considered to be in the same group as SNP and GTN, and appears to offer an alternative to SNP.

URAPIDIL

Urapidil is an aryl piperazine derivative with alpha$_1$-adrenergic blocking activities (Williams *et al.* 1984). It reduces sympathetic tone by a central action and does not cause a reflex tachycardia. In dogs it has no effect on ICP or intracranial compliance, but cerebral perfusion pressure is decreased due to the reduction in arterial pressure (Puchstein *et al.* 1983). The drug is potentially useful in neuroanaesthesia but its effects in profound hypotension are unknown.

PROSTAGLANDIN E₁

Prostaglandin E_1 is effective in reducing mean arterial pressure to 70 mmHg in patients undergoing clipping of cerebral aneurysms without reducing local cerebral blood flow (Abe *et al.* 1991). Carbon dioxide reactivity is not affected by prostaglandin E_1 (Abe *et al.* 1992).

Drugs which improve cerebral blood flow

These are drugs which improve the cerebral circulation. In the presence of degenerative vascular disease they are of little benefit and may have a detrimental effect by inducing cerebral steal. Papaverine and betahistine increase flow by arteriolar relaxation, but this can be at the expense of the ischaemic area (Cook & James 1981). Isoxsuprine is an alpha-adrenergic antagonist with some beta-adrenergic stimulant properties. It produces vasodilatation but this is combined with a fall in arterial pressure and CBF.

CALCIUM ANTAGONISTS

Dihydropyridine calcium antagonists combine with voltage-dependent, stereoselective binding sites causing dilatation of the cerebral vessels (Morel & Godfraind 1990). Nicardipine increases cerebral blood flow velocity with maintenance of cerebral vascular reactivity to hypocapnia (Kawaguchi *et al.* 1991) and is effective in preventing circulatory responses to laryngoscopy and tracheal intubation in hypertensive patients (Omote *et al.* 1992).

Nimodipine causes an increase in CBF but autoregulation remains intact (Schmidt & Waldemar 1990). $CMRO_2$ is not affected and carbon dioxide reactivity is reduced (Schmidt *et al.* 1991).

References

Abdul Rahman A., Dahlgren N., Johansson N. & Siesjo B.K. (1979) Increase in local cerebral blood flow induced by circulating adrenaline: involvement of blood—brain barrier dysfunction. *Acta Physiologica Scandinavica* **107**, 227—232.

Abe K., Demizu A., Kamada K., Morimoto T., Sakak T. & Ikuto Y. (1991) Local cerebral blood flow with prostaglandin E1 or trimetaphan during cerebral aneurysm clip ligation. *Canadian Journal of Anaesthesia* **38**, 831—836.

Abe K., Demizu A., Kamada K., Shimada Y., Sakaki T. & Yoshiya I. (1992) Prostaglandin E1 and carbon dioxide reactivity during cerebral aneurysm surgery. *Canadian Journal of Anaesthesia* **39**, 247—252.

Adams R.W., Gronert G.A., Sundt T.M., Jr. & Michenfelder J.D. (1972) Halothane, hypocapnia and cerebrospinal fluid pressure in neurosurgery. *Anesthesiology* **37**, 510—517.

Adams R.W., Cucchiara R.F., Gronert G.A., Messick J.M. & Michenfelder J.D. (1981) Isoflurane and cerebrospinal fluid pressure in neurosurgical patients. *Anesthesiology* **54**, 97—99.

Alad L.J., Croughwell N., Smith L.R. & Reves J.G. (1991) Cerebral blood flow autoregulation is preserved during cardiopulmonary bypass in isoflurane-anesthetized patients. *Anesthesia and Analgesia* **72**, 48—52.

Alexander S.C., James F.M., Colton E.T., Gleaton H.R. & Wollman H. (1968) Effects of cyclopropane anesthesia on cerebral blood flow and carbohydrate metabolism in man. *Anesthesiology* **29**, 170.

Alexander S.C., Wollman H., Cohen P.J., Chase P.E. & Behar M. (1964) Cerebro-vascular response to $Paco_2$ during halothane anesthesia in man. *Journal of Applied Physiology* **19**, 561—565.

Algotsson L., Messeter K., Nordstroom C.H. & Ryding E. (1988) Cerebral blood flow and oxygen consumption during isoflurane and halothane anesthesia in man. *Acta Anaesthesiologica Scandinavica* **32**, 15—20.

Algotsson L., Messeter K., Rosen I. & Holmin T. (1992) Effects of nitrous oxide on cerebral haemodynamics and metabolism during isoflurane anaesthesia in man. *Acta Anaesthesiologica Scandinavica* **36**, 46—52.

Artru A.A. (1984) Effects of enflurane and isoflurane on resistance to reabsorption of cerebrospinal fluid in dogs. *Anesthesiology* **61**, 529—533.

Artru A.A. (1988) Dose-related changes in the rate of cerebrospinal fluid formation and resistance to reabsorption of cerebrospinal fluid following administration of thiopental, midazolam and etomidate in dogs. *Anesthesiology* **69**, 541—546.

Artru A.A. (1989) Intracranial volume—pressure relationship following thiopental or etomidate. *Anesthesiology* **71**, 763—768.

Artru A.A., Steen P.A. & Michenfelder J.D. (1980) Cerebral metabolic effects of naloxone administered with anesthetic and subanesthetic concentrations of halothane in the dog. *Anesthesiology* **52**, 217—220.

Astrup J., Sorensen P.M. & Sorensen H.R. (1981) Inhibition of cerebral oxygen and glucose consumption in the dog by hypothermia, pentobarbital, and lidocaine. *Anesthesiology* **55**, 263—268.

Barker J., Miller J.D. & Johnston I.H. (1972) The effect of pentazocine on pupillary size and intracranial pressure. *British Journal of Anaesthesia* **44**, 197—202.

Baughman V.L., Hoffman W.E., Miletich D.J. & Albrecht R.F. (1990) Cerebrovascular and cerebral metabolic effects of N_2O in unrestrained rats. *Anesthesiology* **73**, 269−272.

Baughman V.L., Hoffman W.E., Thomas C., Albrecht R.F. & Miletich D.J. (1989) The interaction of nitrous oxide and isoflurane with incomplete cerebral ischaemia in the rat. *Anesthesiology* **70**, 767−774.

Becker D.P. & Vries J.K. (1971) The alleviation of increased intracranial pressure by the chronic administration of osmotic agents. In: Brock M. & Dietz H. (Eds), *Intracranial Pressure* pp. 309−315. Springer-Verlag, Berlin.

Bedford R.F., Winn H.R., Tyson G., Park T.S. & Jane J.A. (1980) Lidocaine prevents increased ICP after endotracheal intubation. In: Shulman K., Marmaru A., Miller J.D., Becker D.P., Hochwald G.M. & Brock M. (Eds), *Intracranial Pressure*, vol. IV, pp. 595−598. Springer-Verlag, Berlin.

Benthuysen J.L., Kien N.D. & Quam D.D. (1988) Intracranial pressure increases during alfentanil-induced rigidity. *Anesthesiology* **68**, 438−440.

Bingham R.M. & Hinds C.J. (1987) Influence of bolus doses of phenoperidine on intracranial pressure and systemic arterial pressure in traumatic coma. *British Journal of Anaesthesia* **59**, 592−595.

Bovill J.G., Sebel P.S., Wauquier A., Rog P. & Schuyt H.C. (1983) Influence of high-dose alfentanil anaesthesia on the electroencephalogram: correlation with plasma concentrations. *British Journal of Anaesthesia* **55** (Suppl. 2), 199S−209S.

Bowton D.L., Haddon W.S., Prough D.S., Adair N., Alford P.T. & Stump D.A. (1988) Theophylline effect on the cerebral blood flow response to hypoxemia. *Chest* **94**, 371−375.

Brown F.D., Hanlon K. & Mullan S. (1978) Treatment of aneurysmal hemiplegia with dopamine and mannitol. *Journal of Neurosurgery* **49**, 525−529.

Bryson D.D. (1977) Which antidote for cyanide. *Lancet* **ii**, 1167.

Campan L. & Lazorthes Y. (1976) The effects of various neuroleptic drugs and various diazepines on intracranial pressure of the dog. *Annales d'Anaesthesiologie Francaise* **17**, 1193−1198.

Campkin T.V. (1984) Isoflurane and cranial extradural pressure. A study in neurosurgical patients. *British Journal of Anaesthesia* **56**, 1083−1087.

Campkin T.V. & Turner J.M. (1972) Blood pressure and cerebrospinal fluid pressure studies during lumbar air encephalography. *British Journal of Anaesthesia* **44**, 849−853.

Carlsson C., Hagerdal M., Kaasik A.E. & Siesjo B.K. (1976) The effects of diazepam on cerebral blood flow and oxygen consumption in rats and its synergistic interaction with nitrous oxide. *Anesthesiology* **45**, 319−325.

Christensen M.S., Hoedt-Rasmussen K. & Lassen N.A. (1967) Cerebral vasodilatation by halothane anaesthesia in man and its potentiation by hypotension and hypercapnia. *British Journal of Anaesthesia* **39**, 927−934.

Christys A.R., Moss E. & Powell D. (1989) Retrospective study of early postoperative convulsions after intracranial surgery with isoflurane or enflurane anaesthesia. *British Journal of Anaesthesia* **62**, 624–627.

Clifton G.L., Robertson C.S., Kyper K., Taylor A.A., Dhekne R.D. & Grossman R.G. (1983) Cardiovascular response to severe head injury. *Journal of Neurosurgery* **59**, 447–454.

Coates D.P., Monk C.R., Prys-Roberts C. & Turtle M. (1987) Hemodynamic effects of infusions of the emulsion formulation of propofol during nitrous oxide anesthesia in humans. *Anesthesia and Analgesia* **66**, 64–70.

Cold G.E., Eskesen V., Eriksen H., Amtoft O. & Madsen J.B. (1985) CBF and CMRO$_2$ during continuous etomidate infusion supplemented with N$_2$O and fentanyl in patients with supratentorial cerebral tumour. A dose–response study. *Acta Anaesthesiologica Scandinavica* **29**, 490–494.

Cold G.E., Eskesen V., Eriksen H. & Blatt Lyon B. (1986) Changes in CMRO$_2$, EEG and concentration of etomidate in serum and brain tissue during craniotomy with continuous etomidate supplemented with N$_2$O and fentanyl. *Acta Anaesthesiologica Scandinavica* **30**, 159–163.

Cook P. & James I. (1981) Cerebral vasodilators. *New England Journal of Medicine* **305**, 1560–1564.

Cote J., Simard D. & Rouillard M. (1979) Repercussion sur le debit sanguin cerebral d'une perfusion de thiopental. *Canadian Anaesthetic Society Journal* **26**, 269–276.

Cotev S. & Shalit M.N. (1975) Effects of diazepam on cerebral blood flow and oxygen uptake after head injury. *Anesthesiology* **43**, 117–122.

Cottrell J.E., Robustelli A., Post K. & Turndorf H. (1977) Furosemide- and mannitol-induced changes in intracranial pressure and serum osmolality and electrolytes. *Anesthesiology* **47**, 28–30.

Cottrell J.E., Gupta B., Rappaport H., Turndoff H., Ransohoff J. & Flamm E.S. (1980) Intracranial pressure during nitroglycerine-induced hypotension. *Journal of Neurosurgery* **53**, 309–311.

Creiss L., Tremblay N.A.G. & Davies D.W. (1976) The toxicity of sodium nitroprusside. *Canadian Anaesthetists Society Journal* **23**, 480–485.

Cuillerier D.J., Manninen P.H. & Gelb A.W. (1990) Alfentanil, sufentanil and fentanyl effect on cerebral perfusion pressure. *Anesthesia and Analgesia* **70**, S75.

Cunitz G., Danhauser I. & Wickbold J. (1978) Comparative investigations on the influence of etomidate, thiopentone and methohexitone on the intracranial pressure of the patient. *Anaesthesist* **27**, 64–70.

Cutler R.W., Page L., Galicich J. & Watters G.V. (1968) Formation and absorption of cerebrospinal fluid in man. *Brain* **91**, 707–720.

Dahlgren N., Rosen I., Sakabe T. & Siesjo B.K. (1980) Cerebral functional, metabolic and circulatory effects of intravenous infusion of adrenaline in the rat. *Brain Research* **184**, 143–152.

Dawson B., Michenfelder J.D. & Theye R.A. (1971) Effects of ketamine on canine cerebral blood flow and metabolism: modification by prior administration of thiopental. *Anesthesia and Analgesia* **50**, 443−447.

De Rood M., Deloof T., Berre J., Verbist A., Fruhling J. & Dang Phuoc T. (1980) Effect of 1% enflurane anesthesia on cerebral blood flow and metabolism in neurosurgical patients during normo- and hyperventilation. *Acta Anaesthesiologica Belgica* **31** (Suppl.), 3−19.

Desmonts J.M., Bohm G. & Couderc E. (1978) Haemodynamic responses to low doses of naloxone after narcotic-nitrous oxide anesthesia. *Anesthesiology* **49**, 12−16.

Domer F.R. (1969) Effects of diuretics on cerebrospinal fluid formation and potassium movement. *Experimental Neurology* **24**, 54−64.

Donchin Y., Amirav B., Sahar A. & Yarkoni S. (1978) Sodium nitroprusside for aneurysm surgery in pregnancy. Report of a case. *British Journal of Anaesthesia* **50**, 849−851.

Donegan M.F. & Bedford R.F. (1980) Intravenously administered lidocaine prevents intracranial hypertension during endotracheal suctioning. *Anesthesiology* **52**, 516−518.

Drummond J.C. & Todd M.M. (1985) The response of the feline cerebral circulation to $Paco_2$ during anesthesia with isoflurane and halothane and during sedation with nitrous oxide. *Anesthesiology* **62**, 268−273.

Drummond J.C., Scheller M.S. & Todd M.M. (1987) The effect of nitrous oxide on cortical cerebral blood flow during anesthesia with halothane and isoflurane, with and without morphine, in the rabbit. *Anesthesia and Analgesia* **66**, 1083−1089.

Edvinsson L. & Mackenzie E.T. (1976) Amine mechanisms in the cerebral circulation. *Pharmacological Reviews* **28**, 275−348.

Eger E.I. (1981) Isoflurane: A review. *Anesthesiology* **55**, 559−576.

Fahmy N.R. (1978) Nitroglycerine as a hypotensive drug during general anesthesia. *Anesthesiology* **49**, 17−20.

Fahmy N.R. & Soter N.A. (1985) Effects of trimetaphan on arterial blood histamine and systemic hemodynamics in humans. *Anesthesiology* **62**, 562−566.

Fahmy N.R., Sunder N., Moss J., Slater E. & Lappas D.G. (1979) Tachyphylaxis to nitroprusside: role of the renin−angiotensin system and catecholamines in its development. *Anesthesiology* **51**, S72.

Farrar J.K., Gamache F.W. Jr., Ferguson G.G., Barker J., Varkey G.P. & Drake C.G. (1981) Effects of profound hypotension on cerebral blood flow during surgery for intracranial aneurysms. *Journal of Neurosurgery* **55**, 857−864.

Fisher B. & Rodarte A. (1987) Use of doxapram to increase respirations without a concomitant increase in ICP. *Critical Care Medicine* **15**, 1072−1073.

Fitch W. & McDowall D.G. (1971) Effect of halothane on intracranial pressure gradients in the presence of intracranial space-occupying lesions. *British Journal of Anaesthesia* **43**, 904−912.

Fitch W., Barker J., Jennett W.B. & McDowall D.G. (1969) The influence of neuroleptanalgesic drugs on cerebrospinal fluid pressure. *British Journal of*

Anaesthesia **41**, 800–806.

Fitch W., Ferguson G.G., Sengupta D., Garibi J. & Murray Harper A. (1976) Autoregulation of cerebral blood flow during controlled hypotension in baboons. *Journal of Neurology, Neurosurgery and Psychiatry* **39**, 1014–1022.

Forster A., Juge O. & Morel D. (1982) Effects of midazolam on cerebral blood flow in human volunteers. *Anesthesiology* **56**, 453–455.

Forster A., Juge O., Louis M. & Nahory A. (1987) Effects of a specific benzodiazepine antagonist (RO 15-1788) on cerebral blood flow. *Anesthesia and Analgesia* **66**, 309–313.

Fragen R.J., Weiss H.W. & Molteni A. (1987) The effect of propofol on adrenocortical steroidogenesis: a comparative study with etomidate and thiopental. *Anesthesiology* **66**, 839–842.

Freedman M. & Levy E.R. (1988) Propofol intravenous anaesthesia for neurosurgery. *South African Medical Journal* **74**, 10–12.

Gagnon R.L., Marsh M.L., Smith R.W. & Shapiro H.M. (1979) Intracranial hypertension caused by nitroglycerine. *Anesthesiology* **51**, 86–87.

Gardner A.E., Dannemiller F.J. & Dean D. (1972) Intracranial cerebrospinal fluid pressure in man during ketamine anesthesia. *Anesthesia and Analgesia* **51**, 741–745.

Gelb A.W., Boisvert D.P., Tang C. *et al.* (1989) Primate brain tolerance to temporary focal cerebral ischemia during isoflurane- or sodium nitroprusside-induced hypotension. *Anesthesiology* **70**, 678–683.

Gibbs J.M. (1972) The effect of intravenous ketamine on cerebrospinal fluid pressure. *British Journal of Anaesthesia* **44**, 1298–1302.

Giffin J.P., Cottrell J.E., Shwirby B., Hartung J., Epstein J. & Lim K. (1984) Intracranial pressure, mean arterial pressure, and heart rate following midazolam or thiopental in humans with brain tumours. *Anesthesiology* **60**, 491–494.

Gomez-Sainz J.J., Elexpuru-Camiruaga J.A., Fernandez-Cano F. & De La Herran J.L. (1988) Effects of isoflurane on intraventricular pressure in neurosurgical patients. *British Journal of Anaesthesia* **61**, 347–349.

Gordon E. (1970) The action of drugs on intracranial contents. In: Boulton T.B., Bryce-Smith R., Sykes M.K., Gillett G.B. and Revell A.L. (Eds), *Progress in Anesthesiology*, pp. 60–68. Excerpta Medica, Amsterdam.

Gray H.StJ., Holt B.L., Whitaker D.K. & Eadsforth P. (1992) Preliminary study of a pregnanolone emulsion (Kabi2213) for iv induction of general anaesthesia. *British Journal of Anaesthesia* **68**, 272–276.

Greenbaum R., Cooper R., Hulme A. & Mackintosh I.P. (1975) The effect of induction of anaesthesia on intracranial pressure. In: Arias A. (Ed.), *Recent Progress in Anaesthesiology and Rescuscitation*, International Congress Series no. 347, pp. 794–801. Excerpta Medica, Amsterdam.

Greenfield J.C., Jr. & Tindall G.T. (1968) Effect of norepinephrine, epinephrine and angiotensin on blood flow in the internal carotid artery of man. *Journal of Clinical Investigation* **47**, 1672–1684.

Griffiths D.P.G., Cummins B.H., Greenbaum R. *et al.* (1974) Cerebral blood flow and metabolism during hypotension induced with sodium nitroprusside. *British Journal of Anaesthesia* **46**, 671−679.

Grummit R.M. & Goat V.A. (1984) Intracranial pressure after phenoperidine. *Anaesthesia* **39**, 565−567.

Guggiari M., Dagreou F., Lienhart A. *et al.* (1985) Use of nitroglycerine to produce controlled decreases in mean arterial pressure to less than 50 mmHg. *British Journal of Anaesthesia* **57**, 142−147.

Hagnevik K., Gordon E., Lins L-E., Wilhelmsson S. & Forster D. (1974) Glycerol-induced haemolysis with haemoglobinuria and acute renal failure. Report of three cases. *Lancet* **i**, 75−77.

Halldin M. & Wahlin A. (1959) Effect of succinylcholine on the intraspinal fluid pressure. *Acta Anaesthesiologica Scandinavica* **3**, 155−161.

Hansen H.C. & Drenck N.E. (1988) Generalized seizures after etomidate anaesthesia. *Anaesthesia* **43**, 805−806.

Hansen T.D., Warner D.S., Todd M.M. & Vust L.J. (1989) Effects of nitrous oxide and volatile anaesthetics on cerebral blood flow. *British Journal of Anaesthesia* **63**, 290−295.

Hansen T.D., Warner D.S., Todd M.M., Vust L.J. & Trawick D.C. (1988) Distribution of cerebral blood flow during halothane versus isoflurane anesthesia in rats. *Anesthesiology* **69**, 332−337.

Henriksen H.T. & Jorgensen P.B. (1973) The effect of nitrous oxide on intracranial pressure in patients with intracranial disorders. *British Journal of Anaesthesia* **45**, 486−492.

Henriksen L., Thorshauge C., Harmsen A. *et al.* (1983) Controlled hypotension with sodium nitroprusside: effects on cerebral blood flow and cerebral venous blood gases in patients operated for cerebral aneurysms. *Acta Anaesthesiologica Scandinavica* **27**, 62−67.

Herrschaft H. & Schmidt H. (1974) Changes in the global and regional cerebral blood flow under the influence of methohexitone in man. *Anaesthesist* **23**, 340−344.

Hodkinson B.P., Frith R.W. & Mee E.W. (1987) Propofol and the electroencephalogram. *Lancet* **ii**, 1518.

Hoien A.O. (1984) Another case of grand mal seizure after fentanyl administration [letter]. *Anesthesiology* **60**, 387−388.

Horsley J.S. (1937) The intracranial pressure during barbital narcosis. *Lancet* **i**, 141−143.

Hunter A.R. (1972a) Thiopentone supplemented anaesthesia for neurosurgery. *British Journal of Anaesthesia* **44**, 506−510.

Hunter A.R. (1972b) Methohexitone as a supplement to nitrous oxide during intracranial surgery. *British Journal of Anaesthesia* **44**, 1188−1190.

Hymes J.A. (1985) Seizure activity during isoflurane anesthesia. *Anesthesia and Analgesia* **64**, 367−368.

Ishikawa T. & McDowall D.G. (1981) Electrical activity of the cerebral cortex during induced hypotension with sodium nitroprusside and trimetaphan in the cat. *British Journal of Anaesthesia* **53**, 605−611.

Jabaily J. & Davis J.N. (1984) Naloxone administration to patients with acute stroke. *Stroke* **15**, 36−39.

James D.J. & Bedford R.F. (1982) Hydralazine for controlled hypotension during neurosurgical operations. *Anesthesia and Analgesia* **61**, 1016−1019.

Javid M. (1958) Urea a new use of an old agent. Reduction of intracranial, intraocular pressure. *Surgical Clinics of North America* **38**, 907−928.

Jennett W.B., Barker J., Fitch W. & McDowall D.G. (1969) Effect of anaesthesia on intracranial pressure in patients with space-occupying lesions. *Lancet* **i**, 61−64.

Jensen K., Bunemann L., Riisager S. & Thomsen L.J. (1989) Cerebral blood flow during anaesthesia: influence of pretreatment with metoprolol or captopril. *British Journal of Anaesthesia* **62**, 321−323.

Jensen N.F., Todd M.M., Kramer D.J., Leonard P.A. & Warner D.S. (1992) A comparison of the vasodilating effects of halothane and isoflurane on the isolated rabbit basilar artery with and without intact endothelium. *Anesthesiology* **76**, 624−634.

Jobes D.R., Kennell E., Bitner R., Swenson E. & Wollman H. (1975) Effects of morphine−nitrous oxide anesthesia on cerebral autoregulation. *Anesthesiology* **42**, 30−34.

Jobes D.R., Kennell E.M., Bush G.L. *et al.* (1977) Cerebral blood flow and metabolism during morphine−nitrous oxide anesthesia in man. *Anesthesiology* **47**, 16−18.

Jorgensen P.B. & Henriksen H.T. (1973) The effects of fluroxene on intracranial pressure in patients with intracranial space-occupying lesions. *British Journal of Anaesthesia* **45**, 599−603.

Jung R., Shah N., Reinsel R. *et al.* (1990) Cerebrospinal fluid pressure in patients with brain tumours: impact of fentanyl versus alfentanil during nitrous oxide/oxygen anesthesia. *Anesthesia and Analgesia* **71**, 419−422.

Karlsson B.R., Forsman M., Roald O.K., Heier M.S. & Steen P.A. (1990) Effect of dexmedetomidine, a selective and potent alpha$_2$-agonist, on cerebral blood flow and oxygen consumption during halothane anesthesia in dogs. *Anesthesia and Analgesia* **71**, 125−129.

Kassell N.F., Hitchon P.W., Gerk M.K., Sokol M.D. & Hill T.R. (1980) Alterations in cerebral blood flow, oxygen metabolism and electrical activity produced by high dose sodium thiopental. *Neurosurgery* **7**, 598−603.

Kavan E.M., Julien R.M. & Lucero J.L. (1974) Persistent electroencephalographic alterations following administration of some volatile anaesthetics. *British Journal of Anaesthesia* **46**, 714−721.

Kawaguchi M., Furuya H., Kurehara K. & Yamada M. (1991) Effects of nicardipine on cerebral vascular responses to hypocapnia and blood flow velocity in the middle cerebral artery. *Stroke* **22**, 1170−1171.

Kazama T. & Ikeda K. (1985) The comparative cardiovascular effects and induction time of sevoflurane with isoflurane and halothane in dogs. *Anesthesiology* **63**, A17.

Keaney N., McDowall D.G., Turner J.M., Lane J.R. & Okuda Y. (1973) The effects of profound hypotension induced with sodium nitroprusside on cerebral blood flow and metabolism in the baboon. *British Journal of Anaesthesia* **45**, 639.

Keats A.S. & Mithoefer J.C. (1955) The mechanism of increased intracranial pressure induced by morphine. *New England Journal of Medicine* **252**, 1110−1113.

Kelman G.R. & Kennedy B.R. (1971) Cardiovascular effects of pancuronium in man. *British Journal of Anaesthesia* **43**, 335−338.

Khambatta H.J., Stone J.G. & Khan E. (1979) Hypertension during anesthesia on discontinuation of sodium nitroprusside-induced hypotension. *Anesthesiology* **51**, 127−130.

Khambatta H.J., Stone J.G. & Khan E. (1981) Propranolol alters renin release during nitroprusside-induced hypotension and prevents hypertension on discontinuation of nitroprusside. *Anesthesia and Analgesia* **60**, 569−573.

King B.D., Sokoloff L. & Wechsler R.L. (1952) The effects of l-epinephrine and l-nor-epinephrine upon cerebral circulation and metabolism in man. *Journal of Clinical Investigation* **31**, 273−279.

Knudsen L., Cold G.E., Holdgard H.O., Johansen U.T. & Jensen S. (1991) Effects of flumazenil on cerebral blood flow and oxygen consumption after midazolam anaesthesia for craniotomy. *British Journal of Anaesthesia* **67**, 277−280.

Kochs E., Werner C., Hoffman W.E., Mollenberg O. & Schulte Am Esch J. (1991) Concurrent increases in brain electrical activity and intracranial blood flow velocity during low-dose ketamine anaesthesia. *Canadian Journal of Anaesthesia* **38**, 826−830.

Kochs E., Hoffman W.E., Werner C., Thomas C., Albrecht R.F. & Schulte Am Esch J. (1992) The effects of propofol on brain electrical activity, neurologic outcome, and neuronal damage following incomplete ischemia in rats. *Anesthesiology* **76**, 245−252.

Lagekrauser M., Sollevi A., Irestedt L., Tidgren B. & Andreen M. (1985) Renin release during controlled hypotension with sodium nitroprusside, nitroglycerin and adenosine: a comparative study in the dog. *Acta Anaesthesiologica Scandinavica* **29**, 45−49.

Lambert A., Mitchell R. & Robertson W.R. (1985) Effect of propofol, thiopentone and etomidate on adrenal steroidogenesis *in vitro*. *British Journal of Anaesthesia* **57**, 505−508.

Lanier W.L., Milde J.H. & Michenfelder J.D. (1985) The cerebral effects of pancuronium and atracurium in halothane-anesthetised dogs. *Anesthesiology* **63**, 589−597.

Lanier W.L., Milde J.H. & Michenfelder J.D. (1986) Cerebral stimulation following succinylcholine in dogs. *Anesthesiology* **64**, 551−559.

Little J.R. (1978) Modification of acute focal ischemia by treatment with mannitol and high-dose dexamethasone. *Journal of Neurosurgery* **49**, 517—524.

Lofgren J. & Zwetnow N.N. (1973) Cranial and spinal components of the cerebro-spinal fluid pressure—volume curve. *Acta Neurologica Scandinavica* **49**, 575—585.

Lowson S., Gent J.P. & Goodchild C.S. (1990) Anticonvulsant properties of propofol and thiopentone: comparison using two tests in laboratory mice. *British Journal of Anaesthesia* **64**, 59—63.

Lutz L.J., Milde J.H. & Milde L.N. (1990) The cerebral functional, metabolic, and hemodynamic effects of desflurane in dogs. *Anesthesiology* **73**, 125—131.

McDowall D.G. & Harper A.M. (1965) Blood flow and oxygen uptake of the cerebral cortex of the dog during anaesthesia with different volatile agents. *Acta Neurologica Scandinavica* **41** (Suppl. 14), 146—151.

MacGillivray R.G. (1982) Pneumocephalus as a complication of posterior fossa surgery in the sitting position. *Anaesthesia* **37**, 722—725.

McLeskey C.H., Cullen B.F., Kennedy R.D. & Galindo A. (1974) Control of cerebral perfusion pressure during induction of anesthesia in high-risk neurosurgical patients. *Anesthesia and Analgesia* **53**, 985—992.

McPherson R.W., Briar J.E. & Traystman R.J. (1989) Cerebrovascular responsive-ness to carbon dioxide in dogs with 1.4% and 2.8% isoflurane. *Anesthesiology* **70**, 843—850.

McPherson R.W., Krempasanka E., Eimerl D. & Traystman R.J. (1985) Effects of alfentanil on cerebral vascular reactivity in dogs. *British Journal of Anaesthesia* **57**, 1232—1238.

Macrae W.R., Wildsmith J.A.W. & Dale B.A.B. (1981) Induced hypotension with a mixture of sodium nitroprusside and trimetaphan camsylate. *Anaesthesia* **36**, 312—315.

Maekawa T., McDowall D.G. & Okuda Y. (1979) Brain-surface oxygen tension and cerebral cortical blood flow during hemorrhagic and drug-induced hypo-tension in the cat. *Anesthesiology* **51**, 313—320.

Mann J.D., Cookson S.L. & Mann E.S. (1980) Differential effects of pentobarbital, ketamine hydrochloride, and enflurane anesthesia on CSF formation rate and outflow resistance in the rat. In: Shulman K., Marmarou A., Miller J.D., Becker D.P., Hochwald G.M. & Brock M. (Eds), *Intracranial Pressure*, vol. IV, pp. 466—471. Springer-Verlag, Berlin.

Marsh M.L., Dunlop B.J., Shapiro H.M., Gagnon R.L. & Rockoff M.A. (1980) Succinylcholine—intracranial pressure effects in neurosurgical patients. *Anesthesia and Analgesia* **59**, 550—551.

Marshall L.F., Smith R.W., Rauscher L.A. & Shapiro H.M. (1978) Mannitol dose requirements in brain-injured patients. *Journal of Neurosurgery* **48**, 169—172.

Marx W., Shah N., Long C. *et al.* (1988) Sufentanil, alfentanil and fentanyl: impact on CSF pressure in patients with brain tumours. *Anesthesiology* **69**, A627.

Mayer N., Weinstabl C., Podreka I. & Spiss C.K. (1990) Sufentanil does not increase cerebral blood flow in healthy human volunteers. *Anesthesiology* **73**, 240–243.

Mazzarella B., Mastronardi P., Cafiero T., Gargiulo G., Frangiosa A. & Stella L. (1987) Effects of propofol (Diprivan) on intracranial pressure. A preliminary controlled study versus thiopentone. *Minerva Anestesica* **53**, 311–314.

Melby J.M., Miner L.C. & Reed D.J. (1982) Effect of acetazolamide and furosemide on the production and composition of cerebrospinal fluid from the cat choroid plexus. *Canadian Journal of Physiology and Pharmacology* **60**, 405–409.

Merckx L., Van Hemelrijck J., Van Aken H., Plets C. & Goffin J. (1988) Total intravenous anesthesia using propofol and alfentanil infusion in neurosurgical patients. *Anesthesiology* **69**, A576.

Messick J.M., Jr. & Theye R.A. (1969) Effects of pentobarbital and meperidine on canine cerebral and total oxygen consumption rates. *Canadian Anaesthetists Society Journal* **16**, 321–330.

Michenfelder J.D. & Milde J.H. (1988) The interaction of sodium nitroprusside, hypotension, and isoflurane in determining cerebral vasculature effects. *Anesthesiology* **69**, 870–875.

Michenfelder J.D. & Theye R.A. (1971) Effects of fentanyl, droperidol, and innovar on canine cerebral metabolism and blood flow. *British Journal of Anaesthesia* **43**, 630–636.

Michenfelder J.D. & Theye R.A. (1972) Effects of cyclopropane on canine cerebral blood flow and metabolism: modification by catecholamine suppression. *Anesthesiology* **37**, 32–39.

Michenfelder J.D. & Theye R.A. (1975) *In vivo* toxic effects of halothane on canine cerebral metabolic pathways. *American Journal of Physiology* **229**, 1050–1055.

Michenfelder J.D. & Tinker J.H. (1977) Cyanide toxicity and thiosulfate protection during chronic administration of sodium nitroprusside in the dog. *Anesthesiology* **47**, 441–448.

Michenfelder J.D., Sundt T.M., Fode N. & Sharbrough F.W. (1987) Isoflurane when compared to enflurane and halothane decreases frequency of cerebral ischaemia during carotid endarterectomy. *Anesthesiology* **67**, 336–340.

Mikawa K., Maekawa N., Kaetsu H., Goto R., Yaku H. & Obara H. (1991) Effects of adenosine triphosphate on the cardiovascular response to tracheal intubation. *British Journal of Anaesthesia* **67**, 410–415.

Milde L.N. & Milde J.H. (1989) Cerebral effects of sufentanil in dogs with reduced intracranial compliance. *Anesthesia and Analgesia* **68**, S196.

Milde L.N. & Milde J.H. (1991) Cerebral and systemic hemodynamic and metabolic effects of desflurane-induced hypotension in dogs. *Anesthesiology* **74**, 513–518.

Milde L.N., Milde J.H. & Gallagher W.J. (1990) Effects of sufentanil on cerebral circulation and metabolism in dogs. *Anesthesia and Analgesia* **70**, 138–146.

Miletich D.J., Gil K.S.L., Albrecht R.F. & Zahed B. (1980) Intracerebral blood flow distribution during hypotensive anesthesia in the goat. *Anesthesiology* **53**, 210–214.

Miller J.D. & Leech P. (1975) Effects of mannitol and steroid therapy on intracranial volume–pressure relationships in patients. *Journal of Neurosurgery* **42**, 274–281.

Minton M.D., Grosslight T.K., Stirt J.A. & Bedford R.F. (1986) Increases in intracranial pressure from succinylcholine: prevention by prior non-depolarising block. *Anesthesiology* **65**, 165–169.

Misfeldt B.B., Jorgensen P.B. & Rishoj M. (1974) The effect of nitrous oxide and halothane upon the intracranial pressure in hypocapnic patients with intracranial disorders. *British Journal of Anaesthesia* **46**, 853–858.

Misfeldt B.B., Jorgensen P.B., Spotoft H. & Ronde F. (1976) The effects of droperidol and fentanyl on intracranial pressure and cerebral perfusion pressure in neurosurgical patients, *British Journal of Anaesthesia* **48**, 963–968.

Modica P.A. & Tempelhoff R. (1992) Intracranial pressure during induction of anaesthesia and tracheal intubation with etomidate-induced EEG burst suppression. *Canadian Journal of Anaesthesia* **39**, 236–241.

Moore R.A., Allen M.C., Wood P.J., Rees L.H. & Sear J.W. (1985) Peri-operative endocrine effects of etomidate. *Anaesthesia* **40**, 124–130.

Morel N. & Godfraind T. (1990) Cerebrovascular effect of calcium antagonists. *European Neurology* **30** (Suppl. 2), 10–15.

Morita H., Nemoto E.M., Bleyaert A.L. & Stezoski S.W. (1977) Brain blood flow autoregulation and metabolism during halothane anesthesia in monkeys. *American Journal of Physiology* **233**, H670–676.

Morris P.J., McDowall D.G. & Heuser D. (1982a) Comparison of changes in ECF potassium concentration and pH of the brain between trimetaphan- and nitroprusside-induced hypotension. *British Journal of Anaesthesia* **54**, 257.

Morris P.J., Todd M. & Philbin D. (1982b) Changes in canine intracranial pressure in response to infusions of sodium nitroprusside and trinitroglycerin. *British Journal of Anaesthesia* **54**, 991–995.

Moss E. (1992) Alfentanil increases intracranial pressure when intracranial compliance is low. *Anaesthesia* **47**, 134–136.

Moss E. & McDowall D.G. (1979) ICP increases with 50% nitrous oxide in oxygen in severe head injuries during controlled ventilation. *British Journal of Anaesthesia* **51**, 757–760.

Moss E. & Price D.J. (1990) The effect of propofol on brain retraction pressure and cerebral perfusion pressure. *British Journal of Anaesthesia* **65**, 823–825.

Moss E., Dearden N.M. & McDowall D.G. (1983) Effects of 2% enflurane on intracranial pressure and cerebral perfusion pressure. *British Journal of Anaesthesia* **55**, 1083–1088.

Moss E., Powell D., Gibson R.M. & McDowall D.G. (1978a) Effects of tracheal intubation on intracranial pressure following induction of anaesthesia with thiopentone or Althesin in patients undergoing neurosurgery. *British Journal of Anaesthesia* **50**, 353−360.

Moss E., Powell D., Gibson R.M. & McDowall D.G. (1978b) Effects of fentanyl on intracranial pressure and cerebral perfusion pressure during normocapnia. *British Journal of Anaesthesia* **50**, 779−784.

Moss E., Powell D., Gibson R.M. & McDowall D.G. (1979) Effect of etomidate on intracranial pressure and cerebral perfusion pressure. *British Journal of Anaesthesia* **51**, 347−352.

Moyer J.H., Pontius R., Morris G. & Hershberger R. (1957) Effect of morphine and n-allylnormorphine on cerebral haemodynamics and oxygen metabolism. *Circulation* **15**, 379−384.

Muizelaar J.P., Lutz H.A. & Becker D.P. (1984) Effect of mannitol on ICP and CBF and correlation with pressure autoregulation in severely head-injured patients. *Journal of Neurosurgery* **61**, 700−706.

Muizelaar J.P., Wei E.P., Kontos H.A. & Becker D.P. (1983) Mannitol causes compensatory cerebral vasoconstriction and vasodilation in response to blood viscosity changes. *Journal of Neurosurgery* **59**, 822−828.

Murphy P.G., Myers D.S., Davies M.J., Webster N.R. & Jones J.G. (1992) The antioxidant potential of propofol (2,6-diisopropylphenol). *British Journal of Anaesthesia* **68**, 613−618.

Musella L., Wilder B.J. & Schmidt R.P. (1971) Electroencephalographic activation with intravenous methohexital in psychomotor epilepsy. *Neurology* **21**, 594−602.

Mutch W.A.C., Patel P.M. & Ruta T.S. (1990) A comparison of the cerebral pressure−flow relationship for halothane and isoflurane at haemodynamically equivalent end-tidal concentrations in the rabbit. *Canadian Journal of Anaesthesia* **37**, 223−230.

Neigh J.L., Garman J.K. & Harp J.R. (1971) The electroencephalograhic pattern during anesthesia with ethrane: effects of depth of anesthesia, $PaCO_2$, and nitrous oxide. *Anesthesiology* **35**, 482−487.

Newberg L.A., Milde J.H. & Michenfelder J.D. (1983) The cerebral metabolic effects of isoflurane at and above concentrations that suppress cortical activity. *Anesthesiology* **59**, 23−28.

Newberg L.A., Milde J.H. & Michenfelder J.D. (1984) Systemic and cerebral effects of isoflurane-induced hypotension in dogs. *Anesthesiology* **60**, 541−546.

Nilsson A. & Persson M.P. (1988) Total intravenous anaesthesia − is there a future for midazolam? *Acta Anaesthesiologica Scandinavica* (Suppl.), **87**, 6−10.

Nilsson A., Persson M.P., Hartvig P. & Wide L. (1988) Effect of total intravenous anaesthesia with midazolam/alfentanil on the adrenocortical and hyperglycaemic response to abdominal surgery. *Acta Anaesthesiologica Scandinavica* **32**, 379−382.

Nugent M., Artru A.A. & Michenfelder J.D. (1982) Cerebral metabolic, vascular and protective effects of midazolam maleate. *Anesthesiology* **56**, 172−176.

Olesen J. (1972) The effect of intracarotid epinephrine, norepinephrine and angiotensin on the regional cerebral blood flow in man. *Neurology* **22**, 978−987.

Omote K., Kirita A., Namiki A. & Iwasaki H. (1992) Effects of nicardipine on the circulatory responses to tracheal intubation in normotensive and hypertensive patients. *Anaesthesia* **47**, 24−27.

Overgaard J. & Skinhoj E. (1975) A paradoxical cerebral haemodynamic effect of hydralazine. *Stroke* **6**, 402.

Pappius H.M. & Dayes L.A. (1965) Hypertonic urea. Its effect on the distribution of water and electrolytes in normal and edematous brain tissues. *Archives of Neurology (Chicago)* **13**, 395−402.

Paul R. & Harris R. (1970) A comparison of methohexitone and thiopentone in electrocorticography. *Journal of Neurology, Neurosurgery and Psychiatry* **33**, 100−104.

Pettinger W.A. (1978) Anesthetics and the renin−angiotensin−aldosterone axis. *Anesthesiology* **48**, 393−396.

Pierce E.C., Jr., Lambertsen C.J., Deutsch S. *et al.* (1962) Cerebral circulation and metabolism during thiopental anesthesia and hyperventilation in man. *Journal of Clinical Investigation* **41**, 1664−1671.

Pollay M., Fullenwider C., Roberts A. & Stevens F.A. (1983) Effect of mannitol and furosemide on blood−brain osmotic gradient and intracranial pressure. *Journal of Neurosurgery* **59**, 945−950.

Poulton T.J. & Ellingson R.J. (1984) Seizures associated with induction of anesthesia with isoflurane. *Anesthesiology* **61**, 471−476.

Puchstein C., Van Aken H., Anger C. & Hidding J. (1983) Influence of urapidil on intracranial pressure and intracranial compliance in dogs. *British Journal of Anaesthesia* **55**, 443−448.

Rampil I.J., Weiskopf R.B., Brown J.G. *et al.* (1988) I-653 and isoflurane produce similar dose-related changes in the electroencephalogram of pigs. *Anesthesiology* **69**, 298−302.

Rao T.L., Mummaneni N. & El-Etr A.A. (1982) Convulsions: an unusual response to intravenous fentanyl administration. *Anesthesia and Analgesia* **61**, 1020−1021.

Ravussin P., Archer D.P., Meyer E., Abou-Madi M., Yamamoto D.T. & Trep D. (1985) The effects of rapid infusions of saline and mannitol on cerebral blood volume and intracranial pressure in dogs. *Canadian Anaesthetists Society Journal* **32**, 506−515.

Renou A.M., Macrez P., Vernhier J., Constant P., Billerey J. & Caille J.M. (1978) The effects of etomidate on cerebral blood flow and oxygen metabolism in man. *Annales de l'Anaesthesiologie Francaise* **19**, 201−205.

Roald O.K., Forsman M., Heier M.S. & Steen P.A. (1991) Cerebral effects of nitrous oxide when added to low and high concentrations of isoflurane in the dog. *Anesthesia and Analgesia* **72**, 75−79.

Roberts F.L., Dixon J., Lewis G.T.R., Tackley R.M. & Prys-Roberts C. (1988) Induction and maintenance of propofol anaesthesia. A manual infusion scheme. *Anaesthesia* **43** (Suppl.), 14—17.

Roberts P.A., Pollay M., Engles C., Pendleton B., Reynolds E. & Stevens F.A. (1987) Effect on intracranial pressure of furosemide combined with varying doses and administration rates of mannitol. *Journal of Neurosurgery* **66**, 440—446.

Rockoff M.A., Naughton K.V.H., Shapiro H.M. *et al.* (1980) Cerebral circulatory and metabolic responses to intravenously administered lorazepam. *Anesthesiology* **53**, 215—218.

Rosa G., Sanfilippo M., Vilardi V., Orfei P. & Gasparetto A. (1986) Effects of vecuronium bromide on intracranial pressure and cerebral perfusion pressure. A preliminary report. *British Journal of Anaesthesia* **58**, 437—440.

Rosenorn J. & Diemer N.H. (1982) Reduction of regional cerebral blood flow during brain retraction pressure in the rat. *Journal of Neurosurgery* **56**, 826—829.

Rubin R.C., Henderson E.S., Ommaya A.K., Walker M.D. & Rall D.P. (1966) The production of cerebrospinal fluid in man and its modification by acetazolamide. *Journal of Neurosurgery* **25**, 430—436.

Safwat A.M. & Daniel D. (1983) Grand mal seizure after fentanyl administration. *Anesthesiology* **59**, 78.

Sakabe T., Kuramoto T., Kumagae S. & Takeshita H. (1976) Cerebral responses to the addition of nitrous oxide to halothane in man. *British Journal of Anaesthesia* **48**, 957—962.

Sakabe T., Maekawa T., Ishikawa T. & Takeshita H. (1974) The effects of lidocaine on canine cerebral metabolism and circulation related to the electroencephalogram. *Anesthesiology* **40**, 433—441.

Sari A., Okuda Y. & Takeshita H. (1972a) The effect of ketamine on cerebrospinal fluid pressure. *Anesthesia and Analgesia* **51**, 560—565.

Sari A., Okuda Y. & Takeshita H. (1972b) The effects of Thalamonal on cerebral circulation and oxygen consumption in man. *British Journal of Anaesthesia* **44**, 330—334.

Sari A., Maekawa T., Tohjo M., Okuda Y. & Takeshita H. (1976) Effects of Althesin on cerebral blood flow and oxygen consumption in man. *British Journal of Anaesthesia* **48**, 545—550.

Sato M., Niiyama K., Kuroda R. & Ioku M. (1991) Influence of dopamine on cerebral blood flow, and metabolism for oxygen and glucose under barbiturate administration in cats. *Acta Neurochirurgica Wien,* **110**, 174—180.

Scheller M.S., Tateishi A., Drummond J.C. & Zornow M.H. (1988) The effects of sevoflurane on cerebral blood flow, cerebral metabolic rate for oxygen, intracranial pressure, and the electroencephalogram are similar to those of isoflurane in the rabbit. *Anesthesiology* **68**, 548—551.

Scheller M.S., Todd M.M., Drummond J.C. & Zornow M.H. (1987) The intracranial pressure effects of isoflurane and halothane administered following cryogenic brain injury in rabbits. *Anesthesiology* **67**, 507−512.

Schettini A., Stahurski B. & Young H.F. (1982) Osmotic and osmotic-loop diuresis in brain surgery. Effects on plasma and CSF electrolytes and ion excretion. *Journal of Neurosurgery* **56**, 679−684.

Schleien C.L., Koehler R.C., Gervais H. *et al.* (1989) Organ blood flow and somatosensory evoked potentials during and after cardiopulmonary rescuscitation with epinephrine and phenylephrine. *Circulation* **79**, 1332−1342.

Schmidt J.F. & Waldemar G. (1990) Effect of nimodipine on cerebral blood flow in human volunteers. *Journal of Cardiovascular Pharmacology* **16**, 568−571.

Schmidt J.F., Waldemar G. & Paulson O.B. (1990) The acute effect of captopril on cerebral blood flow, its CO_2 reactivity, and cerebral oxygen metabolism in human volunteers. *Journal of Cardiovascular Pharmacology* **16**, 1007−1010.

Schmidt J.F., Waldemar G. & Paulson O.B. (1991) The acute effect of nimodipine on cerebral blood flow, its CO_2 reactivity, and cerebral oxygen metabolism in human volunteers. *Acta Neurochirurgica Wien,* **111**, 49−53.

Schroeder T., Schierbeck J., Howardy P., Knudsen L., Skafte-Holme P. & Gefke K. (1991) Effect of labetalol on cerebral blood flow and middle cerebral arterial flow velocity in healthy volunteers. *Neurological Research* **13**, 10−12.

Schulte Am Esch J. & Kochs E. (1990) Midazolam and flumazenil in neuroanaesthesia. *Acta Anaesthesiologica Scandinavica* (Suppl.) **92**, 96−102.

Scott D.B., Stephen G.W., Marshall R.L., Jenkinson J.L. & Macrae W.R. (1972) Circulatory effects of controlled arterial hypotension with trimetaphan during nitrous oxide/halothane anaesthesia. *British Journal of Anaesthesia* **44**, 523−527.

Scremin O.U. (1991) Pharmacological control of the cerebral circulation. *Annual Review of Pharmacology and Toxicology* **31**, 229−251.

Shafer A., Doze V.A., Shafer S.L. & White P.F. (1988) Pharmacokinetics and pharmacodynamics of propofol infusions during general anesthesia. *Anesthesiology* **69**, 348−356.

Shapiro H.M., Wyte S.R. & Harris A.B. (1972) Ketamine anaesthesia in patients with intracranial pathology. *British Journal of Anaesthesia* **44**, 1200−1204.

Shapiro H.M., Galindo A., Wyte S.R. & Harris A.B. (1973) Rapid intraoperative reduction of intracranial pressure with thiopentone. *British Journal of Anaesthesia* **45**, 1057−1062.

Simpson K.H., Halsall P.J., Carr C.M.E. & Stewart K.G. (1988) Propofol reduces seizure duration in patients having anaesthesia for electroconvulsive therapy. *British Journal of Anaesthesia* **61**, 343−344.

Smith A.L. & Marque J.J. (1976) Anesthetics and cerebral oedema. *Anesthesiology* **45**, 64−72.

Smith A.L. & Wollman H. (1972) Cerebral blood flow and metabolism. Effects of anesthetic drugs and techniques. *Anesthesiology* **36**, 378−400.

Smith A.L., Neufeld G.R., Ominsky A.J. & Wollman H. (1971) Effect of arterial

CO_2 tension on cerebral blood flow, mean transit time and vascular volume. *Journal of Applied Physiology* **31**, 701−707.

Smith H.P., Kelly D.L., Jr., McWhorter J.M. *et al.* (1986) Comparison of mannitol regimens in patients with severe head injury undergoing intracranial monitoring. *Journal of Neurosurgery* **65**, 820−824.

Sokrab T-E.O. & Johansson B.B. (1989) Regional cerebral blood flow in acute hypertension induced by adrenaline, noradrenaline and phenylephrine in the conscious rat. *Acta Physiologica Scandinavica* **137**, 101−106.

Sollevi A., Lagerkranser M., Irestedt L., Gordon E. & Lindquist C. (1984) Controlled hypotension with adenosine in cerebral aneurysm surgery. *Anesthesiology* **61**, 400−405.

Sondergard W. (1961) Intracranial pressure during general anaesthesia. *Danish Medical Bulletin* **8**, 18−25.

Stange K., Lagerkranser M. & Sollevi A. (1991) Nitroprusside-induced hypotension and cerebrovascular autoregulation in the anesthetised pig. *Anesthesia and Analgesia* **73**, 745−752.

Steen P.A., Newberg L., Milde J.H. & Michenfelder J.D. (1983) Hypothermia and barbiturates: individual and combined effects on canine cerebral oxygen consumption. *Anesthesiology* **58**, 527−532.

Stephan H., Sonntag H., Schenk H.G. & Kohlhausen S. (1987) Effects of disoprivan (propofol) on cerebral blood flow, cerebral oxygen consumption, and cerebral vascular reactivity. *Anaesthesist* **36**, 60−65.

Stirt J.A., Maggio W., Haworth C., Minton M.D. & Bedford R.F. (1987) Vecuronium: Effect on intracranial pressure and hemodynamics in neurosurgical patients. *Anesthesiology* **67**, 570−573.

Stuart F.P., Torres E., Fletcher R., Crocker D. & Moore F.D. (1970) Effects of single, repeated and massive mannitol infusion in the dog: structural and functional changes in kidney and brain. *Annals of Surgery* **172**, 190−204.

Stuart-Taylor M.E. & Sleigh J.W. (1987) Alfentanil infusions. Comparison of bolus administration of fentanyl with three alfentanil infusion regimens. *Anaesthesia* **42**, 1218−1222.

Takeshita M., Okuda Y. & Sari A. (1972) The effects of ketamine on cerebral circulation and metabolism in man. *Anesthesiology* **36**, 69−75.

Takasaki M., Shirai O., Namiki A., Doi S. & Takahashi N. (1973) Effects of ultrashort acting IV anesthetics, CT 1341, methohexital and propanidid on csf pressure. *Masui* **22**, 778−784.

Tarkkanen L., Laitinen L. & Johansson G. (1974) Effects of d-tubocurarine on intracranial pressure and thalamic electrical impedance. *Anesthesiology* **40**, 247−251.

Tateishi A., Maekawa T., Takeshita H. & Wakuta K. (1981) Diazepam and intracranial pressure. *Anesthesiology* **54**, 335−337.

Theye R.A. & Michenfelder J.D. (1972) The effects of nitrous oxide on canine cerebral metabolism. *Anesthesiology* **29**, 1119−1124.

Thomsen L.J., Riisager S., Jensen K.A. & Bunemann L. (1989) Cerebral blood flow and metabolism during hypotension induced with sodium nitroprusside and captopril. *Canadian Journal of Anaesthesia* **36**, 392−396.

Turner J.M., Coroneos N.J., Gibson R.M. Powell D., Ness M.A. & McDowall D.G. (1973) The effect of althesin on intracranial pressure in man. *British Journal of Anaesthesia* **45**, 168−171.

Turner J.M., Powell D., Gibson R.M. & McDowall D.G. (1977) Intracranial pressure changes in neurosurgical patients during hypotension induced with sodium nitroprusside or trimetaphan. *British Journal of Anaesthesia* **49**, 419−425.

Unni V.K.N., Gray W.J. & Young H.S.A. (1986) Effects of atracurium on intra-cranial pressure in man. *Anaesthesia* **41**, 1047−1049.

Van Aken J. & Rolly G. (1976) Influence of etomidate, a new short acting anesthetic agent on cerebral blood flow in man. *Acta Anaesthesiologica Belgica* **27** (Suppl.), 175−180.

Van Aken H., Puchstein C., Schweppe M-L & Heinecke A. (1982) Effect of labetalol on intracranial pressure in dogs with and without intracranial hypertension. *Acta Anaesthesiologica Scandinavica* **26**, 615−619.

Van Aken H., Puchstein C., Anger C., Heinecke A. & Lawin P. (1984) Changes in intracranial pressure and compliance during adenosine triphosphate induced hypotension in dogs. *Anesthesia and Analgesia* **63**, 381−385.

Vandesteene A., Trempont V., Engelman E. *et al.* (1988) Effect of propofol on cerebral blood flow and metabolism in man. *Anaesthesia* **43** (Suppl.), 42−43.

Van Hemekrijck J., Van Aken H., Plets C., Goffin J. & Vermaut G. (1989) The effects of propofol on intracranial pressure and cerebral perfusion pressure in patients with brain tumours. *Acta Anaesthesiologica Belgica* **40**, 95−100.

Van Hemelrijck J., Fitch W., Mattheussen M., Van Aken H., Plets C. & Lauwers T. (1990) Effect of propofol on cerebral circulation and autoregulation in the baboon. *Anesthesia and Analgesia* **71**, 49−54.

Vernhiet J., Macrez P., Renou A.M., Constant P., Billerey J. & Caille J.M. (1977) The effects of large doses of morphinomimetics (fentanyl and fentathienyl) on the cerebral circulation in the normal subject. *Annales de l'Anesthesiologie Francaise* **18**, 803−810.

Vesey C.J. & Cole P.V. (1985) Blood cyanide and thiocyanate concentrations produced by long-term therapy with sodium nitroprusside. *British Journal of Anaesthesia* **57**, 148−155.

Vesey C.J., Cole P.V. & Simpson P.J. (1976) Cyanide and thiocyanate concentra-tions following sodium nitroprusside infusion in man. *British Journal of Anaes-thesia* **48**, 651−660.

Vickers M.D., O'Flaherty D., Szekely S.M., Read M. & Yoshizumi J. (1992) Tramadol: pain relief by an opioid without depression of respiration. *Anaes-thesia* **47**, 291−296.

Victory R.A.P. & Magee D. (1988) A case of convulsion after propofol anaesthesia [letter]. *Anaesthesia* **43**, 904.

Wardley-Smith B., Little H.J. & Halsey M.J. (1988) Lack of correlation between the anaesthetic and anti-convulsant potencies of althesin, ketamine and methohexitone. *British Journal of Anaesthesia* **60**, 140−145.

Watt I. & Ledingham I.M. (1984) Mortality amongst multiple trauma patients admitted to an intensive therapy unit. *Anaesthesia* **39**, 973−981.

Wauquier A. (1983) Profile of etomidate. A hypnotic, anticonvulsant and brain protective compound. *Anaesthesia* **38**, 26−33.

Weiskopf R.B., Cahalan M.K., Eger E.I. *et al.* (1991) Cardiovascular actions of desflurane in normocarbic volunteers. *Anesthesia and Analgesia* **73**, 143−156.

Werner C., Hoffman W.E., Baughman V.L., Albrecht R.F. & Schulte Am Esch J. (1991) Effects of sufentanil on cerebral blood flow, cerebral blood velocity, and metabolism in dogs. *Anesthesia and Analgesia* **72**, 177−181.

Wilkinson I.M. & Browne D.R. (1970) The influence of anaesthesia and arterial hypocapnia on regional blood flow in the normal human cerebral hemisphere. *British Journal of Anaesthesia* **42**, 472−482.

Williams D.J.M., Morgan R.J.M. & Major E. (1984) Urapidil in the treatment of hypertension following coronary bypass surgery. *British Journal of Anaesthesia* **56**, 427P.

Wollman H., Alexander S.C., Cohen P.J., Chase P.E., Melman E. & Behar M.G. (1964) Cerebral circulation of man during halothane anesthesia. *Anesthesiology* **25**, 180−184.

Wollman H., Alexander S.C., Cohen P.J., Smith T.C., Chase P.E. & Van Der Molen R.A. (1965) Cerebral circulation during general anesthesia and hyper-ventilation in man. Thiopental induction to nitrous oxide and d-tubocurarine. *Anesthesiology* **26**, 329−334.

Young W.L., Prohovnik I., Correll J.W., Ostapkovich N., Ornstein E. & Quest D.O. (1991) A comparison of cerebral blood flow reactivity to CO_2 during halothane versus isoflurane anesthesia for carotid endarterectomy. *Anesthesia and Analgesia* **73**, 416−421.

Zornow M.H., Fleischer J.E., Scheller M.S., Nakakimura K. & Drummond J.C. (1990) Dexmedetomidine, an alpha$_2$-adrenergic agonist, decreases cerebral blood flow in the isoflurane-anesthetized dog. *Anesthesia and Analgesia* **70**, 624−630.

5

Electrical monitoring of the brain and spinal cord

JIM L. JENKINSON

Introduction

Methods available to monitor the electrical activity and functional integrity of the brain and spinal cord may be subdivided into two categories — the electroencephalogram (EEG), and evoked potentials (EPs). The EEG is a monitor of the activity on the surface of the cerebral cortex, whereas EPs monitor the deeper brain pathways and pathways in the spinal cord subserving both sensory and motor functions.

The electroencephalogram

The EEG was first recorded in humans in 1929 by Hans Berger. It is generated in the pyramidal cells in the superficial laminae (I, II and V) of the cerebral cortex and is the summation of excitatory and inhibitory postsynaptic potentials in nerve pathways running from thalamic nuclei to the cerebral cortex. It is the summation of these potentials which produces the waveforms of the EEG which are subdivided into four categories.

The EEG waveforms

Beta waves are the fastest and smallest waves of the EEG, having a frequency of 14–30 Hz and an amplitude of less than 20 µV. They occur when the patient is awake, alert, has his or her eyes open and is seeing patterned vision, and are most frequently found in the precentral cortex. However, beta waves also occur if the patient is given barbiturates, phenytoin, benzodiazepines, low concentrations of halothane or iso-flurane, or has ingested alcohol. These drug-produced beta waves may be misleading. For example, if a severely comatose patient in the intensive-care unit (ICU) is commenced on a benzodiazepine infusion for sedation·

122

the increase in beta activity which follows may make the observer think, incorrectly, that the patient's neurological status is improving, or if anaesthesia is deepened from a light plane by the introduction of a small concentration of isoflurane the ensuing beta waves may give the false impression that the patient is wakening.

Alpha waves are slower and larger than beta waves, having a frequency of 8−13 Hz and an amplitude of 20−50 μV. They occur when the patient is awake, but is relaxed and has his or her eyes closed, and are found mainly over the occipital cortex.

Theta waves have a frequency range of 4−7 Hz and an amplitude of 20−50 μV. They are normal in children and the elderly, and in adults during sleep, but otherwise indicate some neuronal dysfunction either by hypothermia, disease or medication.

Delta waves are the slowest and largest of the EEG waves having a frequency of less than 4 Hz and an amplitude greater than 50 μV. They are normal during sleep, but otherwise are abnormal indicating neuronal dysfunction by disease or medication.

The amplitude and frequency of the EEG is the resultant of the postsynaptic potentials. If these potentials are synchronized, as for example in deep sleep or coma, high-amplitude slow waves will be produced, but if the potentials are desynchronized, as in a state of alertness, the amplitude will be small and the frequency fast.

Electrodes

The electrodes are normally chlorided silver domes which are retained in position on the scalp with collodion and are filled with conductive jelly. The use of collodion can be difficult for the inexperienced, and platinum needle electrodes may be more convenient in anaesthetic practice. For best results these needles should be kept in saline for 24 h before use, and should not be touched by hand or wiped with a spirit swab. Despite these precautions the signal may deteriorate after 4 h monitoring because of an accumulation of ions on the platinum needle. Recently, a combined fixative and conductive jelly which can be used with the chlorided silver domes has been introduced, and this makes their use more convenient.

In a neurophysiology department 21 electrodes are used, and accurately placed according to an international Ten Twenty system. This montage is too cumbersome for anaesthetic practice and it is customary to use only two or four recording electrodes and an additional reference electrode. The common positions for electrodes used for monitoring are shown in Fig. 5.1. Fz is the position of the reference electrode, and P3 and P4 are frequently used positions as they are over the areas of cortex which is perfused by the limits of blood supply from anterior, middle and posterior cerebral arteries. These positions are known as the common boundary zones of blood supply from the three cerebral arteries. C3/P3 and C4/P4 lie above cortex at the boundary of blood supply between middle and anterior cerebral arteries, and are useful areas to monitor if it is possible to compare two areas of brain at the same time. As the electrodes receive the signal from an area of 2.5 cm^2 around them their correct placement is vital in monitoring. If the electrodes are placed over healthy brain adjacent to an area of pathology the EEG will be normal and give no indication of the adjacent pathology.

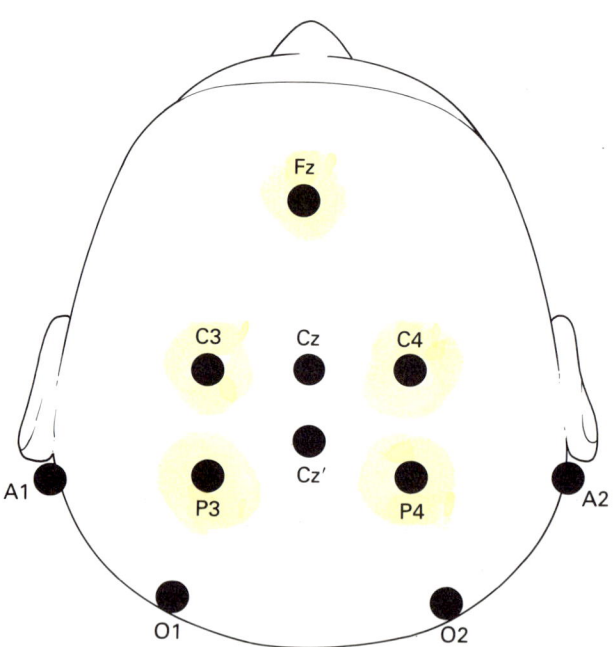

Fig. 5.1 The commonly used positions for electrodes for monitoring the electrical activity of the brain and spinal cord. F is frontal, C is central, P is parietal, O is occipital and A is auditory on the mastoid process or ear lobe. Z refers to the midline electrodes; the ones on the left have odd numbers and those on the right have even numbers.

Electrical interference

The EEG signal is very small, and recording it may not be easy in the electrically 'hostile' environment of the operating theatre or ICU. Leakage current from other equipment attached to the patient can interfere with recording the EEG, as can the use of monopolar diathermy. Other physiological signals such as the electrocardiogram (ECG) or muscle tone can give interference.

EEG monitors

The EEG is difficult to interpret without training and experience, and the EEG recorder produces vast amounts of bulky paper trace. To overcome these difficulties EEG monitors are available which analyse the EEG and present the data in a more readily understood form.

The first of these monitors to be introduced was the cerebral function monitor (CFM) (Maynard *et al.* 1969). It uses one pair of recording electrodes and gives an indication of the total electrical activity of the area of brain being monitored. The printout is the product of the frequency and logarithm of the amplitude of the waves. As slow waves have high amplitudes the CFM decreases the contribution of these waves to the final printout by using the logarithm of the amplitude (Fig. 5.2).

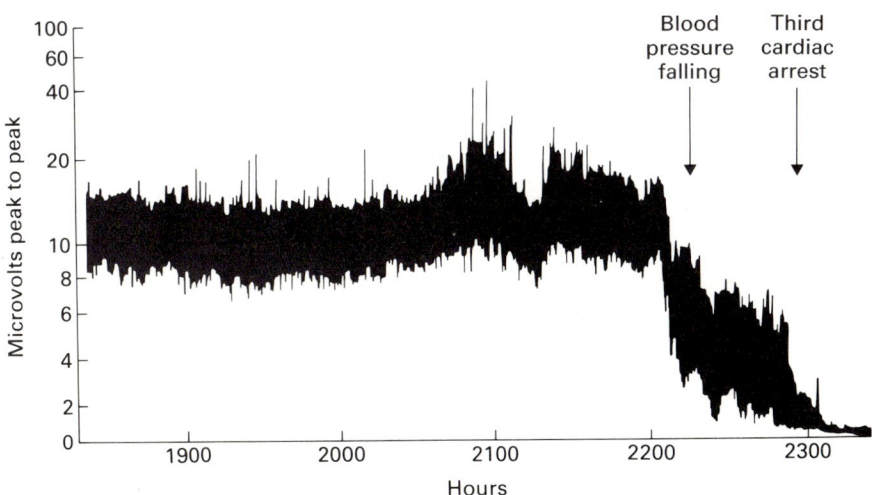

Fig. 5.2 Cerebral function monitor recording during cardiac arrest.

The cerebral function analysing monitor (CFAM) is a development of the CFM (Maynard & Jenkinson 1984). It displays, in 2-s epochs, an analysis of the amplitude of the waves and the amount of activity in each of the four classical wavebands. It can analyse from four recording electrodes, produce a trace of the EEG, and compute evoked potentials (Fig. 5.3).

The compressed spectral array (CSA) was described by Bickford *et al.* (1971) and displays the analysis of the EEG as a series of mountains and valleys. The more activity there is in any frequency the higher is the 'mountain', and as the pen traces from left to right it traces the activity

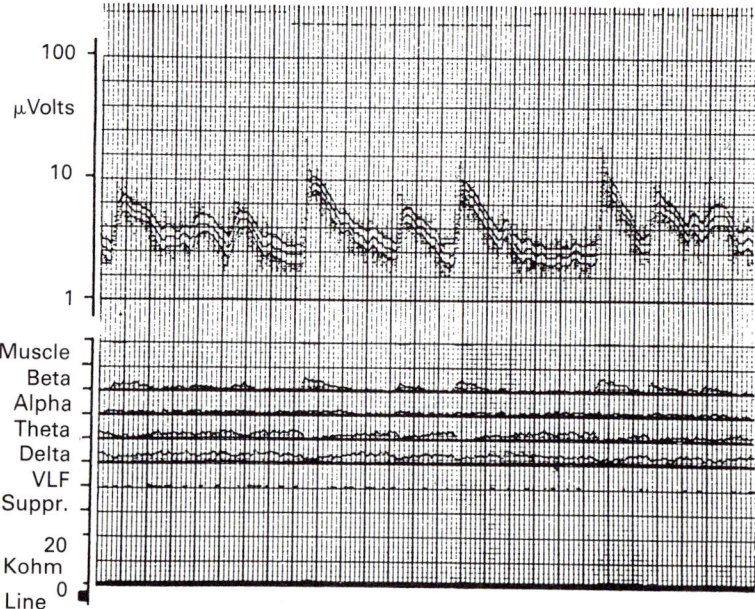

Fig. 5.3 Trace from the CFAM showing status epilepticus. The markings along the top of the upper trace are at 1-min intervals. The upper trace records analysis of the amplitude of the EEG in 2-s epochs. The scale is logarithmic in microvolts peak to peak. The lower trace records the frequency analysis. From the top downwards is the display of the amount of activity in: muscle, beta band, alpha band, theta band, delta band, very low frequency, suppression and impedence in kohms. The overall amplitude of the trace is low as the patient had sustained a cardiac arrest. During each fit there is a rise in beta activity and a fall in theta and delta activity. There is also a small amount of muscle activity which could have contributed to the beta band activity, but in fact beta band activity outlasts muscle activity. From Maynard and Jenkinson (1984).

in increasing frequency bands. The problem with this display is that after a period of high activity in a frequency band subsequent lesser activity may get lost from view for some time behind the 'mountain' (Fig. 5.4).

The density spectral array (DSA) (Fleming & Smith 1979) overcomes this problem by displaying each analysis as a single horizontal line and increasing activity in a frequency band by broadening the width of the line.

Rampil *et al.* (1979) introduced the concept of spectral edge frequency, which is a mark put on to the CSA or DSA at the highest frequency with a significant amount of energy. When the major activity of the EEG moves from high to low frequencies the spectral edge mark moves from right to left.

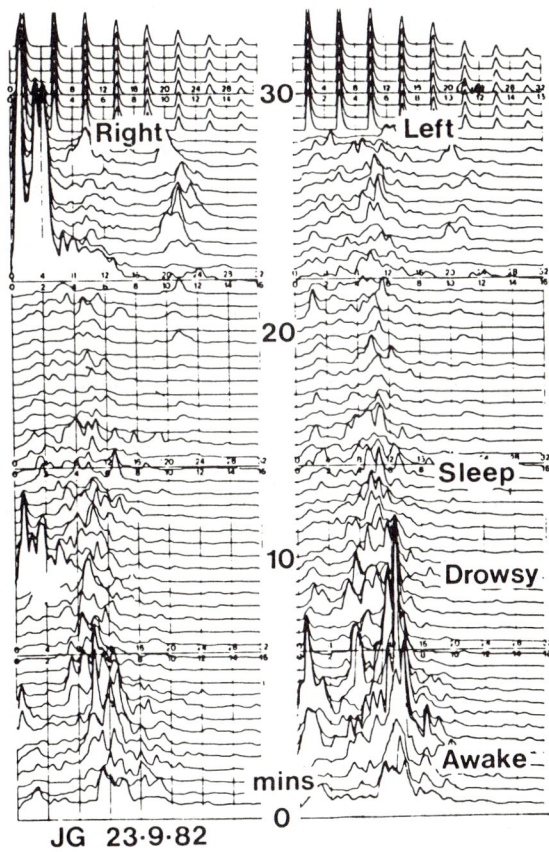

Fig. 5.4 Compressed spectral array in normal circumstances.

Demetrescu (1975) described the aperiodic technique, in which the EEG analysis is displayed by a series of vertical lines and the final display resembles a 'bed of nails'. An aperiodic algorithm which measures the time between the high and low peaks in the EEG is used to calculate the frequency. The more activity there is in a frequency band the more and higher will be the number of vertical lines.

The role of EEG monitoring in neuroanaesthesia and neurointensive care

The EEG gives a good indication of the adequacy of oxygenation of the cerebral cortex. Of the total consumption of oxygen by the brain 60% is required to generate the signals which produce the EEG and the other 40% is required to maintain cellular integrity. If the oxygen supply is compromised the oxygen which would have been used in the production of the EEG is diverted to maintain cellular integrity. A decrease in oxygen supply to the brain will therefore result in depression of EEG activity before irreversible brain damage occurs. The oxygen supply is the product of cerebral blood flow, oxygen saturation and haemoglobin concentration. A reduction in oxygen supply by a decrease in any of these parameters, which can be controlled by the anaesthetist, will be detected by alteration in the EEG. The initial response to an acute ischaemic episode is an increase in high-amplitude beta band waves, and if the ischaemia is not corrected low-amplitude theta and delta waves will follow.

Cerebral blood flow (CBF) may be reduced from the normal $50 \, ml \, 100 \, g^{-1} \, min^{-1}$ to $30 \, ml \, 100 \, g^{-1} \, min^{-1}$ before changes are seen in the EEG in the non-anaesthetized patient, to $20 \, ml \, 100 \, g^{-1} \, min^{-1}$ when volatile anaesthetic agents are being administered, and Michenfelder *et al.* (1987) found that value to be even lower when isoflurane was used. Irreversible brain damage occurs during the use of these agents when the blood flow is reduced to $12 \, ml \, 100 \, g^{-1} \, min^{-1}$.

There is a good correlation between cerebral blood flow and the amplitude analysis of the EEG with mean arterial pressure (MAP). As the CBF decreases when the MAP decreases below the lower limit of auto-regulation, so also does the amplitude of the EEG (Prior 1985). EEG monitoring is therefore very useful during controlled hypotension.

The reduction in oxygen supply resulting from cerebral artery vaso-constriction associated with hypocarbia less than 25 mmHg produced by hyperventilation increases the delta band activity (Fig. 5.5).

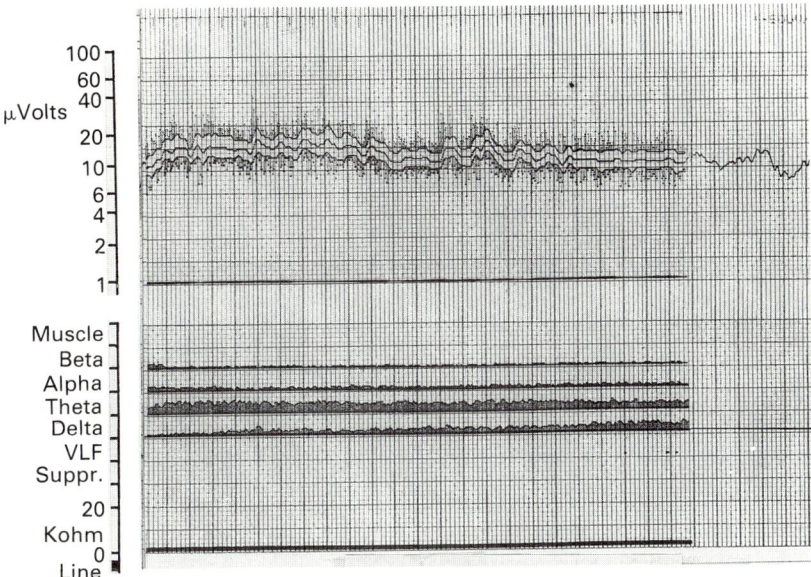

Fig. 5.5 CFAM trace of decreasing Pa_{CO_2} by hyperventilation. As the Pa_{CO_2} decreases the cerebral blood vessels vasoconstrict and there is an increase in the delta band activity.

Some neuroanaesthetists administer an infusion of thiopentone or propofol during clipping of cerebral artery aneurysms. The aim is to reduce cerebral metabolic rate for oxygen (CMRO$_2$) so that if the aneurysm should rupture during surgery the oxygen demand of the brain will be reduced, allowing the neurosurgeon greater time to achieve control of the haemorrhage. Monitoring the EEG during the infusion will indicate the degree of CMRO$_2$ reduction which has been achieved. It is customary to reduce the EEG activity to burst suppression, but even greater reduction in CMRO$_2$ will be achieved by producing an isoelectric EEG (Fig. 5.6). Infusions of intravenous anaesthetic agents may be used in the ICU to reduce intracranial pressure (ICP). However, there is evidence that this is unlikely to be effective if the amplitude of the EEG is less than 6 μV peak to peak (Bingham *et al.* 1985).

The EEG has been used to determine the need for the insertion of a shunt during clamping of the carotid artery during carotid artery endarterectomy. Monitoring the EEG for this short period of time has not proved reliable at predicting nueorological deficits postoperatively. Better results are obtained if the processed EEG is monitored continuously from

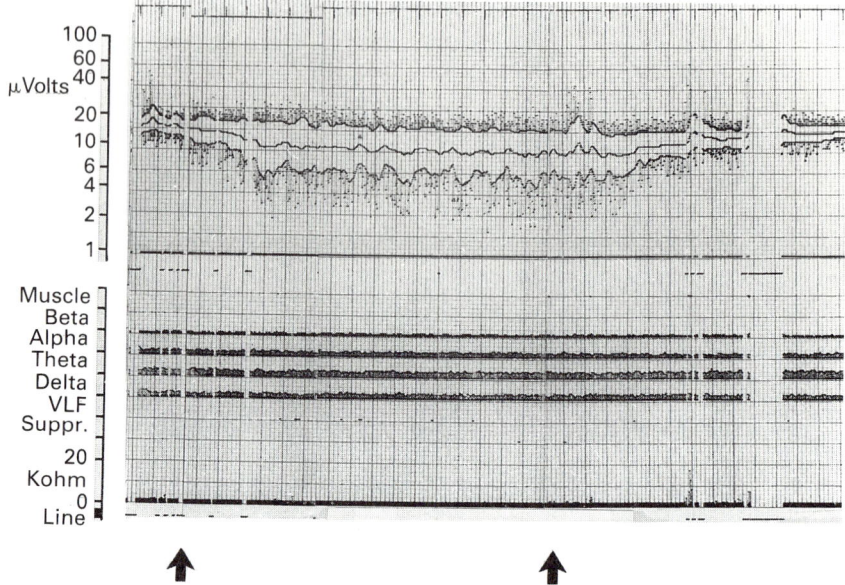

Fig. 5.6 CFAM trace of burst suppression during an infusion of thiopentone for clipping of an aneurysm. The burst suppression is indicated by the widening of amplitude analysis in the upper trace. The infusion was commenced at the left arrow and stopped at the right one. The EEG was no longer in burst suppression 8 min after stopping the infusion.

the preoperative period through to postoperative care, but even here the predictability of outcome is poor because of the limitations of the number of recording electrodes which can be used. Observing the spectral edge on CSA monitors has proved to be unreliable also (Bowdle *et al.* 1988). To be able to demonstrate any perioperative ischaemic episode during carotid artery surgery it is best to use at least a 16-lead montage and record unprocessed EEG.

When a patient is receiving muscle relaxants and positive-pressure ventilation in the ICU neurological observations are difficult to make, and observing the EEG is a useful alternative. There should be a rhythmic variation in the amplitude occurring about two or three times per minute. Absence of this variation or absence of EEG response to stimulation, is indicative of a poor prognosis. Hutchison *et al.* (1991) noted that head-injured patients with an isoelectric EEG or repeated periods of an isoelectric EEG died, but if there was reactivity of the EEG to external stimuli the patient tended to make a favourable outcome. Observing the

EEG in paralysed patients in the ICU is the only way of noting the occurrence of epileptic fits and adequately suppressing them (Fig. 5.3), because the clinical features of the fit will be obtunded. As benzodiazepines increase the beta band activity, monitoring the EEG will demonstrate their adequate use for sedation in the ICU. Barbiturates also increase beta band activity, and Klein *et al.* (1988) demonstrated that if a head-injured patient responded with a short increase in beta activity following a bolus of thiopentone the outcome was favourable. The EEG will demonstrate alpha coma in those patients who have sustained a discrete brainstem haemorrhage, whose cortex is functioning, but transmission through the brain stem is blocked and who are 'locked in'. The indications for monitoring EEG in neuroanaesthesia or neurointensive care are listed in Table. 5.1.

Table 5.1 Indications for EEG monitoring in neuroanaesthesia and neurointensive care

The EEG may be used
1 To monitor the adequacy of cerebral oxygenation
2 To monitor the adequacy of cerebral blood flow
3 The reduction in cerebral metabolic rate during infusions of intravenous anaesthetic agents for cerebral protection
4 To monitor the neurological status of the patient in the ICU
5 To monitor the response to stimulating the patient in the ICU
6 To monitor the occurrence of epileptic fits in paralysed patients in the ICU
7 To give an indication of the value of administering intravenous anaesthetic agents to reduce ICP
8 To monitor the effectiveness of sedation in the ICU
9 To give a prediction of outcome from coma

Evoked potentials

Evoked potentials monitor the deeper brain pathways and pathways in the spinal cord, and can monitor sensory and motor pathways. Visual, somatosensory and brainstem auditory are the commonly employed sensory evoked potentials. The recording electrodes are placed on the appropriate position on the scalp and pick up not only the EEG but also the responses to the sensory stimulus. Repeated sensory stimuli have to be given to allow the monitor to subtract the EEG from the sensory evoked response and record only the sensory evoked potential. A series of waves is obtained and the amplitude and latency of the waves after the stimulus are studied. The response can be affected by anaesthetic agents and so a steady-state anaesthetic, rather than one which employs incremental boli of agents, should be used. The amplitude of the waves is decreased and the latency increased in visual, somatosensory and brainstem auditory evoked potentials by halothane, enflurane and iso-flurane. Nitrous oxide decreases the amplitude of the waves of somato-sensory and visual evoked potentials, increases the latency of the visual evoked potential waves, but has no effect on the latency of somatosensory responses, and no effect on the amplitude or latency of brainstem auditory responses. Thiopentone, etomidate and propofol have no effect on these evoked responses. Analgesics decrease the amplitude and increase the latency of the waves of the somatosensory evoked potential. The responses are affected by alteration in blood pressure, blood gases, haematocrit, cerebral blood flow, hypothermia, hypoglycaemia and diathermy.

Visual evoked potential (VEP)

In a neurophysiology department the signal generator for this potential is an electronic checker-board, somewhat similar to a chess-board, where the black and white squares can alternate. Obviously in the operating theatre or ICU this is not practicable, and a pair of goggles with light-emitting diodes can be used instead. The recording electrodes are pos-itioned at O1 and O2 (Fig. 5.1) and 100 flashes of light are administered. A typical VEP is shown in Fig. 5.7.

The VEP is of limited value during anaesthesia as it is very sensitive to anaesthetic agents; the pupils may also deviate or constrict during anaesthesia so that the optimal response to the stimulus is not obtained. It can, however, be used as a monitor during surgery near the optic nerve, optic chiasm, pituitary gland or sphenoidal wing. Pfurtscheller *et al.* (1985) demonstrated that as a patient becomes less comatose following a head injury, the VEP can be recorded over a greater area of cerebral cortex. One of the main uses of VEP is in the diagnosis of multiple sclerosis.

Brainstem auditory evoked potential (BAEP)

The recording electrodes for this potential are positioned over the mastoid processes or ear lobes and at Cz (Fig. 5.1). The stimuli, which are auditory clicks, can be given through small ear-pieces, similar to those which are used for personal radios, as they are not bulky and should not

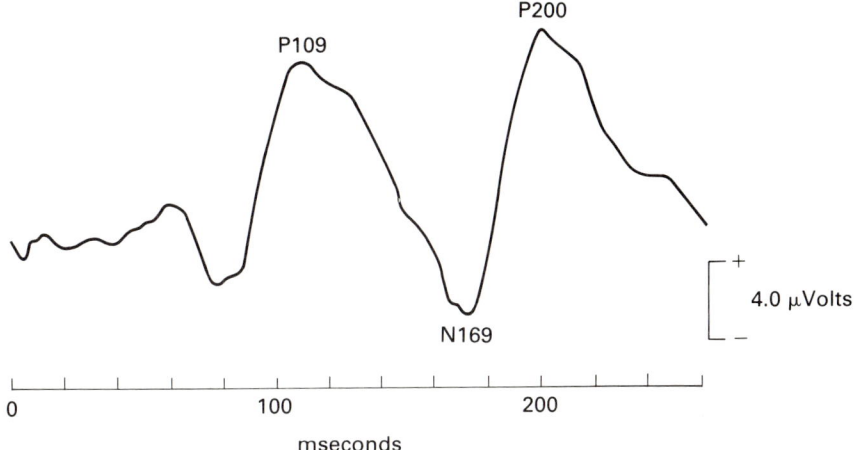

Fig. 5.7 An example of a normal visual evoked potential. P refers to a positive deflection, N to a negative one, and the numbers to the number of milliseconds after the stimulus when the deflection normally occurs.

interfere with the surgical approach. However they must be magnetically sealed and preferably give alternating positive and negative clicks to reduce the amount of signal artifact which will be picked up by the recording electrode which is on the mastoid process and near to the ear-pieces. To be able to get a clear BAEP trace, 2000 stimuli have to be administered, and during this time other electrical signals in the operating theatre or ICU could give interference, making it difficult to obtain a good trace. A typical BAEP trace is shown in Fig. 5.8.

The BAEP is a useful monitor during the removal of an acoustic neuroma or posterior fossa surgery. During surgery on the fifth or seventh cranial nerves (Janetta procedure) it is possible to damage the eighth cranial nerve by incorrect placement of the retractors. Monitoring the BAEP will give an early indication of this, allowing the retractors to be replaced and avoiding possible postoperative deafness.

Kawahara *et al.* (1989) found that the interpeak latency I–V was significantly increased if the ICP was greater than 50 mmHg for 4 h, or greater than 45 mmHg for 8 h, or greater than 40 mmHg for 24 h. Wave III was lost if the ICP was greater than 50 mmHg. There was no significant correlation between cerebral perfusion pressure (CPP) and the interpeak latencies, but wave I was lost if the ICP was greater than 50 mmHg or CPP was less than 40 mmHg.

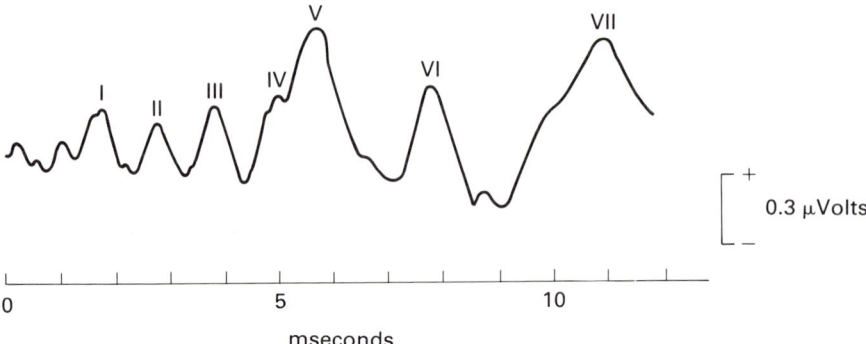

Fig. 5.8 An example of a normal brainstem auditory evoked potential. The waves are numbered I–VII and are generated by the passage of the stimuli along the auditory pathway from the ear to the cortex. Wave I comes from the acoustic nerve, II from the cochlear nucleus in the pons, III from the superior olive in the pons, IV from the lateral lemniscus in the pons, V from the inferior colliculus in the midbrain, VI from the medial geniculate body in the thalamus, and VII from thalamocortical radiations.

Auditory evoked responses (AER)

The recording montage and stimuli for these responses are exactly the same as for BAEP. The BAEP responses occur in 12 ms after the stimulus, but the AER responses are observed much later and are thought to represent cortical responses to the auditory clicks. The first of these waves is a positive deflection (Pa) which occurs at 26 ms after the stimulus, the second is a negative deflection (Nb) at 35 ms, and a series of waves to 300 ms have been studied. With increasing concentrations of anaesthetic agents, either intravenous or inhalational, the amplitude of the waves decreases and the latency increases. It is thought that the AER may give an indication of the depth of anaesthesia (Thornton *et al.* 1989), and in particular if Nb has a latency of less than 44.5 ms the patient may be aware of the surgery. As neuroanaesthetics are usually administered at a light plane of anaesthesia the AER may be a useful monitor to know that the patient is not aware of the procedure. The AER has also been studied in comatose patients, and as the conscious level improves so the amplitudes and latencies of the AER waves return to normal (Ottaviani *et al.* 1986). Sneyd *et al.* (1992) have demonstrated that the latency of the first negative wave of the AER is decreased during chest physiotherapy on patients in the ICU who are sedated with propofol, fentanyl and atracurium, presumably as an arousal response to the physiotherapy.

Somatosensory evoked potentials (SEP)

The stimuli for this potential is a series of 100 electric shocks which can be given over the posterior tibial nerve at the ankle, or the median nerve at the wrist. As the signal travels along the posterior columns in the spinal cord, unfortunately SEP cannot be relied upon to monitor the integrity of the lateral or anterior columns. The trace which is recorded differs between the two sites of stimulation.

A typical SEP trace from posterior tibial stimulation is shown in Fig. 5.9. The recording electrodes should be placed at Cz and Cz' (Fig. 5.1) which is 1 cm behind Cz. When the median nerve is used the signal is recorded as it passes Erb's point in the brachial plexus (which is at the level of the junction of the lateral and middle thirds of the clavicle) the seventh cervical vertebra (CV7), the second cervical vertebra (CV2) and at C3' or C4' (Fig. 5.1) which are 1 cm behind C3 and C4 and are over the sensory cortex. A typical median nerve SEP is shown in Fig. 5.10.

The posterior tibial SEP is a useful monitor during operations on the spinal cord such as the removal of an arteriovenous malformation, drainage of a syrinx, or excision of an intramedullary tumour. It also indicates the integrity of the posterior columns during spinal operations, but unfortunately will not demonstrate the integrity of the anterior

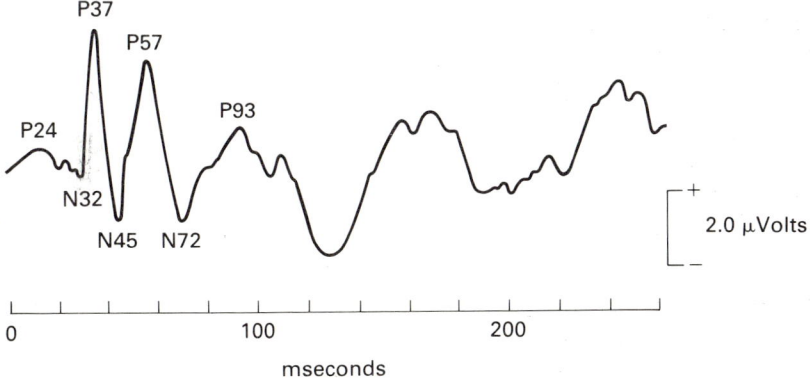

Fig. 5.9 An example of a normal posterior tibial somatosensory evoked potential. P refers to positive deflections, N to negative ones, and the numbers are milliseconds after the stimulus.

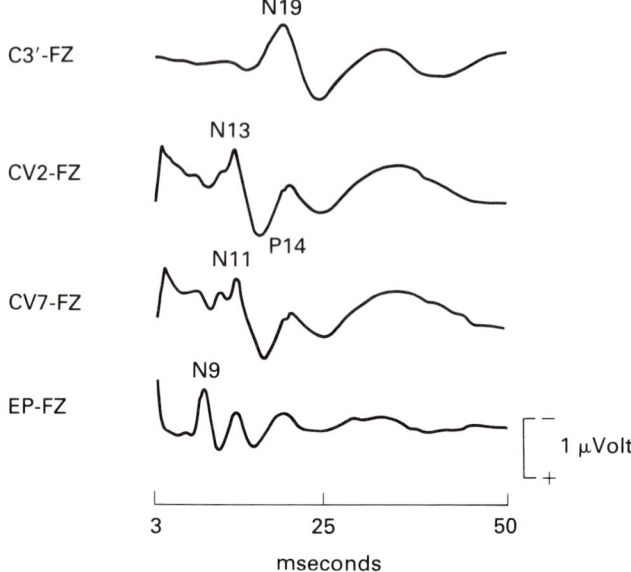

Fig. 5.10 An example of a right median nerve somatosensory evoked potential. One electrode is always positioned at Fz, and the other one is used to trace the passage of the signal from the wrist to the sensory cortex. EP is Erb's point over the brachial plexus and the response is normally recorded at 9 ms after the stimulus, CV7 is recorded over the seventh cervical vertebra at 11 ms, CV2 is at the second cervical vertebra and gives a negative deflection at 13 ms and a positive one at 14 ms. C3' is recorded 1 cm behind C3 over the contralateral sensory cortex at 19 ms after the stimulus. The time which the response takes to travel from CV2 to the sensory cortex is the central conduction time (CCT).

motor columns. The need for a 'wake-up' test is not completely removed therefore by the use of the SEP, but motor evoked potentials, which are described later, are now available and probably monitor the integrity of the anterior columns of the cord.

Astrup *et al.* (1977) found that the SEP was a good indicator of cerebral blood flow. The amplitudes of the waves decreased and the latencies increased when CBF decreased to 20 ml 100 g^{-1} min^{-1}, and the waveforms were absent when the CBF decreased to 15 ml 100 g^{-1} min^{-1}. Irreversible brain damage does not occur until the CBF decreases to 12 ml 100 g^{-1} min^{-1}, and so the SEP will give an indication of decreasing CBF before it has reached dangerous levels.

The SEP correlates well with the patient's clinical status as assessed by the Glasgow Coma Scale, and is a good predictor of outcome from head injury (Pfurtscheller *et al.* 1985). If the SEP is present bilaterally the outcome should be good provided no further secondary insult occurs in the ICU, but if the SEP is absent bilaterally the outcome is poor (Judson *et al.* 1990, Hutchinson *et al.* 1991).

The median nerve evoked potential can be used to monitor operations on the spinal cord and spine above the eighth cervical vertebra, and also posterior fossa operations as it monitors a different pathway from the BAEP. The time taken for the signal to pass from CV2 to the sensory cortex is known as the central conduction time (CCT) and is normally of the order of 5.4 ms. This value is increased immediately after a subarachnoid haemorrhage from a rupture of a cerebral artery aneurysm, but returns to normal as the patient's condition improves and can be used to indicate the optimum time for clipping the aneurysm (Rosenstein *et al.* 1985). The CCT is also increased if the CBF is less than $30 \, \text{ml} \, 100 \, \text{g}^{-1} \, \text{min}^{-1}$. Lindsay *et al.* (1990) demonstrated quite a good correlation with outcome from head injury and CCT recorded 2–3 days after the injury.

Motor evoked potential (MEP)

As the presence of a SEP does not guarantee the integrity of the motor pathway in the spinal cord, methods of monitoring that pathway have been developed. It is possible to stimulate the motor cortex by the application of an electrical shock through the skull, somewhat similar to administering electroconvulsive therapy, or to electrically stimulate the motor anterior columns of the spinal cord during surgery on the cord. Recently it has become possible to apparently stimulate the motor pathway by the use of repeated applications of a powerful magnetic field. However, there is some doubt that this is specific for the motor pathway. The MEP is affected by thiopentone, propofol, etomidate, midazolam and isoflurane, but not by nitrous oxide or fentanyl (Kalkman *et al.* 1992, Schmidt *et al.* 1992). The motor response can be observed if the patient is not paralysed during the anaesthetic, otherwise the response has to be recorded as it passes down the anterior compartment of the spinal cord or along the appropriate peripheral nerve. Despite these anaesthetic challenges it has been possible to record meaningful MEP intraoperatively (Jellinek *et al.* 1991, Owen *et al.* 1991).

Eighth nerve action potential

During some posterior fossa explorations, especially during the excision of an acoustic neuroma, the neurosurgeon will try to identify both the auditory and vestibular components of the eighth nerve, and also the facial nerve. By observing that wave I is present in the BAEP the integrity of the eighth nerve can be assumed, but the BAEP takes some time to record and does not give an instant result. It is possible to stimulate directly the eighth nerve under direct vision with a Teflon-coated stimulating needle. One single stimulation on the auditory part of the nerve will give an action potential response which can be detected by the BAEP electrodes, whereas stimulation of the vestibular portion will give no response. Unfortunately it is possible to get a false-positive result if the stimulation is transmitted from another structure to the auditory part of the nerve through cerebrospinal fluid.

Facial nerve electromyography

Identifying the facial nerve can be done in a similar fashion. The recording needles are placed in the orbicularis oculi and orbicularis oris muscles, and for best responses the patient should not be paralysed during the anaesthetic.

Conclusion

Electrical monitoring of the brain and spinal cord is not easy in the 'hostile' environment of the operating theatre or ICU because of the possibility of interference from electrical equipment which is connected to or is in the vicinity of the patient. The EEG electrodes record from a small area, and if they are not placed accurately pathological changes may not be monitored. The evoked potentials monitor specific pathways in the cord or brain and the correct potential must be chosen for each monitoring purpose. Many factors can produce similar alterations in the EEG or EP and their interpretation must be done in conjunction with the clinical condition of the patient. Despite these limitations monitoring the EEG or EP does give useful information about the functional integrity of the brain or spinal cord, whereas CT or MRI scans give anatomical information. More useful information will be gained if more than one parameter is monitored at any one time.

References

Astrup J., Symon L., Branston N.M. & Lassen N.A. (1977) Cortical evoked potential and extracellular K+ and H+ at critical levels of brain ischemia. *Stroke* **8**, 51–57.

Bickford R.G., Fleming N.I. & Billinger T.W. (1971) Compression of EEG data by isometric power spectral plots. *Electroencephalography and Clinical Neurophysiology* **31**, 63P.

Bingham R.M., Procaccio F., Prior P.F. & Hinds C.J. (1985) Cerebral electrical activity influences the effects of etomidate on cerebral perfusion pressure in traumatic coma. *British Journal of Anaesthesia* **57**, 843–848.

Bowdle T.A., Rooke A. & Kaziners A. (1988) Intraoperative stroke during carotid endarterectomy without a change in spectral edge frequency of the compressed spectral array. *Journal of Cardiothoracic Anaesthesia* **2**, 204–206.

Demetrescu M. (1975) The aperiodic character of the electroencephalogram (EEG): A new approach to data analysis and condensation. *Physiologist* **18**, 189.

Fleming R.A. & Smith N.T. (1979) An inexpensive device for analyzing and monitoring the electroencephalogram. *Anesthesiology* **50**, 456–460.

Hutchinson D.O., Frith R.W., Shaw N.A., Judson J.A. & Cant B.R. (1991) A comparison between electroencephalography and somatosensory evoked potentials for outcome prediction following severe head injury. *Electroencephalography and Clinical Neurophysiology* **78**, 228–233.

Jellinek D., Jewkes D. & Symon L. (1991) Noninvasive intraoperative monitoring of motor evoked potentials under propofol anaesthesia: effects of spinal surgery. *Neurosurgery* **29**, 551–557.

Judson J.A., Cant B.R. & Shaw N.A. (1990) Early prediction of outcome from cerebral trauma by somatosensory evoked potentials. *Critical Care Medicine* **18**, 363–368.

Kalkman C.J., Drummond J.C., Ribberink A.A., Patel P.M., Sano T. & Bickford R.G. (1992) Effects of propofol, etomidate, midazolam and fentanyl on motor evoked responses to transcranial electrical or magnetic stimulation in humans. *Anesthesiology* **76**, 502–509.

Kawahara N., Sasaki M., Mii K., Tsuzuki M. & Takakura K. (1989) Sequential changes of auditory brain stem responses in relation to intracranial and cerebral perfusion pressure and initiation of secondary brain stem damage. *Acta Neurochirurgica (Wien)* **100**, 142–149.

Klein H.J., Rath S.A. & Goppel F. (1988) The use of EEG spectral analysis after thiopental bolus in the prognostic evaluation of comatose patients with brain injuries. *Acta Neurochirurgica Supplement (Wien)* **42**, 31–34.

Lindsay K., Pasaoglu A., Hirst D., Allardyce G., Kennedy I. & Teasdale G. (1990) Somatosensory and auditory brain stem conduction after head injury: a comparison with clinical features in prediction of outcome. *Neurosurgery* **26**, 278–285.

Maynard D.E. & Jenkinson J.L. (1984) The Cerebral Function Analysing Monitor. Initial clinical experience, application and further development. *Anaesthesia* **39**, 678–690.

Maynard D., Prior P.F. & Scott D.F. (1969) Device for continuous monitoring of cerebral activity in resuscitated patients. *British Medical Journal* **4**, 545–546.

Michenfelder J.D., Sundt T.M., Fode N. & Sharbrough F.W. (1987) Isoflurane when compared to enflurane and halothane decreases the frequency of cerebral ischemia during carotid endarterectomy. *Anesthesiology* **67**, 336–340.

Ottaviani F., Almadori G., Calderazo A.B., Frenguelli A. & Paludetti G (1986) Auditory brain-stem (ABRs) and middle latency auditory responses (MLRs) in the prognosis of severely head injured patients. *Electroencephalography and Clinical Neurophysiology* **65**, 196–202.

Owen J.H., Bridwell K.H., Grubb R. *et al.* (1991) The clinical application of neurogenic motor evoked potentials to monitor spinal cord function during surgery. *Spine* **16** (Suppl.), 385–390.

Pfurtscheller G., Schwarz G. & Gravenstein N. (1985) Clinical relevance of long latency SEPs and VEPs during coma and emergence from coma. *Electro-encephalography and Clinical Neurophysiology* **62**, 88–98.

Prior P.F. (1985) EEG monitoring and evoked potentials in brain ischaemia. *British Journal of Anaesthesia* **57**, 63–81.

Rampil I.J., Sasse F.J., Smith N.T., Hoff B.H., Rusy B.F. & Fleming D.C. (1979) A new method for testing the response to an inhalational agent. *Anesthesiology* **51** (Suppl.), S26.

Rosenstein J., Wang A.D., Symon L. & Suzuki M. (1985) Relationship between hemispheric cerebral blood flow, central conduction time, and clinical grade in aneurysmal subarachnoid hemorrhage. *Journal of Neurosurgery* **62**, 25–30.

Schmid U.D., Boll J., Ljechti S., Schmid J. & Hess C.W. (1992) Influence of some anaesthetic agents on muscle responses to transcranial magnetic cortex stimulation: a pilot study in humans. *Neurosurgery* **30**, 85–92.

Sneyd J.R., Wang D.Y., Edwards D. *et al.* (1992) Effect of physiotherapy on the auditory evoked response of paralysed, sedated patients in the intensive care unit. *British Journal of Anaesthesia* **68**, 349–351.

Thornton C., Barrowcliffe M.P., Konieczko K.M. *et al.* (1989) The auditory evoked response as an indicator of awareness. *British Journal of Anaesthesia* **63**, 113–115.

6
Anaesthesia for neuroradiology

STEVEN CRUICKSHANK

Introduction

Enormous changes have taken place over the past two decades in the practice of neuroradiology. A glance at a standard textbook of neuro-anaesthesia in use some 20 years ago (McComish & Bodley 1971) gives an idea of the advances which have been made. Then there was extensive discussion on general anaesthesia for air encephalography, ventriculo-graphy and cerebral angiography. Angiography was frequently performed by direct carotid artery puncture and procedures were often extended by the need to develop and assess X-ray plates before the next series of films could be taken.

Recent developments in imaging have had a huge impact and advances in catheter technology and contrast media have altered the nature of work in the neuroradiology department. The introduction of CT in 1973 was a major advance allowing speedy, non-invasive and accurate locali-zation of tumours, detection of blood in the subarachnoid space and assessment of trauma. Rapid improvements in the technology soon allowed better and better image quality and more detailed diagnostic information.

MRI, which became fairly widely available in the late 1980s, has exceeded initial expectations and can produce images in many cases superior to those of CT. The increasing demands for this technology will continue to generate challenges for the anaesthetist.

The principles of cerebral angiography and its value in delineating the precise anatomy of vascular lesions and tumour blood supply are unchanged. However, the availability of superior contrast media and the introduction of digital angiographic equipment resulting in shorter pro-cedure times have reduced the requirement for general anaesthesia. Cerebral angiography can be performed satisfactorily in the majority of cases with a technique involving local anaesthesia and minimal sedation.

Air encephalography is now virtually obsolete and is not performed where CT and MRI are available.

141

Ultrasound plays an important role in investigation of neonates, especially for hydrocephalus, or parenchymal or intraventricular haemorrhage. This investigation does not involve anaesthesia as it is non-invasive, and patient movement does not seriously interfere with its performance.

The investigation of spinal problems frequently involves myelography, although increasingly MRI is becoming the technique of choice.

Finally, developments in catheter technology have enabled the advance of interventional radiology. This field is developing rapidly and involvement of the anaesthetist as part of the team is advisable (Mazziotta & Gilman 1992).

The involvement of the anaesthetist in neuroradiology

The anaesthetist's role in the neuroradiology department involves some or all of the following:

1 Care of patients during angiography. Practice varies in the United Kingdom with some units employing anaesthesia for most angiograms and others using sedation techniques almost entirely.

2 Care of severely injured patients and patients from the intensive care unit (ICU) requiring life support during investigations, principally CT scanning and angiography.

3 Administration of anaesthesia for patients unsuitable for sedation techniques, such as children or demented, confused adults. This may be required for angiography, CT scanning, MRI scanning or myelography.

4 Interventional radiology. This new field is involving neuroanaesthetists increasingly and is considered in detail later.

Any technique of sedation or anaesthesia in neuroradiology must be based on the same principles of control of intracranial pressure and dynamics as for any neurosurgical procedure. Careful assessment of the patient before the procedure should reveal the extent of problems of lack of cooperation, airway protection and intracranial dynamics, and how they may be handled.

Environment

The environment for administering general anaesthesia in the neuroradiology department is seldom ideal. Space is often limited by large, bulky imaging equipment, anaesthetic assistance and the availability of equipment may not be adequate, and the use of normal monitoring equipment may be restricted in the MRI suite. Computer-based equipment needs to be kept in air-conditioned accommodation and patients, especially small children, can become hypothermic during long investigations. High noise levels, especially in the MRI suite, and low ambient lighting are additional problems. Chronic exposure of staff to ionizing radiation is, of course, a well-known hazard.

Contrast media

All water-soluble agents are derivatives of tri-iodobenzoic acid. The ionic agents which dissociate in solution have largely been superseded by non-ionic agents which are less toxic and less liable to give rise to hypersensitivity reactions. Neurotoxicity is related in part to the osmotic effects of the agent. The non-ionic media, which have alcohol or glucose moieties added to the tri-iodobenzoic acid base, have a lower osmolality for each iodine molecule and hence are less toxic. The non-ionic media used commonly in neuroradiology are iopamidol and iohexol, both of which are alcohol-substituted. They are used, in different formulations and strengths for angiography, myelography and contrast-enhanced CT. Care must be exercised in their use in patients who are dehydrated, who have hepatic or renal impairment or myelomatosis. Anticonvulsant medication should be maintained in epileptic patients.

Metrizamide, which was used from the 1970s until recently, was associated with a higher incidence of convulsions and arachnoiditis. The incidence of convulsions was increased by the concurrent use of phenothiazines.

CONTRAST MEDIA TOXICITY

Adverse reactions to radiological contrast media (Goldberg 1984) can be divided into chemotoxic and idiosyncratic.

Chemotoxic effects are directly related to the osmolality of the agent and have become less of a problem since the introduction of the newer non-ionic media. The media may permeate an already damaged blood–brain barrier after trauma, infarction or in tumours, and increase local oedema by osmotic effects. This can lead to seizures.

Idiosyncratic effects may be minor or serious and life-threatening reactions. Rashes or minor vasomotor symptoms of flushing and dizziness may occur and require only reassurance. The incidence of serious anaphylactoid reactions is now very low. The incidence is increased in the following groups of patients:

1   History of prior reaction to contrast media.
2   Cardiovascular disease.
3   Allergic diathesis, asthma or hay fever.
4   Age less than 1 year or greater than 60 years.

MANAGEMENT OF CONTRAST MEDIA REACTION (CMR)

Patients with a previous history of CMR are best treated prophylactically with antihistamines and steroids starting 18 h prior to the investigation. Oral prednisolone 10 mg 6-hourly for three doses and chlorpheniramine 10 mg intramuscularly 1 h beforehand should suffice for the typical adult patient. Such regimens have been shown to reduce the incidence and severity of CMR. Skin testing is not worthwhile.

A full anaphylactoid reaction is a rarity but can appear with alarming rapidity. The patient may exhibit collapse, cyanosis, wheezing, diarrhoea, rash and urticaria, nausea, vomiting or facial swelling.

IMMEDIATE THERAPY
(doses for 70 kg patient)

1   Discontinue contrast injection.
2   Establish clear airway and administer 100% oxygen. Consider intubation if reaction is severe; oral and pharyngeal swelling may cause rapid obstruction.
3   Give adrenaline $50-100\,\mu g$ ($0.5-1$ ml. $1:10\,000$) intravenously. Repeat if necessary and establish infusion if reaction persists ($5-8\,\mu g\,kg^{-1}\,min^{-1}$).
4   Establish large-bore intravenous line and give $500-1000$ ml fluid, preferably colloid.
5   If bronchospasm persists in spite of adrenaline, consider aminophylline $250-500$ mg slowly intravenously or terbutaline $250-500\,\mu g$ intravenously.
6   Give intravenous hydrocortisone 500 mg and an antihistamine such as chlorpheniramine 20 mg.
7   Check arterial blood gases and coagulation screen.
8   If appropriate, transfer to ICU for further therapy.

Computerized tomography (CT)

The introduction of CT scanning in the early 1970s revolutionized the diagnosis of neurosurgical conditions, and by demonstrating the possibilities of non-invasive, computer-based imaging systems, paved the way for the development of magnetic resonance imaging and positron emission tomography (PET).

CT scanning is now widely used all over the world. In some respects MRI scanning can produce better images, but the two techniques should be seen as complementary. They are compared in Table 6.1. Technical developments have led to better CT image quality and shorter scanning times, and there is a prospect that individual scan cut times can be made short enough so that requirement for anaesthesia or sedation in small children undergoing CT will diminish (Boyer 1992).

CT is extensively used in the assessment of patients with multiple injuries. Many of these need life support, continuation of invasive monitoring, and inotropic support during the scan, and this can be difficult within the confines of the CT suite. In view of the non-invasive nature of the investigation there are no special anaesthetic considerations

Table 6.1 CT and MRI compared

CT	MRI
Wide availability	Restricted availability
Less expensive	Expensive
More experience in interpretation	Limited experience
Compatible with full life support	Not available for patients with clips, pacemakers, etc. Difficulties with anaesthetic and monitoring equipment
Rapid acquisition times	Long procedures
Ionizing radiation used	No ionizing radiation
Good demonstration of:	
Subarachnoid blood	Tumours
Calcification in tumours	Soft tissue lesions, e.g. disc prolapse
Trauma — fractures, etc.	White matter lesions, e.g. post-trauma, multiple sclerosis. Good grey vs white matter differentation

applying to CT. Anaesthetic management follows the principles discussed for other diagnostic procedures.

Magnetic resonance imaging (MRI)

MRI is becoming widely available. After initial development during the 1970s, clinical trials started in Nottingham, Aberdeen and London in 1980, and by the late 1980s commercially available machines had been installed in many centres.

The principles of the imaging method

A detailed explanation of the physics of nuclear magnetic resonance (NMR) is not possible in a short space. A brief description will, however, illuminate the problems encountered by the anaesthetist.

The signal for NMR imaging arises in nuclei and depends upon those nuclei having both an odd number of nucleons (protons or neutrons) and also the property called spin. Such nuclei possess a magnetic moment and behave like miniature bar magnets, and when placed in a strong external magnetic field these nuclei align themselves with the magnetic field. Hydrogen, with a single proton in the nucleus, has these properties and is abundant in tissues and forms the basis of clinical imaging.

Nuclei with spin, aligned in an external magnetic field, exhibit the phenomenon of precession; that is their axis of spin 'wobbles' in its alignment with the applied field. The application of an oscillating radio-frequency (RF) pulse of a particular frequency at right angles to the field causes the protons to absorb the energy and change the orientation of their vector of rotation. The frequency of radiation (resonant or Larmor frequency) which will cause this depends upon the strength of the magnetic field and on the nucleus in question. The dependence of resonant frequency on magnetic field strength means that magnetic field gradients can be used for spatial resolution. Following the RF pulse the nuclei 'relax' back to their original orientation with respect to the field, and re-emit the energy absorbed as a RF signal. Processing of this re-emitted signal enables construction of a cross-sectional image of the tissue.

The process is thus completely different from that of CT imaging, which depends upon absorption of radiation by the electron shell of atoms and analysis of the attenuation of applied ionizing radiation. CT is an absorption technique and MRI an emission technique.

The emitted signal dies away as the protons (or other nuclei) relax back to their original alignment. Two times are used to describe this process. The time to restore equilibrium is referred to as $T1$.

Initially after the cessation of the RF pulse the nuclei relax in phase, i.e. all together. However, progressively, individual nuclei are affected by slight inhomogeneities in their immediate magnetic environment and by interaction with neighbouring nuclei such that they become out of phase. The time taken to lose the phase coherence is described as $T2$. $T1$ is always longer than $T2$.

Measurement of the initial signal and its decline characteristics give information on the physical nature of tissues. Application of differing RF pulse sequences enables signals weighted to proton density or different relaxation times to be analysed. Common sequences are termed 'spin echo' (SE) and 'inversion recovery' (IR). Field gradient can be varied across a region so that signals can be isolated to a particular point and thus a two-dimensional image constructed. Since hydrogen is present in water, differing water content of tissues is well displayed, allowing excellent differentiation of grey and white matter for instance.

In vivo biochemical investigation using ^{31}P NMR is a promising research tool in investigation of metabolic muscle disorders. Extension of this principle (magnetic resonance spectroscopy (MRS)) to other nuclei and other tissues will enable investigation of metabolic and pharmacological processes.

CONTRAST MEDIUM

A paramagnetic substance will change the relaxation times of tissues where it is present. Intravenous gadolinium, chelated to render it non-toxic, is used to increase tissue differentiation in distinguishing tumour from surrounding oedema or in vascular lesions such as meningiomas.

These complex matters are dealt with comprehensively by Kean and Smith (1986). A short and admirable review of the physics is given by Pykett (1982).

Anaesthetic problems

Although most MRI scans are performed without general anaesthesia, when it is required, considerable difficulties are posed for the anaesthetist (Nixon *et al.* 1986, Burk 1989). Some of the problems presented are:

1   In common with other sites in the neuroradiology department, the suite is often in an isolated location, with little provision of space for

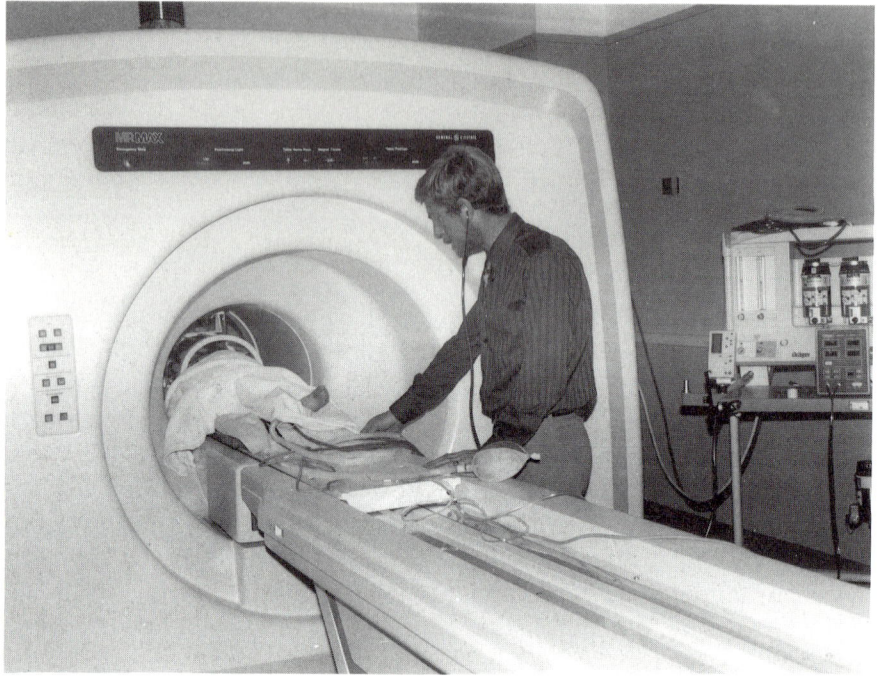

Fig. 6.1 MRI scanner. The patient is situated in a long tunnel restricting access and observation. The anaesthetic machine has no ferromagnetic components.

induction and recovery of patients. The air-conditioned accommodation and prolonged scanning time can lead to hypothermia. The machines may be very noisy in operation.

2   The patient is enclosed in a long, narrow tube during imaging, restricting both observation and access (Fig. 6.1).

3   The strong magnetic field (present even when a patient is not being scanned) attracts ferromagnetic objects which can become lethal projectiles. Keys, metal badges, etc., must be left outside the suite. Magnetic storage media, e.g. floppy discs and credit cards, can be wiped clear. Items of anaesthetic equipment which are magnetic, e.g. cylinders, anaesthetic machine, laryngoscopes, or ventilators need to be kept well clear of the magnetic field, or substitutes found which are non-magnetic.

4   Monitoring equipment may not function in the presence of strong magnetic field and RF radiation.

5   Image quality is degraded by ferromagnetic objects within range of the scanner. These disturb the homogeneity of the magnetic field and interfere with the imaging process. Conductive leads from monitoring equipment may act as antennae and capture stray RF signals with consequent image degradation.

6 Patients with surgically implanted clips of magnetic materials, e.g. older aneurysm clips, cannot be imaged. Patients with cardiac pacemakers are also excluded because the pacemaker may malfunction, or physical motion of the pacemaker itself may occur.

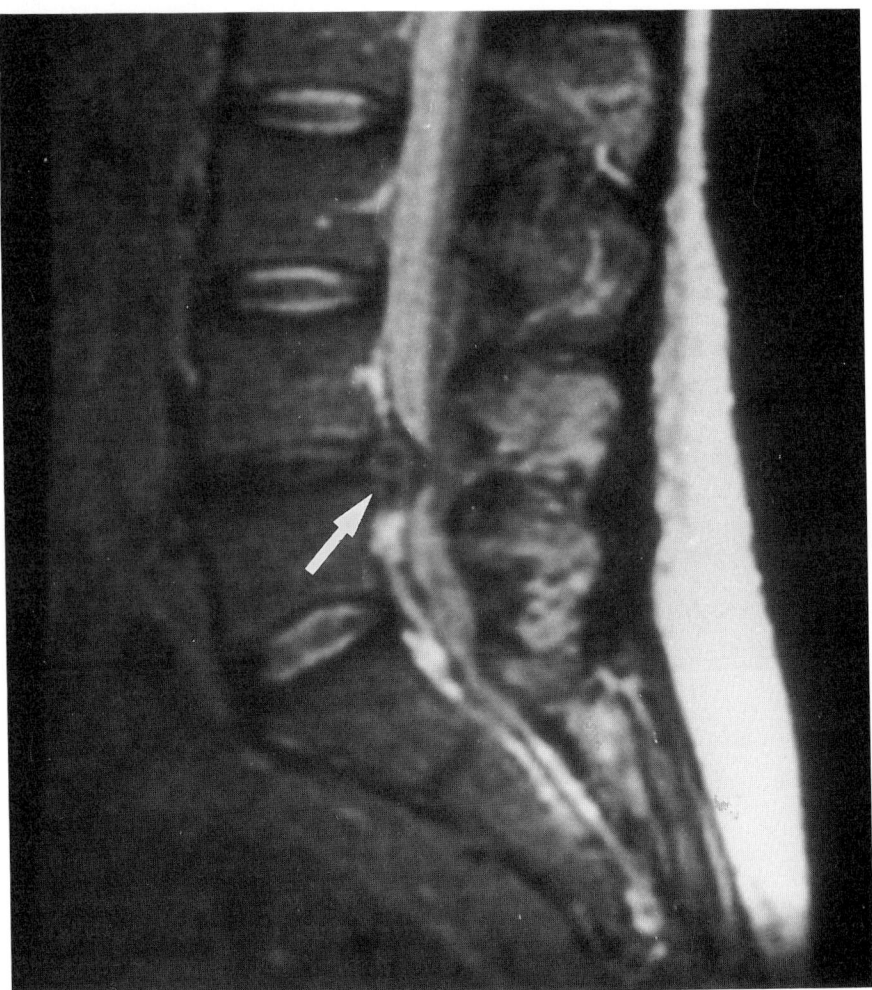

Fig. 6.2 MRI image. *T*2 weighted sagittal image showing L4–5 prolapsed disc.

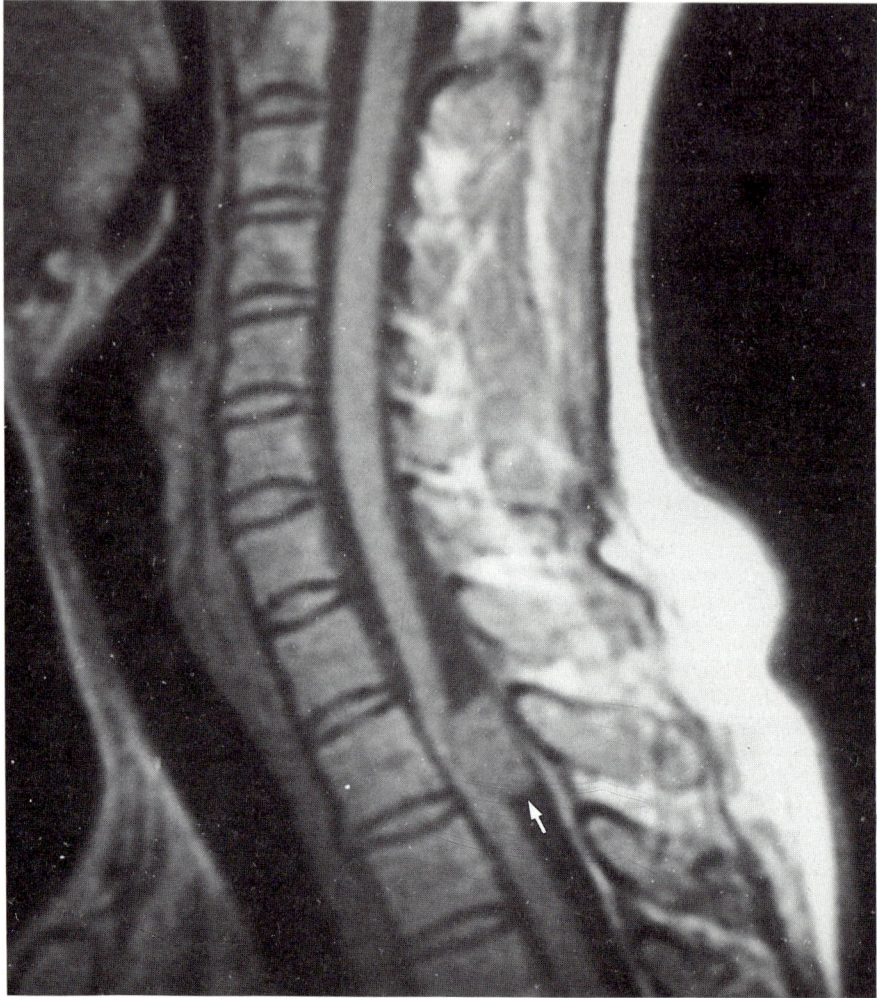

Fig. 6.3 MRI image. *T*1 weighted sagittal image showing extramedullary spinal tumour (meningioma) at level of second thoracic vertebra.

General anaesthesia

Wherever possible, sedation rather than general anaesthesia should be employed. Scan times are 5–10 min, during which the patient must lie still and a complete brain MRI study may take up to 90 min. However, small children, patients with psychiatric disorders, those who cannot

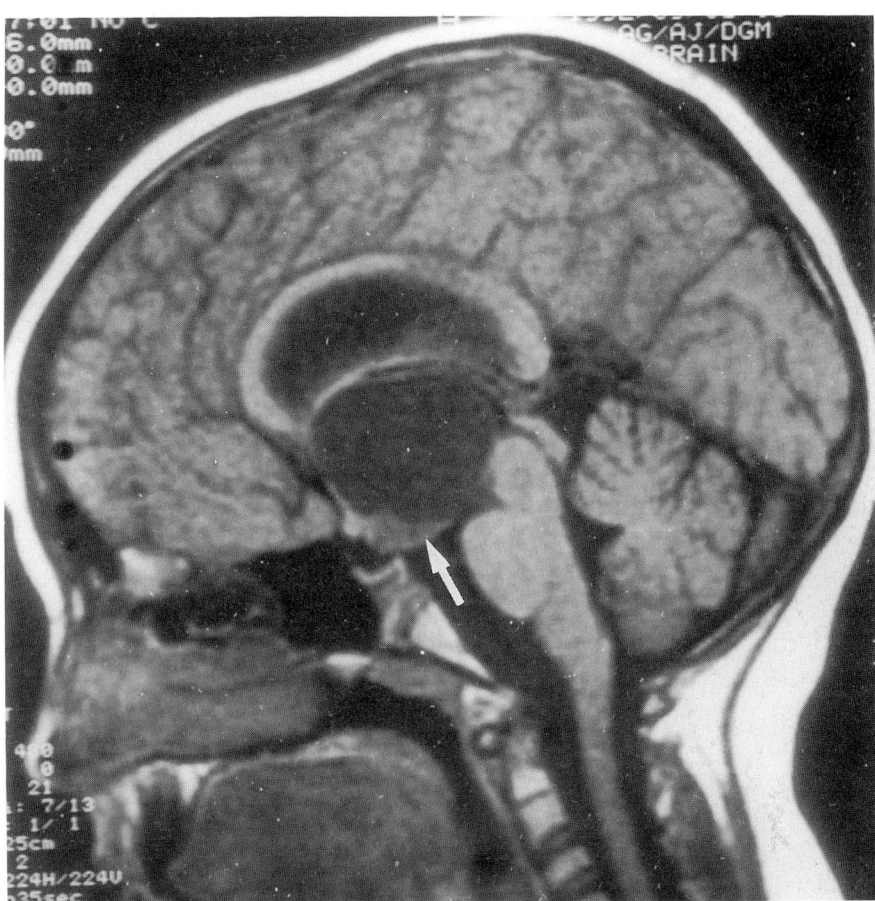

Fig. 6.4 MRI image. Sagittal *T*1 weighted midline image showing cranio-pharyngioma.

tolerate being confined in the enclosed tunnel of the scanner, have movement disorders or painful conditions and are unable to lie still, will usually require anaesthesia.

The anaesthetic technique must be chosen with the general condition of the patient in mind. In addition the particular problems of the MRI suite have to be tackled. In many cases a technique involving spontaneous respiration will be preferable, although suitable mechanical ventilators without magnetic components are available. Hand ventilation, though tedious and restrictive, allows detection of disconnection and assessment of airway resistance and pulmonary compliance. Anaesthetic machines made from aluminum are safe, or a wall-mounted machine at a sufficient distance to the side of the scanner is satisfactory. Standard machines have been modified by replacing ferromagnetic components.

Endotracheal intubation is probably preferable to the use of the laryngeal mask, since the noise of the scanner and difficulty of access to the patient make assessment of laryngeal spasm and airway problems difficult. Endotracheal tubes armoured with a metal spiral must not be employed, and anaesthesia should be induced well away from the scanner; even plastic laryngoscopes are higly magnetic because of the batteries. Long breathing circuits are required and coaxial circuits are generally satisfactory, although expiratory resistance can be high. The anaesthetist may find it difficult to maintain vigilance throughout the duration of the scan, and the restricted access to and availability of suitable monitoring equipment can be dangerous. Good lighting is essential to allow assessment of the patient's colour, since oximetry may be impossible.

In an emergency, scanning can be stopped quickly and the patient removed from the tunnel. Resuscitation, however, must be conducted away from the scanner because, although the magnet can be turned off instantly, re-establishment of the field may take 72 h.

MONITORING

The problems of patient monitoring during MRI scanning are manifold (Roth *et al.*, 1985, Rejger *et al.* 1989, Sellden *et al.* 1990). The monitoring instruments themselves may contain ferromagnetic materials and be attracted towards the scanner if too close, and degradation of image quality may be caused by conductive leads, even if they are not magnetic. ECG signals may be lost in 'noise' created by the oscillating magnetic field. Currents induced in the patient may cause artifact and the oscilloscope display itself be distorted by the magnetic field. These problems may be largely overcome by telemetric transmission of the signal at a frequency well away from that of the RF output of the scanner.

Precordial stethoscopes must be of plastic construction but their usefulness is limited by the noise of the scanner in operation. Plethysmography of finger or toe can be transmitted by fibreoptic means and a useful pulse display obtained.

Non-invasive blood pressure machines function well if all metal connections are replaced with plastic ones, and the monitor placed a safe distance from the scanner.

Capnography is possible if connectors are plastic and the monitor kept distant from the scanner, but long sampling tubes are required and readings must be interpreted with caution.

Oximetry is difficult or impossible. MRI image distortion occurs and the monitor does not function satisfactorily. There have been reports of the successful use of oximetry during MRI scanning but the problems are considerable.

Arterial monitoring is too invasive to justify for most patients, but if indicated or already established can work satisfactorily either with long pressure lines or fibreoptic signal transmission.

Cerebral angiography

It might be thought that the introduction of CT and MRI has led to a reduction in cerebral angiography, and it is true that tumour localization by angiography has been superseded by CT and MRI. However, the undisputed place of angiography in the investigation of subarachnoid haemorrhage, the increasing frequency of carotid endarterectomy and the advent of interventional techniques, have ensured that angiography remains a common investigation. Details of tumour circulation are still best displayed by angiography.

Direct carotid or vertebral artery puncture is rarely required nowadays. Introduction of a catheter via the femoral artery in the groin allows selective cannulation of each carotid and vertebral artery with greater patient safety and acceptability. Difficulties in negotiating the arterial tree occasionally necessitate a direct carotid artery puncture.

Indications for cerebral angiography

Common indications are the investigation of subarachnoid haemorrhage (SAH), carotid artery disease, demonstration of arteriovenous malformations (AVM), tumour circulation and the assessment of the feasibility of interventional methods.

Complications of cerebral angiography

Complications of cerabral angiography are listed in Table 6.2, and fortunately the serious ones are now rare. When direct carotid puncture is performed, neck haematoma can lead to tracheal compression. Newer non-ionic contrast media are much less likely to produce neurological

Table 6.2 Complications of cerebral angiography

Haematoma at puncture site
Arterial dissection
Arterial occlusion distal to puncture site
Intracranial vascular spasm
Aneurysm rupture
Embolus — air, thrombus or atheroma
Contrast medium reaction
Neurological deficit — blindness, hemiparesis, dysphasia

sequelae since their osmolality is much less than the old-fashioned ionic media. Some units administer dextran 70 after angiography in children to reduce risk of thrombosis in the femoral artery.

Anaesthetic considerations

Cerebral angiography may be performed under sedation or anaesthesia. Some neuroradiologists administer sedation with trained assistants, but most prefer to concentrate their attention and energies on imaging, leaving supervision of the patient to the anaesthetist.

Pre-angiography assessment

This gives an opportunity to assess the neurological and general state of the patient. If a sedative technique is planned, careful and sympathetic explanation to the patient of what will take place will help allay fear. Clues to the pathology, the state of hydration and the likely degree of intracranial compliance should be sought. Any previous history of adverse reaction to contrast medium should also be obtained.

Sedation

In most cooperative patients a combination of light sedation (1–2 mg midazolam intravenously is often enough) and local anaesthesia around the femoral artery puncture site will be all that is required. The investigation is not painful and analgesia is not necessary. Opiates can cause retching or vomiting and may depress respiration and cause an increase in ICP. Over enthusiastic sedation can similarly cause respiratory depression and the patient may become less rather than more cooperative, particularly if hypoxic. In practice, minor degrees of patient movement can be compensated by manipulation of the digitized image (pixel shifting).

General anaesthesia

The anaesthetic and radiological literature of the 1960s and 1970s contained numerous articles demonstrating the superiority of angiography during controlled ventilation (Dallas & Moxon 1969, Campkin 1976). Hyperventilation, causing cerebral vasoconstriction, delayed contrast passage through the cerebral circulation. In areas of unresponsive vessels such as tumour circulation, relative vasodilatation enabled better definition to be obtained. The advent of digital vascular imaging technology has rendered these arguments unimportant; the image can be manipulated on screen to produce the contrast required. Subtraction of the bony 'mask', i.e. the image prior to contrast injection, removes extraneous detail and improves definition.

The decision to opt for anaesthesia rather than sedation now depends upon the condition of the patient and, of course, individual preference of radiologist and anaesthetist. General anaesthesia would be preferred in small children, restless or uncooperative adults, and in those patients where the amount of sedation needed might produce respiratory depression and a critical increase in ICP. The patient already on life-support measures would obviously need anaesthesia. In patients where a direct 'follow-on' to surgery is planned, it might sometimes be considered expedient to induce anaesthesia prior to angiography.

Anaesthesia involves the same considerations as any neurosurgical procedure with due attention to state of hydration, avoidance of elevation of ICP and attenuation of hypertensive response to intubation, especially in those with a suspected aneurysm or vascular disease. Airway provision must be perfect. Pieces of anaesthetic apparatus such as ECG electrodes, metal connections, capnography sampling ports, etc., should be routed so that they do not interfere with images. A technique involving thiopentone, a non-depolarizing muscle relaxant, and mild hyperventilation with oxygen, nitrous oxide and isoflurane is satisfactory in most cases.

Careful note should be taken of volumes of contrast and saline flush used in children, as this may represent a large proportion of their circulatory volume.

Investigation of spinal disease

Myelography

The requirement for general anaesthesia for myelography is confined to small children and uncooperative adults. The problems of anaesthesia involve: the patient, the procedure and the environment.

THE PATIENT

It is important in the pre-anaesthetic assessment of paediatric patients presenting for myelography that note is made of any other features of the child's illness. Presentation may be with an abnormal gait or delayed walking, and the spinal abnormality may be a feature of some developmental disorder involving multiple pathology. It is wise to enquire from the referring paediatrician if a syndrome is suspected which may imply pathology elsewhere. All the usual problems of paediatric anaesthesia apply, and are discussed in Chapter 13.

THE PROCEDURE

Myelography takes place in a room which may be periodically in darkness. Steep head-up and head-down postures will probably be employed, often with rapid movement of the patient table, to see the entire length of the spinal canal and craniocervical junction. Patient position on the table is altered during the examination with lateral position for the lumbar puncture and prone or supine for the imaging. Dislodgement of endotracheal tube or intravenous cannula is possible in these circumstances. Long lengths of fresh-gas tubing on a T-piece circuit or an extended Bain circuit are useful. Although the use of an armoured endotracheal tube can be helpful to avoiding kinking, it may interfere with images of the cervical area.

Anaesthesia usually involves endotracheal intubation and spontaneous ventilation with a volatile agent. Analgesia is unnecessary and small children tolerate the abrupt changes in posture remarkably well. The use of suxamethonium in spinal cord disease can be dangerous because of a possible increase in serum potassium, and the association of malignant hyperpyrexia and neuromuscular disease should also be remembered. Finally the possibility of contrast medium reaction occurring during myelography must be borne in mind.

THE ENVIRONMENT

The myelography room is not ideal for anaesthesia. The lights are frequently dimmed, there is bulky equipment restricting access to the patient, and the wearing of lead aprons further limits easy performance of procedures. The availability of pulse oximetry has improved monitoring during myelography.

Spinal angiography

This investigation is infrequently performed and can be prolonged if selective catheterization of vessels proves difficult. Neurological deterioration can occur during the procedure and a simple sedative technique is usually employed to enable monitoring of neurological signs, although anaesthesia is used in some centres.

Interventional radiology

The rapid development of this branch of radiology is likely to involve the anaesthetist more and more in the near future. Radiology has expanded from its traditional diagnostic function to embrace a therapeutic role. The scope for endovascular attack on certain lesions is enormous, and already interventional radiological techniques are encroaching on some traditional areas of neurosurgery (Lasjuanias & Berenstein 1987).

Indications

The indications for endovascular treatment vary depending upon local experience. Where an experienced interventional radiologist is available, these methods can be used in the management of a wide variety of lesions, some of which would have been approached surgically in the past. Sometimes multiple interventions are required. Examples of some of the areas where these methods are used are listed in Table 6.3.

The interventional radiologist's armamentarium includes a variety of catheters with fixed or detachable balloons and the use of various embolic materials, the choice of which depends upon the indication.

Embolization by particles at capillary bed level is used to reduce the vascularization of tumours such as meningiomas prior to surgical removal. Gelatine foam is often used, but it is absorbable and recanalization may

Table 6.3 Indications for interventional techniques

Tumours

1 Highly vascular intracranial or extracranial tumours may be embolized to reduce their vascularity prior to surgery (Fig. 6.5)
2 Chemotherapeutic agents may be administered close to a tumour by selective catheterization of feeder vessels

Vascular lesions

1 Flow control — temporary or permanent:
   (a) Temporary balloon occlusion of the artery may be used during clipping of a giant aneurysm where proximal control of the blood flow is difficult to achieve surgically
   (b) Temporary occlusion is also used as a 'tolerance test' to assess effects of proposed surgical ligation of a vessel
   (c) Permanent occlusion of blood flow is used in the management of an arteriovenous fistula (Fig. 6.6)
2 Occlusion of vascular lesions as definitive therapy:
   (a) Aneurysms: Endosaccular balloon or coil occlusion (Fig. 6.7); parent vessel occlusion
   (b) Arteriovenous malformations: Embolization of nidus of lesion (Fig. 6.8); parent vessel occlusion
3 Other indications:
   (a) Angioplasty
   (b) Control of traumatic or surgical haemorrhage. This is another example of flow control and is occasionally used where conventional surgical methods have failed

---

occur after a few days. This is unimportant if the procedure is done immediately before surgery. Particles of reconstituted lyophilized dura mater, which is not resorbable, may be used to achieve permanent occlusion, or polyvinyl alcohol (PVA) microemboli are available which are also non-absorbable. Liquid embolic agents, cyanoacrylate 'superglues', are used in certain circumstances. Opacification of the embolic material can be achieved by the addition of tantalum powder which is inert and biocompatible. Ethanol which is cytotoxic may be injected in circumstances where tissue necrosis as well as vascular occlusion is sought in the aggressive management of malignant tumours. Chemotherapeutic agents may be injected directly. Various thrombogenic coils are available for permanent occlusion of larger vessels and vascular lesions.

Catheters with detachable balloons enable definitive treatment of certain lesions, e.g. large, technically difficult or surgically unapproachable lesions, or where operative morbidity and mortality are expected to be high. As experience is gained, and developments in catheter technology progress, more and more lesions become amenable to interventional endovascular radiological attack.

Angioplasty

This may be employed to treat a localized constriction of an artery. Extracranial or intracranial carotid or vertebral artery constrictions may be dilated using some of the recently developed catheters.

Anaesthetic considerations

The anaesthetic contribution to the care of these patients is important. Because acute deterioration of the patient's neurological state or conscious level may occur, an anaesthetist should be present throughout. The need to monitor neurological state demands a conscious and cooperative patient, but the procedure may last a long time and adequate sedation is required to make this tolerable. Lying still for prolonged periods may cause backache, which causes the patient more distress than the procedure itself.

Anaesthetic techniques suitable for these procedures are still being developed. The anaesthetic management for a simple preoperative embolization of a tumour with suitable vascular anatomy presents very few problems, and is similar to that for a straightforward angiogram, but the more complex methods employing detachable balloons, etc., require more intensive involvement by the anaesthetist. Discussion with the radiologist before the procedure should clarify any particular requirements.

Neurological deterioration of the patient may occur at any time (fits, reduced conscious level, acute neurological deficit, aphasia, hemiparesis, etc.) because of rupture of the aneurysm, or migration of the catheter or balloon. This may necessitate urgent resuscitative measures, occasionally proceeding to emergency craniotomy. The need to assess constantly the neurological status of the patient favours a sedative technique, but there are cases which are unsuitable and anaesthesia will be required.

The preoperative visit is a vital part of the procedure. Gaining the patient's confidence, and explanation of the arrangements, will contribute to the success of the intervention. Induced hypotension may be required and a history of transient ischaemic attacks, coronary artery disease or hypertension may influence the management. A history of back pain should be ascertained, because such a patient may become restless during the procedure.

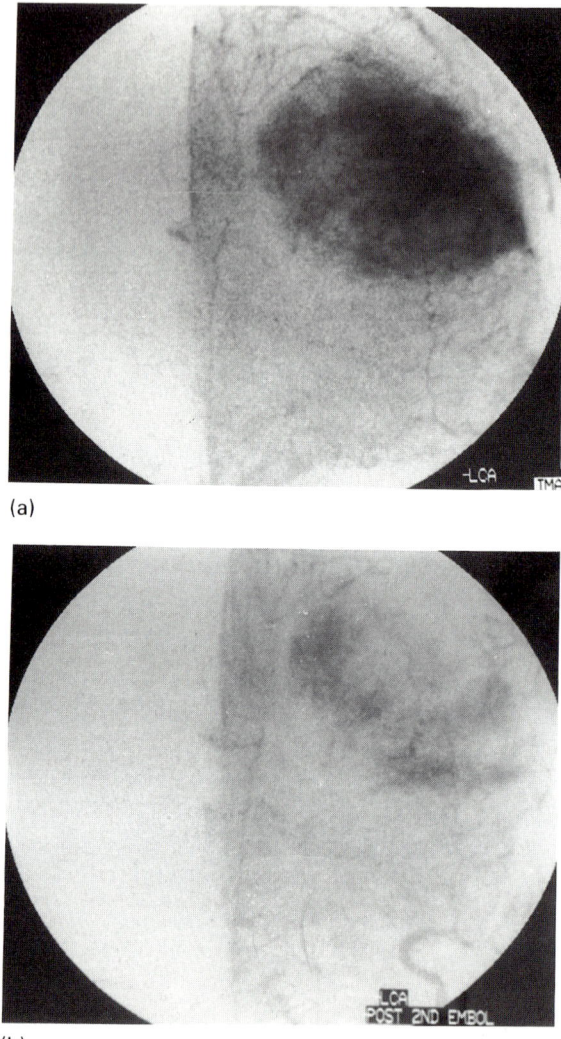

(a)

(b)

Fig. 6.5 Interventional radiology. (a) Pre-embolization angiogram of vascular left parietal meningioma showing prominent tumour blush. (b) Post-embolization angiogram showing marked reduction in vascularity. The tumour was subsequently removed with little surgical haemorrhage. The embolic material was PVA particles.

Sedation

This aims for a comfortable, motionless patient who is readily rousable. This may be achieved with a neuroleptic technique with fentanyl and

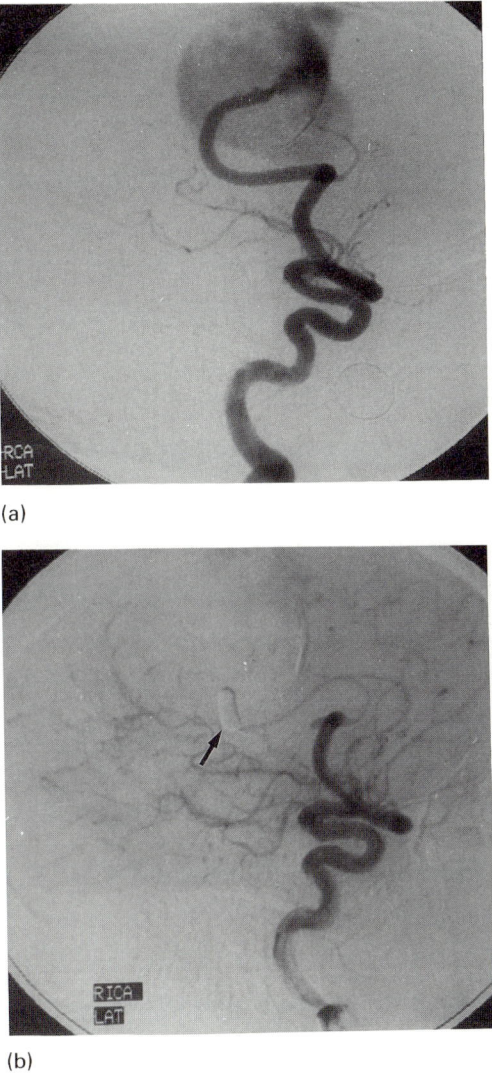

(a)

(b)

Fig. 6.6 Interventional radiology. (a) Pre-embolization angiogram of right parietal arteriovenous fistula. (b) Post-embolization angiogram. A detachable balloon (arrowed) was placed in the feeding vessel.

droperidol, or with a propofol infusion titrated to obtain the desired level. The use of a thick mattress or inflatable lumbar support can contribute greatly to patient comfort and reduce sedative and analgesic requirements. A urinary catheter for longer procedures may be necessary.

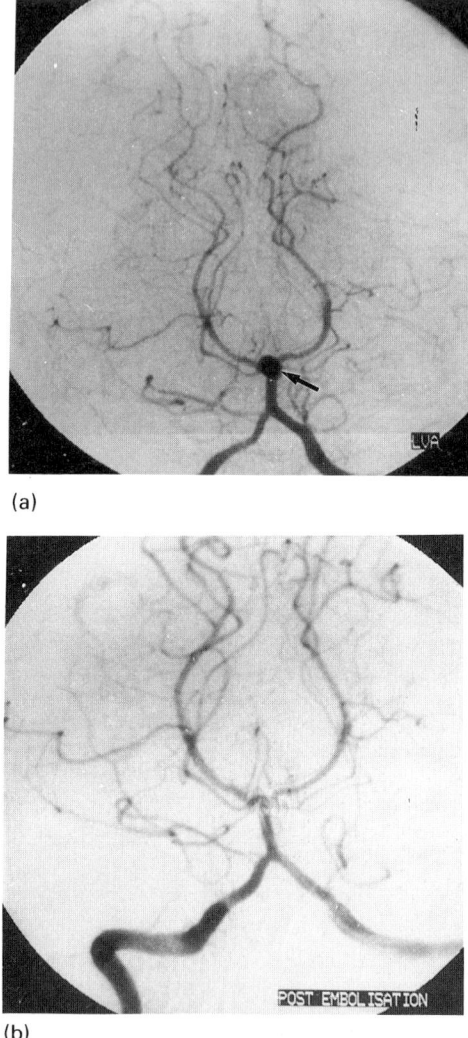

(a)

(b)

Fig. 6.7 Interventional radiology. (a) Pre-embolization angiogram of basilar artery bifurcation aneurysm. (b) Post-embolization angiogram showing occlusion of aneurysm sac with coils.

General anaesthesia

This is not often required and removes the safety factor of continuous neurological assessment. If it is employed, the usual considerations as for any neurosurgical operation will apply in addition to those considered below.

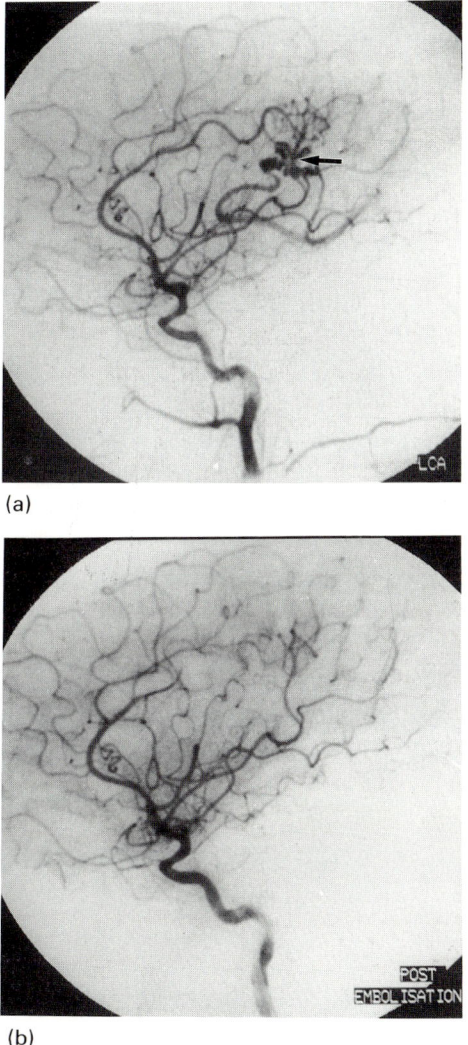

(a)

(b)

Fig. 6.8 Interventional radiology. (a) Parietal arteriovenous malformation. Pre-embolization angiogram. (b) Post-embolization angiogram showing obliteration of AVM nidus. The embolic material was cyanoacrylate glue.

BLOOD PRESSURE CONTROL

To embolize successfully some lesions, AVM for example (O'Mahoney & Bolsin 1988), a moderate decrease in arterial pressure may be required to increase flow time through the lesion. Occlusion of the venous portion of an AVM without occluding the arterial feeders may lead to swelling and haemorrhage. Reduction in non-autoregulated flow by hypotension will enable a cyanoacrylate glue to set in these feeder vessels as well as in the nidus. Invasive arterial monitoring is essential in these cases. Hypotension is induced by labetalol, glyceryl trinitrate or sodium nitroprusside. There is sometimes a hypertensive response to occlusion of the lesion and this must be controlled. The amount of hypotension will depend upon the nature of the lesion and the general condition of the patient, but usually a mean arterial pressure of 55–70 mmHg is required. Supplementary oxygen always be administered to these patients.

OTHER MEDICATIONS

Dexamethasone may be requested where postembolization oedema is expected, such as following occlusion of large AVMs.

Calcium channel blockers may be employed where vascular spasm is a problem. Nimodipine is used for this purpose in the author's unit.

Heparinization is frequently required and activated clotting time (ACT) is monitored routinely during the longer procedures. Baseline ACT for the patient is determined and heparin 5000 units typically given. ACT is maintained at two or three times baseline levels throughout. Protamine may be given at the end of the procedure using ACT as a guide. If a vessel or aneurysm should rupture during the procedure, heparinization must be reversed promptly.

RECOVERY

The patient must be observed and monitored as closely as after any neurosurgical operation. Delayed onset of oedema or vasospasm, or the occurrence of seizures, may require prompt intervention.

Blood pressure (BP) control is important and depends upon the type of intervention. After embolization of a large AVM, the BP may need to be kept lower than normal, whereas after a carotid or vertebral artery occlusion a higher than normal pressure is required to allow cross-circulation.

The important point about this relatively new field is that a team approach involving radiologist, anaesthetist and surgeon is developed. Consultation before the procedure to establish requirements for hypotension or anticoagulation is essential.

Acknowledgement

I wish to thank Dr A. Gholkar, Consultant Neuroradiologist, Newcastle General Hospital, who performed all the interventional procedures shown for supplying the radiographs.

References

Boyer R.S. (1992) Sedation in pediatric neuroimaging: the science and the art. *American Journal of Neuroradiology* **13**, 777−783.

Burk N.S. (1989) Anesthesia for magnetic resonance imaging. *Anesthesiology Clinics of North America* **7**, 707−721.

Campkin T.V. (1976) General anaesthesia for neuroradiology. *British Journal of Anaesthesia* **48**, 783−789.

Dallas S.H. & Moxon C.P. (1969) Controlled ventilation for cerebral angiography. *British Journal of Anaesthesia* **41**, 597−602.

Goldberg M. (1984) Systemic reactions to intravascular contrast media. *Anesthesiology* **60**, 46−56.

Kean D.M. & Smith M.A. (1986) *Magnetic Resonance Imaging. Principles and Applications.* Heinemann, London.

Lasjaunias P. & Berenstein A. (1987) *Surgical Neuroangiography,* vol. 2: *Endovascular Treatment of Craniofacial Lesions.* Springer-Verlag, Berlin.

McComish P.B. & Bodley P.O. (1971) *Anaesthesia for Neurological Surgery.* Lloyd-Luke, London.

Mazziotta J.C. & Gilman S. (Eds) (1992). *Clinical Brain Imaging. Principles and Applications. Contemporary Neurology Series,* vol. 39. F.A. Davis, Philadelphia.

Nixon C., Hirsch N.P., Ormerod I.E.C. & Johnson G. (1986) Nuclear magnetic resonance. Its implications for the anaesthetist. *Anaesthesia* **41**, 131−137.

O'Mahony B.J. & Bolsin S.N.C. (1988) Anaesthesia for closed embolisation of cerebral arteriovenous malformations. *Anaesthesia and Intensive Care* **16**, 318−323.

Pykett I.L. (1982) NMR imaging in medicine: nuclear magnetic resonance, or NMR, can reveal the distribution of atoms in a sample of material. It can do the same in the body, generating images of internal structure without the use of X-rays. *Scientific American* **246**, 54−64.

Rejger V.S., Cohn B.F., Vielvoye G.J. & de Raadt F.B. (1989) A simple anaesthetic and monitoring system for magnetic resonance imaging. *European Journal of Anaesthesiology* **6**, 373−378.

Roth J.L., Nugent M., Gray J.E. *et al.* (1985) Patient monitoring during magnetic resonance imaging. *Anesthesiology* **62**, 80−83.

Sellden H., de Chateau P., Ekman G., Linder B., Saaf J. & Wahlund L-O (1990)

Circulatory monitoring of children during anaesthesia in low-field magnetic resonance imaging. *Acta Anaesthesiologica Scandinavica* **34**, 41−43.

7

Basic anaesthetic technique for intracranial surgery

J.R. DAVID LAYCOCK AND FRANK J.M. WALTERS

Introduction

Anaesthesia for neurosurgery requires an understanding of basic principles of neurophysiology and the effects of anaesthetic agents on intracranial dynamics. The aims in neuroanaesthesia are summarized in Table 7.1. The following sections deal with the practical problems in achieving some of these aims. These are outlined in Table 7.2.

Cerebral volume

The volume of the intracranial contents which determines intracranial pressure is in itself determined by the cerebral blood volume, brain bulk,

Table 7.1 Aims

1 Maintenance of cerebral perfusion
2 Maintenance of oxygenation
3 Control of arterial carbon dioxide
4 Provision of a good surgical field
5 Maintenance of fluid balance
6 Temperature control

Table 7.2 Considerations

Cerebral volume
Cerebral blood volume
Brain bulk
CSF volume
Intracranial pressure
Airway management
Positioning
Vital centres

167

and cerebrospinal fluid (CSF) volume. The volume of these compartments may be affected by anaesthesia, surgery and pathological processes within the brain. Any increase in cerebral volume renders surgery difficult, and raises the risk of trauma or ischaemia due to retraction. The anaesthetic technique should not cause increases in, and should sometimes allow control of, cerebral volume.

CEREBRAL BLOOD VOLUME

The different physiological factors which affect arterial and venous blood volumes are discussed in detail in Chapter 2. Any factor which produces a change in cerebral blood flow will cause a similar alteration in cerebral arterial blood volume. Therefore hypoxia, hypercapnia, hypertension and hyperthermia must all be avoided. As autoregulation may be lost in the presence of cerebral pathology, notably head injury (Cold & Jensen 1978) and tumours (Risberg *et al.* 1969), unpredictable effects on cerebral blood flow can occur even with moderate hypertension within the normal limits of autoregulation. In patients with tumours, prior hyperventilation will prevent increases in intracranial pressure when volatile agents are introduced (Adams *et al.* 1972, 1981). This may not be universally true, and therefore even with hypocapnia it is perhaps unwise to use volatile agents at more than half minimal alveolar concentration (MAC) multiples prior to elevation of the bone flap in the presence of a raised intracranial pressure (ICP).

Coughing and straining will cause surges in venous pressure, engorgement of cerebral veins and increases in cerebral venous blood volume. Obstruction to the free drainage of venous blood will have a similar effect. Therefore close attention should be paid to the position of the head during preparation of the patient for surgery. A clear and unobstructed airway should be maintained, both to ensure as low a mean intrathoracic pressure as possible, and to avoid the application of inadvertent PEEP.

BRAIN BULK

Brain bulk is increased by the presence of either space-occupying lesions or cerebral oedema. The oedema associated with cerebral tumours is usually reduced preoperatively by the administration of steroids. Similarly mannitol ($0.25-1.0\,\mathrm{g\,kg^{-1}}$) may be given at the start of surgery to reduce brain volume. It is given over 10 min, reducing ICP after 4–5 min and exerting its peak effect after 45 min. In addition to its osmotic effects on the brain, mannitol also increases cerebral blood flow (CBF) (Mendelow *et al.* 1985), and cerebral blood volume (Ravussin *et al.* 1988). Of concern is the possibility that mannitol may initially raise ICP in situations where it is already critically raised. It does indeed lead to a slight increase in ICP where ICP is normal, but little increase is seen where the ICP is raised due to tumour (Ravussin *et al.* 1988). Urine output should be monitored in any patient who receives mannitol.

CSF VOLUME

Where there is obstruction to the outflow of CSF by tumour or blood, obstructive hydrocephalus will ensue. This may necessitate the insertion of a ventriculoperitoneal shunt or as a preliminary procedure a ventricular access device.

During craniotomy, surgical access may be improved at the time of operation by a variety of manoeuvres. First, a brain cannula may be inserted into the lateral ventricle on exposure of the brain, and CSF removed until the brain has retracted sufficiently. Secondly, if the surgical approach allows, a retractor can be placed near the basal cisterns and CSF aspirated. Thirdly, a lumbar spinal drain employing an epidural catheter can be inserted following induction of anaesthesia, and CSF allowed to drain by the lumbar route. The catheter is inserted through a Tuohy needle at the L2−L3 interspace and attached to a specifically designed drainage set. This is particularly useful during aneurysm surgery or for tumours of the base of skull. The drain can also be used postoperatively to reduce the risk of, or control, any CSF leaks. Obviously lumbar drainage should not be used before the bone flap is raised where there is a risk of cerebellar impaction and subsequent coning. Whatever method of CSF drainage is used, care should be taken not to remove an excessive volume, otherwise there is a risk of subdural bleeding distant to the craniotomy site, an increase in transmural pressure across an aneurysm site, or rather more commonly a period of reduced conscious level postoperatively. Up to 250 ml can be removed from the lumbar drain but not at a rate exceeding 5 ml min^{-1}.

RAISED INTRACRANIAL PRESSURE

Clinical evaluation of the patient generally will detect those patients with raised ICP. Early signs are morning headache, nausea and vomiting, and the development of papilloedema. As ICP rises conscious level will deteriorate. A Cushing response of hypertension and bradycardia indicate a critically raised ICP, Cheyne-Stokes respiration and unilateral pupillary dilatation are signs of impending coning. In patients with posterior fossa lesions neck stiffness is an important sign.

Radiological investigations should be evaluated together with the clinical symptoms and signs, as on their own they will not provide a reasonable assessment of ICP. Where CT scanning demonstrates enlargement of the lateral ventricles and obstructive hydrocephalus, ICP may be relatively normal in long-standing conditions. In contrast following an acute event such as a subarachnoid haemorrhage, such hydrocephalus is usually associated with a raised ICP. In the presence of an intracranial tumour the degree of peritumour oedema has been found to correlate to some extent with rises in ICP perioperatively (Bedford *et al.* 1982). However, the degree of midline shift and effacement of the lateral ventricles are poor indicators of the likelihood of a critically raised ICP.

Where the conscious level is impaired due to a raised ICP the danger of aspiration pneumonia should be borne in mind, and the patient positioned appropriately. If necessary a nasogastric tube should be inserted.

Airway management

Access to the airway is difficult during craniotomies and operations on the cervical spine. In addition the neck may be flexed, extended or twisted. A clear airway must be guaranteed; this is best achieved by use of a flexometallic tube. Difficulties can arise with the prone position when the endotracheal tube can migrate into a main bronchus. A throat pack is required in all frontal craniotomies, pituitary surgery, and transfacial approaches to base of skull lesions.

Each unit has its own particular method of securing endotracheal tubes. The prime consideration is that it should not allow the tube to 'creep' out of position due to traction on it after the patient is draped. Figure 7.1 shows one method of achieving this.

Positioning and anaesthetic access

For neurosurgical procedures the patient may be in any position from the prone to the sitting. Particular problems with the prone, semiprone, and sitting positions are described in the chapters on posterior fossa and spinal surgery. The supine position is used for pituitary surgery, frontal, transfacial and temporoparietal craniotomies. The lateral position is used for temporoparietal craniotomies, some cervical surgery, and some posterior fossa procedures. The semisitting position is used for some occipital craniotomies. All these positions are fully described by Anderton *et al.* (1988).

SUPINE POSITION

In the supine and lateral positions the patient should be placed in a slight reverse Trendelenberg position with a 15−25° tilt, this promotes cerebral venous drainage while causing the least fall in mean arterial pressure. If the head is turned to the side in the supine position then a sandbag should be placed under the shoulder; this prevents kinking of the jugular veins and reduces traction on the brachial plexus. Compression and kinking of the jugular veins can produce striking increases in ICP (Fig. 7.2). The arms should be placed at the side with particular attention to the ulnar and radial nerves. The head may be placed on a conventional horseshoe or in a three-point fixator (Fig. 7.3). With a three-point fixator care should be taken not to overtighten the pins because of the risk of extradural haematoma (Baerts *et al.* 1984), and to support the neck and head when manoeuvring the patient while the fixator is attached. Air can also enter the circulation through the pin sites of the fixator (Pang 1982).

LATERAL POSITION

In this position care should be exercised to avoid extreme neck flexion or extension, so hindering cerebral venous outflow. In addition particular care must be taken to protect the eyes when the face is turned into the horseshoe headrest. A firm pad should be placed under the axilla to protect the brachial plexus, and pressure points over the shoulder, greater trochanter and peroneal nerves protected. A pillow is placed between the legs with the lower extended and upper flexed. Alternatively the use of inflation boots will support and protect the legs, as well as contributing to the prevention of deep-vein thrombosis. Pressure on the abdomen and chest should be minimal to allow a free rise and fall of the diaphragm. The patient can either be secured with a restraining strap or, if the table is to be rotated, a vacuum bag (Fig. 7.4).

In both these positions a Mayo table may be clamped to the operating

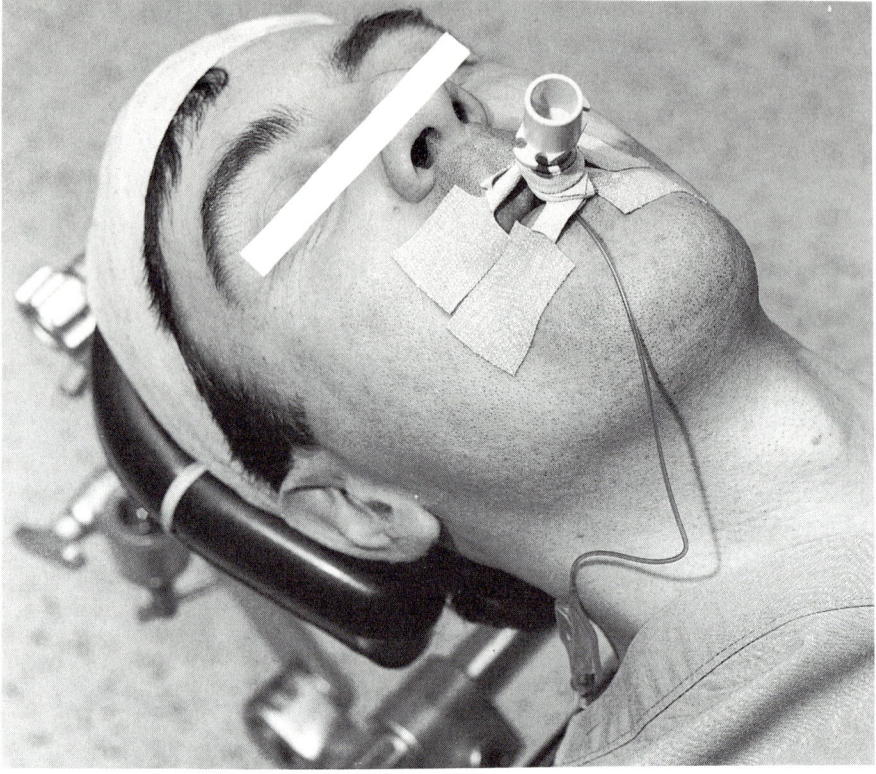

(a)

Fig. 7.1 (a, b) One possible method of securing an endotracheal tube.

table. This generally allows reasonable access to the patient without disturbing the surgical field. Monitoring and lines to the patient can then be arranged logically, avoiding any confusion.

Vital centres

There are two vital centres which, if significantly damaged, will result in the death of the patient. The first is the hypothalamic area, located in the floor of the third ventricle, adjacent to the upper brainstem. Amongst other functions this area is concerned with autonomic activity. Operations in this area include those for pituitary disease, craniopharyngioma, suprasellar and parasellar meningiomas and optic chiasma gliomas.

The other vital centre is in the brainstem in the medulla, and is involved with the automatic control of respiration and the cardiovascular

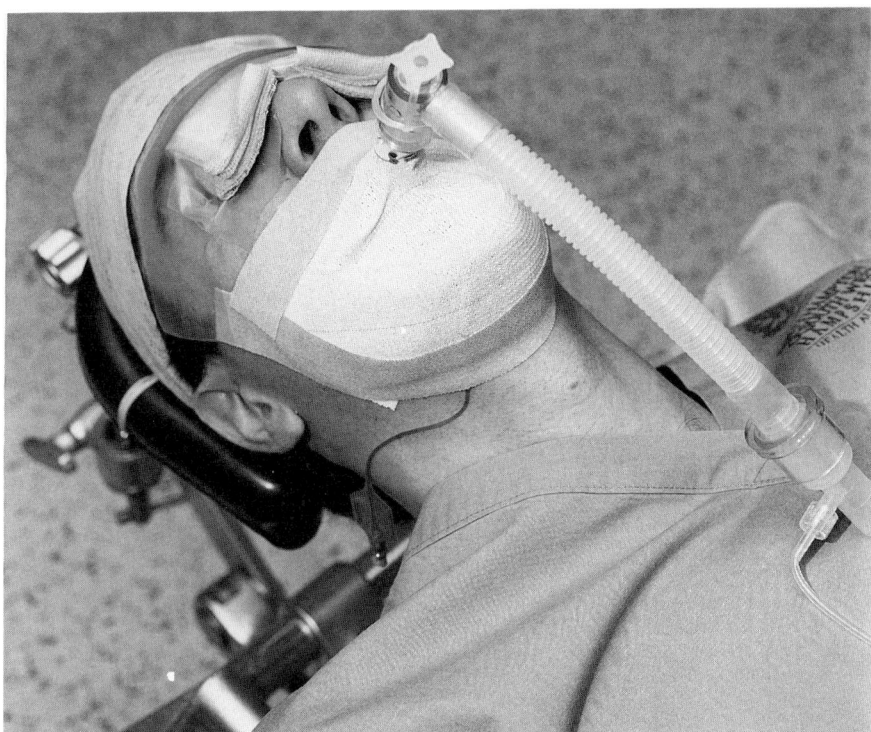

(b)

Fig. 7.1 (*Continued*)

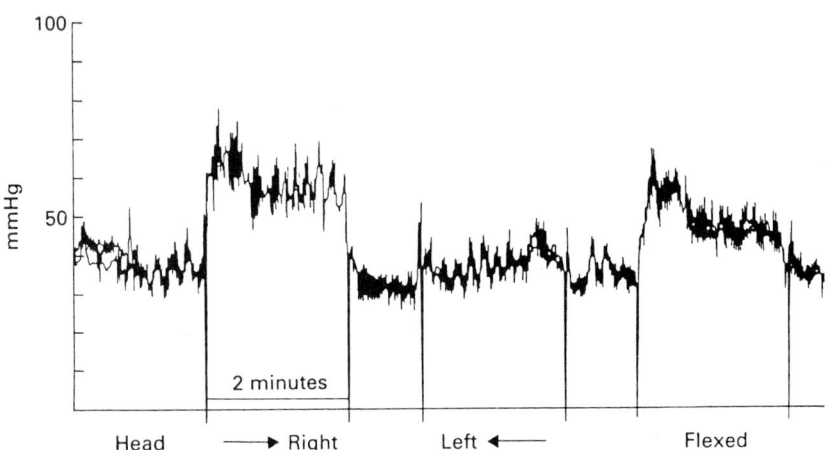

Fig. 7.2 Changes in intracranial pressure in a patient with a frontal tumour when the head and neck position is altered; turning the head to the right, the left and flexing the neck.

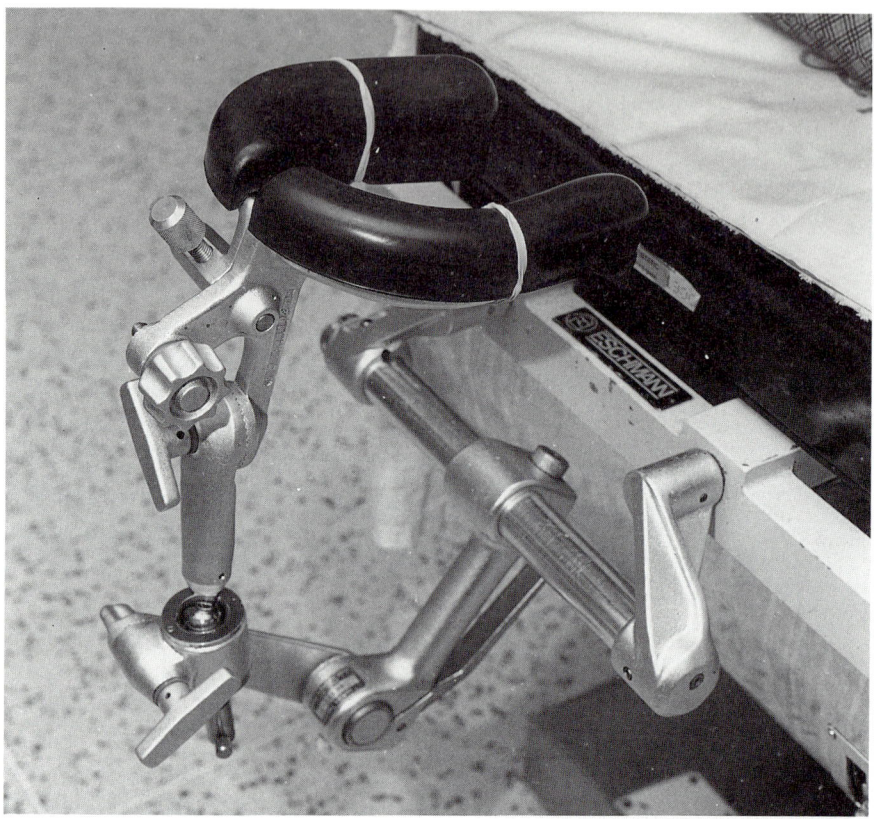

(a)

Fig. 7.3 (a, b) A conventional horseshoe headrest and three point fixator.

system. This area is at risk during surgery to the posterior fossa which is described in more detail in Chapter 9. Patients undergoing surgery in these areas should be closely monitored for sudden changes in either

Table 7.3 Monitoring

1	ECG
2	Blood pressure
3	Central venous pressure
4	Carbon dioxide
5	Oximetry
6	Nerve stimulator
7	Temperature
8	Electrophysiological
9	Other monitoring

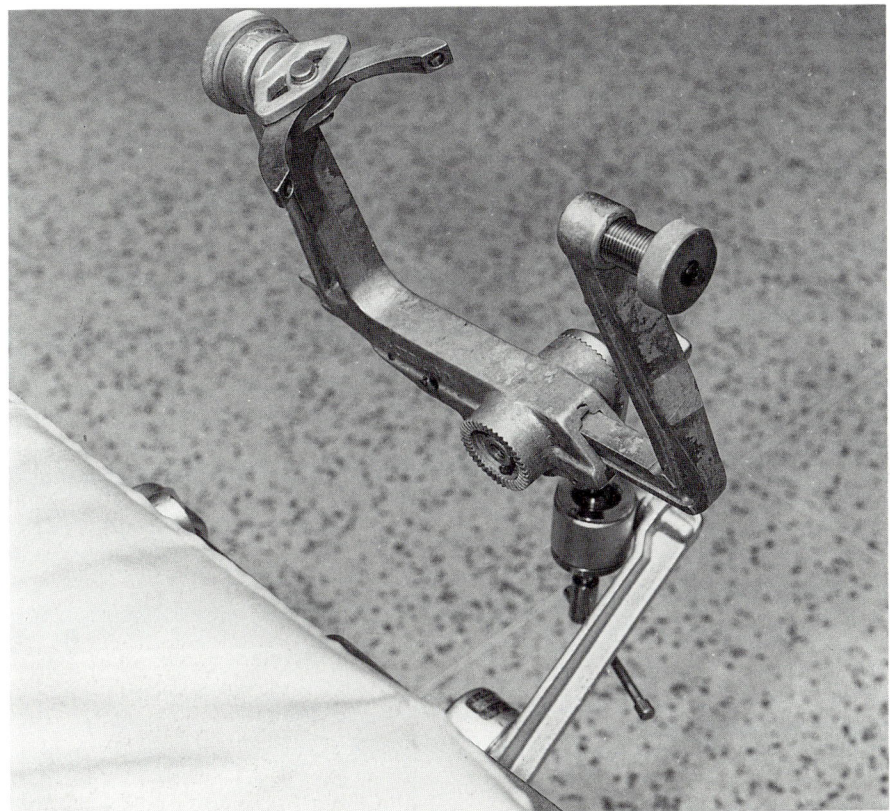

(b)

Fig. 7.3 (*Continued*)

pulse rate or blood pressure so that the surgeon can be informed of proximity to these zones.

Monitoring

ECG

Changes in heart rate and rhythm are common, and particularly relevant during intracranial procedures which involve surgery near the hypothalamus and brainstem, and those which involve manipulation of the orbital contents, trigeminal or vagus nerves. Manipulation of the carotid sinus during carotid endarterectomy also produces dysrhythmias.

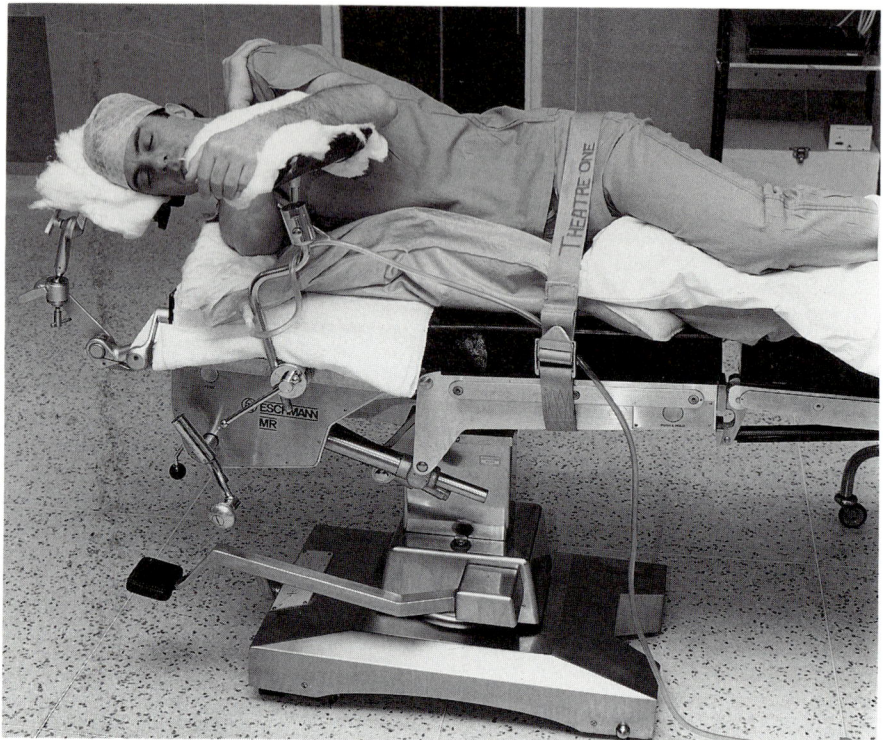

Fig. 7.4 Correct positioning of the patient in the lateral position. Note the pressure pad under the axilla.

Distortion of the brainstem may also result from pressure differentials across the tentorium cerebelli, due, for example, to sudden decompression of a supratentorial lesion, or the rapid application of subatmospheric wound drainage (Wang *et al.* 1991).

During intracranial surgery the surgeon should be advised of any sudden changes in heart rate or rhythm which may indicate possible proximity of a vital structure or excessive retraction on a cranial nerve or the brainstem. In general, release of traction results in restoration of normal heart rate and rhythm. A dysrhythmia should be treated only if absolutely necessary, as otherwise a useful sign to the surgeon is lost.

Blood pressure

The indications for direct intra-arterial monitoring are listed in Table 7.4. In practice this means that the majority of patients undergoing intracranial

Table 7.4 Indications for invasive arterial pressure monitoring

Surgery causing rapid blood pressure changes
Risk of rapid blood loss
Induced hypotension
Coexistent pathology in the patient
Postoperative ventilation anticipated

surgery require the insertion of an arterial line. Suitable sites are the radial and dorsalis pedis artery. Selection of a suitable site will be influenced by the planned position of the patient. In the lateral positions the upward-facing extremity is preferable. As patients are often placed in a head-up position, it is helpful to keep the transducer level with the cranium.

Central venous pressure

The indications for insertion of a central venous line are listed in Table 7.5. The antecubital route is preferred to the subclavian or internal jugular, despite it resulting in a larger number of catheters being incorrectly sited. This is not only because of the risk of pneumothorax or haemothorax, but also because of the danger of piercing the carotid artery. Pressure to the neck in these circumstances may result in serious consequences where venous pressure is raised in the presence of raised intracranial pressure, or where arterial inflow is reduced in the presence of an already compromised cerebral circulation. Similarly the use of the Trendelenberg position to facilitate insertion of a central line will not be appropriate in the presence of raised intracranial pressure. For these reasons, if a central route is to be used, the subclavian vein on the side opposite the lesion is recommended.

Carbon dioxide

Because of the profound effect of carbon dioxide on the cerebral vasculature, monitoring of end-tidal carbon dioxide is mandatory during any

Table 7.5 Indications for central venous pressure measurement

Risk of large blood loss
Assessment of volume status
Sitting position
Route for vasoactive drugs

intracranial procedure. In normal individuals Pe_{CO_2} correlates well with both alveolar and arterial carbon dioxide tensions. However, where there are pulmonary ventilation perfusion inequalities and alveolar dead space is increased, the relationship will not be so close. Typically this occurs in patients with pre-existing lung disease, during hypotension and with the sitting position. In these circumstances blood gas analysis will establish the relationship.

Alveolar P_{CO_2} and thus Pe_{CO_2} are determined by the ratio of carbon dioxide production to alveolar ventilation. Following an air embolus the effective carbon dioxide excretion is reduced because of the fall in cardiac output, and this, together with ventilation perfusion inequalities, accounts for the resultant fall in end-tidal carbon dioxide. It should be stressed that, as many neurosurgical procedures are performed with a head-up tilt, air embolus is not confined to the sitting position.

Oximetry

As with any other anaesthetic, use of an oximeter is mandatory. This is especially so because of the effects of hypoxia on the cerebral circulation. The presence of an oximeter will also aid in the detection of endobronchial intubation when the position of the head is manipulated during positioning or surgery. A decrease in Sa_{O_2} is often also the first sign of developing neurogenic pulmonary oedema following a head injury.

Nerve stimulator

Any sudden movement during neurosurgery can be disastrous. Train-of-four monitoring at the ulnar or the peroneal nerve is routinely employed. During surgery the level of neuromuscular blockade should be maintained such that the first twitch in the train-of-four is just palpable, correlating with a neuromuscular block of 95% or more (Lee 1975). This will avoid coughing and straining, which will impair surgical access for up to 30 min and can most easily be achieved by use of a continuous infusion of vecuronium or atracurium. Towards the end of surgery the infusion can be discontinued, and provided two twitches of the train-of-four are present when the reversal is administered, then adequate reversal is assured (Rupp *et al.* 1986).

Attention should be paid to concurrent drug therapy which may influence the response to muscle relaxants. For instance phenytoin will increase the dose of relaxant required (Hickey *et al.* 1988). If the patient has a motor deficit the nerve stimulator should be applied to a normal limb. This is because the denervated limb will be relatively resistant to relaxants, and if used may result in an inappropriately high relaxant dose, with subsequent difficulties in reversal (Laycock *et al.* 1987).

Electrophysiological monitoring

No method of monitoring the brain during neurosurgery has gained wide acceptance. The EEG, transcranial Doppler and CBF measurements have all been used during carotid endarterectomy and ligation for giant intracerebral aneurysm. Somatosensory evoked potentials have been used during operations on the cervical cord and brainstem. At present, all techniques suffer from difficulties in interpreting the data while the patient is anaesthetized. These are described in Chapter 5.

Other monitoring

Temperature should be monitored in all patients, using an oesophageal probe, as significant rises or falls in temperature can occur during long procedures. Cerebral metabolic rate increases by about 5% for every 1°C rise in temperature (Michenfelder & Theye 1968), and CBF will rise to match this.

Monitoring ICP before and during induction is not common practice in the UK. This may alter in future with the continuing development of devices for non-invasively monitoring ICP. However, ICP monitors are placed in some head-injured and postoperative ventilated patients. If these patients have to be returned to theatre then ICP should be monitored continuously during transfer and initial surgery. This allows the anaesthetist to detect any further deterioration in ICP dynamics and to treat accordingly.

Pulmonary artery monitoring is not common during neuroanaesthesia in the UK. Indications for its use are either on cardiovascular grounds or for fluid management in difficult situations. Its place in the management of air embolism is discussed in Chapter 9.

Preoperative assessment

In addition to routine assessment of patients for anaesthesia and surgery particular attention should be paid towards an assessment of intracranial

Table 7.6 Preoperative assessment

History
Examination
Investigation
CT
MRI
General
Dehydration
Electrolytes
Chest
Drugs

pressure. While clinical signs do not reliably indicate a level of ICP, a history of headache, nausea and drowsiness would indicate a significant disturbance. Examination which reveals papilloedema and unilateral pupillary dilatation with depressed consciousness and irregular respiration indicates an advanced stage of intracranial hypertension. If examination of the MRI or CT scan reveals a midline shift of greater than 0.5 cm, or encroachment on the ventricles or CSF cisterns by an enlarging brain, then there is almost certainly some disturbance in intracranial dynamics.

Patients who have been unconscious may be dehydrated, have electro-lyte disturbances or have aspirated, all of which may require treatment preoperatively. Finally attention should be paid to the effects of concurrent drug therapy, in particular dexamethasone and anticonvulsants.

Anaesthetic technique

Premedication

For most neurosurgical patients a moderate dose of benzodiazepine such as diazepam 5–15 mg or temazepam 10–30 mg will suffice. If desired the benzodiazepine can be accompanied by metoclopramide 5–15 mg to ensure absorption and for its antiemetic effect. Sedative premedication should be avoided in patients with evidence of raised ICP, or those with large posterior fossa lesions potentially interfering with respiration. Anti-convulsant and steroid therapy should be continued up to the time of surgery.

There is little to be gained by the routine use of anticholinergic agents. Indeed the disadvantages of tachycardia and inspissation of secretions would seem to outweigh any advantages.

A few centres employ low-dose heparin deep venous thrombosis (DVT) prophylaxis in neurosurgery, if so it should obviously be commenced with premedication. Because of a perceived increased risk of haemorrhage with intracranial procedures, most do not. There is little published work on the benefits and risk of low-dose heparin during neurosurgical procedures, it may well be that the risk of postoperative haematoma is exaggerated (Barnett *et al.* 1977, Cerrato *et al.* 1978). A consensus view (Risk Factors Consensus Group 1992) is that, for intracranial procedures, stockings and preferably compression boots should be used, and continued on into the postoperative phase if the patient is immobile. For extracranial procedures and spinal work low-dose heparin may be used in addition to compression boots.

Induction and intubation

Induction and intubation should be smooth with no coughing or bucking, no hypotension or hypertension, and no hypoxia or hypercarbia. After the patient arrives in the anaesthetic room, ECG, non-invasive blood pressure, oximeter and nerve stimulator are applied, and intravenous access established. An arterial line may be placed under local anaesthetic prior to induction. The advantage of doing so is continuous monitoring during induction allowing reliable control of arterial pressure. The potential disadvantage is patient distress, leading to transient hypertension. Certainly an arterial line should be placed before induction in unstable patients, those with aneurysms or markedly raised ICP, and in hypovolaemic patients. Anaesthesia may then be induced with a sleep dose of any of the intravenous agents except ketamine. Thiopentone is often used when intracranial pressure is raised. Although there may be some reduction in mean arterial pressure, cerebral perfusion pressure (CPP) is usually maintained or increased because of the reduction in ICP that can be achieved (Shapiro *et al.* 1973). Propofol will also reduce ICP in patients with intracranial hypertension (Herregods *et al.* 1988), and is also used for induction if ICP is raised. The cerebral metabolic effects of propofol appear to be similar to those of thiopentone (Vandesteene *et al.* 1988) and, like thiopentone, propofol does not impair cerebral autoregulation (Van Hemelrijck *et al.* 1990).

Neuromuscular blockade

For cases where no intubation difficulties are expected, or risk of pulmonary aspiration, a non-depolarizing muscle relaxant is administered in the appropriate dose. The airway must be carefully assessed as difficulties in ventilation with a facemask may lead to hypoxia and hypercarbia, with detrimental effects on intracranial dynamics. The neuropharmacology of the different drugs has already been discussed in Chapter 4. Where there is a risk of aspiration as in emergency cases, then succinylcholine should be used even in the presence of a raised ICP. The rise in ICP following succinylcholine administration appears to be due to afferent stimulation from muscle spindles. On the one hand this can be virtually abolished by precurarization with a non-depolarizing relaxant (dose equal to 0.1 of the ED_{95}) (Stirt *et al.* 1987). On the other hand, intubating conditions are less satisfactory, and as the rise in ICP is short-lived it is reasonable to use succinylcholine alone. Following administration of the muscle relaxant, bag and mask ventilation is commenced with oxygen, or oxygen and nitrous oxide if this is to be used for maintenance. Laryngoscopy and intubation may then be performed when no twitches are visible with train-of-four stimulation.

During the procedure neuromuscular blockade can be maintained by intermittent boluses of relaxant or a continuous infusion. For a continuous infusion either vecuronium commencing at $0.1 \, \text{mg} \, \text{kg}^{-1} \, \text{h}^{-1}$ or atracurium at $0.5 \, \text{mg} \, \text{kg}^{-1} \, \text{h}^{-1}$ may be used, adjusting the rate to maintain the first twitch only of a train-of-four.

Prevention of hypertension

Hypertension is associated with intubation and elevation of the bone flap. The two principal situations where hypertension is most dangerous are when ICP is raised and during aneurysm surgery. Various methods have been described to attenuate hypertensive responses to intubation (Table 7.7). Whatever method is used, care should be taken to avoid significant hypotension and the consequent fall in CPP. The most common technique is the administration of rapidly acting, potent opiates with or

Table 7.7 Techniques to attenuate hypertension on intubation

Further dose of induction agent
Narcotics
Lignocaine
Beta-adrenergic blockade
Central alpha$_2$-adrenergic stimulation

before the induction agent (Dahlgren & Messeter 1981). Fentanyl in doses greater than $5 \mu g \, kg^{-1}$, or alfentanil in doses greater than $50 \mu g \, kg^{-1}$ are effective (Black *et al.* 1984) but should be administered cautiously to avoid significant hypotension. Alfentanil crosses the blood–brain barrier much more rapidly than fentanyl, producing a rapid peak effect, and is the more logical agent to employ when used for this purpose (Scott *et al.* 1985). An alternative is the administration of a second but smaller dose of the induction agent just prior to intubation (Unni *et al.* 1984). In this case a reduced initial dose of narcotic will be required.

Beta-adrenergic blockers have been shown to attenuate hypertensive responses to intubation (Prys-Roberts *et al.* 1973). They may either be given orally with the premedication, or intravenously prior to induction. For intravenous use esmolol may be preferable because of its short half-life (Vucevic *et al.* 1992). Some patients for aneurysm surgery are already taking beta-blockers, and these should be continued up to the time of surgery. Beta-adrenergic blockade is contraindicated in patients with asthma and is best avoided in diabetics. Many centres employ the calcium antagonist nimodipine to prevent ischaemia associated with delayed vasospasm following a subarachnoid haemorrhage (Allen *et al.* 1983). There is a theoretical risk of depressant synergistic effects between beta-blockers, nimodipine and volatile agents on the myocardium. However, clinically significant interactions seem to be rare during anaesthesia.

Alternatives to beta-blockers include the central alpha$_2$-adrenergic agonist clonidine (Carabine *et al.* 1991), and the calcium antagonist nifedipine (Puri & Batra 1988). Clonidine given orally as a single dose with the premedication has been investigated during vascular and general surgery. It has been found effective in reducing the response to intubation and in smoothing out peaks in blood pressure during surgery. It also reduces the MAC requirements for volatile agents (Bloor & Flacke 1982), and reduces cerebral metabolic rate for oxygen (CMRO$_2$). Nifedipine is probably an inferior agent for ablating the hypertensive response to intubation.

Lignocaine $1-2 \, mg \, kg^{-1}$ has been given intravenously two or more minutes prior to intubation to attenuate the intubation reflex (Wilson *et al.* 1991), and to reduce ICP directly (Bedford *et al.* 1980). Lignocaine can depress the sinus node and therefore should be given slowly over $20 \, s$ (Demczuk 1984). Lignocaine can be administered as a spray to the larynx and trachea prior to intubation, and has been used for many years to anaesthetize the trachea to prevent coughing and straining. However, when given by this route it appears to be less effective in abolishing the intubation response, and some response to laryngoscopy will still occur (Hamill *et al.* 1981).

Ventilation

Intermittent positive pressure ventilation (IPPV) with humidified gases is routinely used for the majority of patients in all positions. There is a decrease in brain volume, intraventricular and spinal intrathecal pressure within minutes of commencing IPPV. As soon as intubation has been accomplished the patient should be hyperventilated to an end-tidal P_{CO_2} of 29–30 mmHg. This allows a volatile agent to be introduced in up to half MAC multiples without unduly raising CBF.

In the lateral and prone positions mismatches of ventilation and perfusion can occur and physiological dead space may increase. Therefore end-tidal and arterial P_{CO_2} measurements may not correlate as closely, and some hypoxaemia may even occur. If the brain appears tight in these circumstances, the adequacy of ventilation should be confirmed by taking an arterial sample for blood gas analysis.

High-frequency ventilation may possibly have a role in neuroanaesthesia. The advantage is the minimal change in venous pressure which results in minimal movement of the cranial contents with respiration. There appears little surgical demand for it, and the lack of access to the airway creates difficulties if a malfunction occurs.

Maintenance

During maintenance of anaesthesia, which may last anything up to 12 h, the principal aims are prevention of surges in CBF and thus brain volume, and rapid emergence and neurological evaluation. Painful stimuli occur at the beginning of operation during the scalp incision and raising of the bone flap, and at the end during closure. At the beginning of the operation it is helpful if the surgeon infiltrates the scalp incision and pericranium with lignocaine 1% and adrenaline 1 : 200 000. Bupivacaine has been shown to reduce hypertensive episodes during surgical opening (Hillman *et al.* 1987). For similar reasons, local anaesthesia should be used prior to applying the three-point fixator, if it is to be used.

Once the bone flap has been raised a normal brain can be seen pulsating with both arterial pulsations and respiratory movement. When the brain is swollen, or conditions poor, the brain appears tense with no movement. The effect of any physiological manipulation on the brain can be assessed by observing any change in the surface of the brain.

Anaesthesia can be maintained either by a 'conventional' nitrous oxide, narcotic and volatile agent technique or by intravenous infusion. The principal reason for using an intravenous technique is avoidance of nitrous oxide when there is air in the intracranial cavity (Fig. 7.5) (Artru 1982), a risk of air embolus, or a desire to avoid using nitrous oxide under circumstances where intracranial conditions are critical and its administration might provoke an undesirable increase in CBF and ICP (Michenfelder 1988). Figure 7.6 shows such an example where the introduction of nitrous oxide led to an immediate increase in ICP. Otherwise there is no evidence that nitrous oxide is contraindicated in neuroanaesthesia, or that one technique is superior to the other.

Patients may very easily become hypothermic; this may be prevented by the use of warm humidified gases, warming and space blankets and the infusion of warmed intravenous fluids.

BALANCED TECHNIQUE

Following induction anaesthesia is maintained with nitrous oxide, 70%, in oxygen; a narcotic, most commonly fentanyl; and a volatile agent, invariably isoflurane. Fentanyl is probably the best narcotic to use if ICP

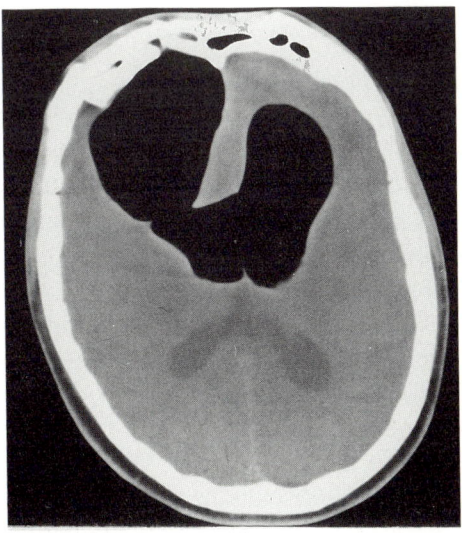

Fig. 7.5 CT scan of a patient with pneumocephalus following head injury.

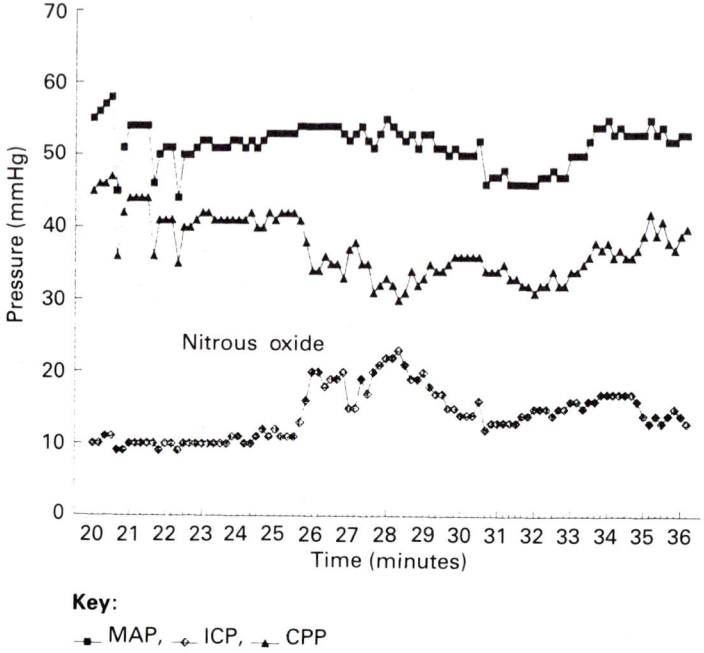

Fig. 7.6 The effect on arterial, intracranial and cerebral perfusion pressures of introducing 50% nitrous oxide in a child receiving 10 mg kg⁻¹ h⁻¹ propofol prior to undergoing craniotomy for evacuation of intracerebral haematoma 16 h following a head injury. Nitrous oxide exposure was limited to 2 min.

is raised, as unlike alfentanil (Moss 1992), and sufentanil (Marx *et al.* 1988), it produces no increase in CBF or ICP (Moss *et al.* 1978). Following the induction dose of fentanyl (1–3 µg kg⁻¹), further doses of 0.5–1.0 µg kg⁻¹ are given hourly. Some anaesthetists supplement this with up to 5 mg of droperidol, which may be useful because of its alpha-blocking and antiemetic properties. No further fentanyl is given once the intracranial part of the operation is completed. Isoflurane is used to fine-tune the anaesthetic, once raising of the bone flap is completed, doses of 0.25–0.6% being usually adequate.

If hypertension occurs during raising of the flap, this should be treated first with further narcotics, e.g. 1–3 µg kg⁻¹ bolus of fentanyl. It is permissible, even in the presence of a raised ICP, to increase inspired isoflurane concentrations to 0.6% provided that hypocapnia has been established. if hypertension persists and tachycardia is a feature then labetalol in 10 mg increments may be given. If tachycardia is not a feature then hydralazine in 2 mg increments may be used. Sodium nitroprusside and glyceryl trinitrate vasodilating agents are also cerebral vasodilators and are contraindicated until the dura is opened.

INTRAVENOUS INFUSION TECHNIQUES

Some anaesthetists prefer this approach because of the long periods where patients must lie 'asleep' with minimal surgical stimulation. It also has the theoretical advantage that, for a given degree of cerebral metabolic depression, CBF and thus brain bulk will be less with a hypnotic as opposed to an inhalation agent.

Central to any discussion of infusional anaesthesia are the concepts of minimal infusion rate (MIR), volume of distribution at steady state (VD$_{ss}$), and clearance (Sear 1989). The MIR is analogous to an inhalational agent's MAC value, in other words the infusion rate at which 50% of subjects move in response to a standard stimulus. The volume of distribution will determine the initial dose of agent which must be administered. The VD$_{ss}$ and clearance determine recovery properties. A low VD$_{ss}$ and high clearance imply rapid recovery; conversely a high VD$_{ss}$ and low clearance imply prolonged recovery.

Thiopentone has been used for continuous intravenous anaesthesia (Hunter 1972); however the plasma levels necessary for anaesthesia ($>40 \, \mu g \, ml^{-1}$) (Becker 1978), mean that amounts in excess of 500 mg h^{-1} must be used. Because of cumulation and the conversion of thiopentone to the active metabolite pentobarbitone, this precludes its use in neuro-anaesthesia except under circumstances where the patient will be ventilated postoperatively. Althesin from a neuroanaesthetic point of view seemed to be an ideal agent before its withdrawal. Etomidate is no longer used for continuous infusion. Methohexitone has been studied as an intravenous anaesthetic (Sear *et al.* 1983), but possible problems with postoperative convulsions preclude its use in neuroanaesthesia.

Propofol is the principal agent used for intravenous anaesthesia, supplemented by a narcotic. Although the volume of distribution of propofol is large (around 300 litres), clearance is rapid (1300–1900 ml min^{-1}), and return to consciousness is prompt on discontinuing the infusion. The MIR for propofol is 2.94 mg kg^{-1}h^{-1}. With an ED$_{95}$ of 4.98 mg kg^{-1}h^{-1} when accompanied by alfentanil and air (Richards *et al.* 1990). A variety of dosing regimens have been described (Kay 1986, Merckx *et al.* 1988, Roberts *et al.* 1988, Van Hemelrijck *et al.*

1991). It is also possible to interface a portable computer with infusion devices and deliver a preset regimen which can be varied, based on the patient's age, weight and sex (White & Kenny 1990). The following is one regimen which may be used in practice. Anaesthesia is induced with propofol 1.0 mg kg^{-1} and fentanyl 2–3 µg kg^{-1} or alfentanil 30–50 µg kg^{-1} administered cautiously. A syringe driver is then set to deliver propofol 10 mg kg^{-1} h^{-1} for 10 min, 8 mg kg^{-1} h^{-1} for a further 10 min, then a maintenance rate of 6 mg kg^{-1} h^{-1}. Meanwhile fentanyl is infused at 1.0 µg kg^{-1} h^{-1}, or alfentanil at 50 µg kg^{-1} h^{-1}. If hypertension occurs it can be treated either with boluses or increased rate of infusion of narcotic agent or propofol, by the judicious use of small quantities of volatile agent or, if the patient is felt to be adequately anaesthetized, by the administration of antihypertensives as detailed above. Fentanyl is discontinued 1 h and alfentanil ½ h before the end of surgery, and the propofol when the head dressing has been applied.

Obviously the use of a pure intravenous technique for a long neurosurgical case can use large doses and become very costly. The need for avoiding nitrous oxide usually diminishes either once the brain is decompressed in situations where ICP is acutely raised, or when the major part of the dissection has been completed where there is a risk of air embolus. At this point it is reasonable to introduce nitrous oxide or a volatile agent in order to reduce or halt the propofol infusion.

Fluid management

All fluid and blood losses must be replaced adequately during a neurosurgical procedure to maintain blood volume and cerebral perfusion. Attention should also be paid to third space losses, particularly following cranial trauma, and especially if there are multiple injuries.

The blood–brain barrier acts like an osmometer, as opposed to peripheral capillary beds which behave more like oncometers (Zornow *et al.* 1987). Therefore fluid fluxes across normal brain are determined primarily by osmotic forces, whereas fluxes across the peripheral capillary beds are determined by differences in colloid oncotic pressure. Thus a fall in plasma osmolality by as little as 5–10 mosmol kg^{-1} can have a marked effect on water movement across the blood–brain barrier and result in cerebral oedema. This can be contrasted with hypoalbumenaemic states, where cerebral oedema is not a feature, but the reduction in plasma oncotic pressure results in peripheral oedema. When the blood–brain barrier is disrupted neither an osmotic nor an oncotic gradient can be

[handwritten marginal note:] Queen's Square – low-dose nimodipine (0.02 mg/kg/min?) to ↑↑↑ vasodilator effect of propofol/opiates TIVA + O₂/air – treat acute falls: BP c̄ gelatine

established, and water movement becomes dependent on hydrostatic forces. A reduction in plasma oncotic pressure in these circumstances again does not result in brain oedema (Zornow *et al.* 1988). Fluid therapy should thus be directed at maintaining plasma osmotic pressure. There may be reasons for 'favouring' a colloid over a crystalloid in a trauma patient, for example, but the maintenance of a normal osmotic rather than oncotic gradient is all-important to the brain.

Intraoperative maintenance fluid should be lactated Ringer's or 0.9% saline. Saline may be preferable if large volumes of fluid are adminis-tered, because although Ringer's lactate has a calculated osmolality of $273 \, \text{mosmol kg}^{-1}$, the tendency of sodium particles to aggregate produces a real osmotic force of $250 \, \text{mosmol kg}^{-1}$. Therefore the equivalent of as much as 110 ml free water is given with each litre of Ringer's lactate when the patient's osmolality is normal. If the patient is dehydrated this may rise to as much as 300 ml of free water with each litre (Pfenninger & Himmelseher 1991). Dextrose-containing solutions should be avoided, not only because of their hypo-osmolality, but because of the danger that hyperglycaemia may exacerbate cerebral ischaemia (Nakakimura *et al.* 1990).

There is little published work on the effect of haemodilution on cerebral blood flow or the 'optimum' haematocrit for oxygen delivery to the brain. Although oxygen delivery to peripheral tissues may improve at a haemoglobin of $10 \, \text{g dl}^{-1}$, this may not be true of the cerebral circulation. Isovolaemic haemodilution will produce an increase in CBF (Henrikson *et al.* 1981); however, an increased CBF will not necessarily lead to an increase in brain oxygen transport (Kusunoki *et al.* 1981). It is the author's policy to replace fully any losses in excess of 20% of the patient's circulating volume. Cell-saving techniques have not found wide usage as yet, principally because of obvious concerns during tumour surgery and the high concentration of thromboplastins in brain tissue. Aprotinin has yet to be formally evaluated in cranial operations. Initial experience suggests that reductions in the amount of blood lost can be achieved, particularly from large raw areas in craniofacial procedures.

Emergence

Following completion of surgery, closure of scalp and dura takes at least ½ h. Closure of the scalp, removal of pins from the three-point fixator, and manipulation of the head during application of the head dressing, all provide significant stimulation to the end of the anaesthetic.

Hypertension during this phase of surgery is common, and may be dangerous in situations where ICP is raised or an aneurysm has been left unclipped. Rapid gentle emergence, as opposed to sudden awakening, is desirable at the end of anaesthesia. Strategies include incremental doses of propofol (20−40 mg), labetalol (10 mg) or hydralazine (2 mg), or an infusion of propofol. With longer-acting agents such as labetalol or hydrallazine care should be taken that the patient does not become hypotensive in recovery once the painful stimulus is removed. In the rare circumstances where this is anticipated an infusion of esmolol may be used (Gibson *et al.* 1988).

For reversal of neuromuscular blockade glycopyrrolate is preferable to atropine as an anticholinergic agent. This is not only because of smaller changes in heart rate with glycopyrrolate, but also because CNS recovery is more rapid with this drug (Sheref 1985). There is also the risk of development of a central anticholinergic syndrome with atropine − a risk not present with glycopyrrolate, which does not pass through the blood−brain barrier because of its quaternary ammonium structure.

Coughing and bucking on the endotracheal tube must be avoided at the end of surgery. The advantage of a propofol infusion may be evident at this stage, as there is some evidence that it decreases laryngeal reactivity, allowing patients to tolerate an endotracheal tube (McKeating *et al.* 1988).

Due to variations in individual pharmacokinetics and pharmaco-dynamics, occasional patients will be found to be excessively narcotized at the end of the procedure. Naloxone should not be given if there is concern about the occurrence of hypertension (Estilo & Cottrell 1981). Naloxone has also been reported as causing an increase in cerebral blood flow (Turner *et al.* 1984), and should not be given in situations where an increase in CBF and ICP is undesirable. It is preferable to continue to ventilate the patient in the recovery area till narcotic effects have worn off, and then extubate the patient. In other circumstances naloxone may be used; small increments of 40−80 µg should be given every 5 min until the desired reversal of narcotic activity is achieved.

Recovery

All patients should be closely monitored in recovery; detailed management will be described in Chapter 15. The principal problems are those of hypertension and the insidious development of a subdural or extradural haematoma.

References

Adams R.W., Gronert G.A., Sundt T.M. & Michenfelder J.D. (1972) Halothane, hypocapnia and cerebrospinal fluid pressure in neurosurgery. *Anesthesiology* **37**, 510–517.

Adams R.W., Cucchiara R.F., Gronert G.A., Messick J.M. & Michenfelder J.D. (1981) Isoflurane and cerebrospinal fluid pressure in neurosurgical patients. *Anesthesiology* **54**, 97–99.

Allen G.S., Ahn H.S., Preziosi T.J. *et al.* (1983) Cerebral arterial spasm — A controlled trial of nimodipine in patients with subarachnoid hemorrhage. *New England Journal of Medicine* **308**, 619–624.

Anderton J.M., Keen R.I. & Neave R. (1988) *Positioning the Surgical Patient.* Butterworths, London.

Artru A.A. (1982) Nitrous oxide plays a direct role in the development of tension pneumocephalus intraoperatively. *Anesthesiology* **57**, 59–61.

Baerts W.D.M., De Lange J.J., Booij L.H.D.J. & Broere G. (1984) Complications of the Mayfield skull clamp. *Anesthesiology* **61**, 460–461.

Barnett H.G., Clifford J.R. & Llewellyn R.C. (1977) Safety of mini-dose heparin administration for neurosurgical patients. *Journal of Neurosurgery* **47**, 27–30.

Becker K.E. (1978) Plasma levels of thiopental necessary for anesthesia. *Anesthesiology* **49**, 192–196.

Bedford R.F., Morris L. & Jane J.A. (1982) Intracranial hypertension during surgery for supratentorial tumor; correlation with pre-operative computed tomography scans. *Anesthesia and Analgesia* **61**, 430–433.

Bedford R.F., Persing J.A., Pobereskin L. & Butler A. (1980) Lidocaine or thiopental for rapid control of intracranial hypertension? *Anesthesia and Analgesia* **59**, 435–437.

Black T.E., Kay B. & Healy T.E.J. (1984) Reducing the haemodynamic responses to laryngoscopy and intubation. A comparison of alfentanil with fentanyl. *Anaesthesia* **39**, 883–887.

Bloor B.C. & Flacke W.E. (1982) Reduction in halothane anesthetic requirement by clonidine, an alpha-adrenergic agonist. *Anesthesia and Analgesia* **61**, 741–745.

Carabine U.A., Wright P.M.C., Howe J.P. & Moore J. (1991) Cardiovascular effects of intravenous clonidine — Partial attenuation of the pressor response to intubation by clonidine. *Anaesthesia* **46**, 634–637.

Cerrato D., Ariano C. & Fiacchino R. (1978) Deep vein thrombosis and low-dose heparin prophylaxis in neurosurgical patients. *Journal of Neurosurgery* **49**, 378–381.

Cold G.E. & Jensen F.T. (1978) Cerebral autoregulation in unconscious patients with brain injury. *Acta Anaesthesiologica Scandinavica* **22**, 270–280.

Dahlgren N. & Messeter K. (1981) Treatment of stress response to laryngoscopy and intubation with fentanyl. *Anaesthesia* **36**, 1022−1026.

Demczuk R.J. (1984) Significant sinus bradycardia following intravenous lidocaine injection. *Anesthesiology* **60**, 69−70.

Estilo A.E. & Cottrell J.E. (1981) Naloxone, hypertension and ruptured cerebral aneurysm. *Anesthesiology* **54**, 352.

Gibson B.E., Black S., Maass L. & Cucchiara R.F. (1988) Esmolol for the control of hypertension after neurologic surgery. *Clinical Pharmacology and Therapeutics* **44**, 650−653.

Hamill J.F., Bedford R.F., Weaver D.C. & Colohan A.R. (1981) Lidocaine before endotracheal intubation: intravenous or laryngotracheal? *Anesthesiology* **55**, 578−581.

Henrikson L., Paulson O.B. & Smith R.J. (1981) Cerebral blood flow following normovolemic hemodilution in patients with high hematocrit. *Annals of Neurology* **9**, 454−457.

Herregods L., Verbeke J., Rolly G. & Colardyn F. (1988) Effect of propofol on elevated intracranial pressure. Preliminary results. *Anaesthesia* **43** (Suppl.), 107−109.

Hickey D.R., Sangwan S. & Bevan J.C. (1988) Phenytoin-induced resistance to pancuronium. Use of atracurium infusion in management of a neurosurgical patient. *Anaesthesia* **43**, 757−759.

Hillman D.R., Rung G.W., Thompson W.R. & Davis N.J. (1987) The effect of bupivacaine scalp infiltration on the hemodynamic response to craniotomy under general anaesthesia. *Anesthesiology* **67**, 1001−1003.

Hunter A.R. (1972) Thiopentone supplemented anaesthesia for neurosurgery. *British Journal of Anaesthesia* **44**, 506−510.

Kay B. (1986) Propofol and alfentanyl infusion. A comparison with methohexitone and alfentanyl for major surgery. *Anaesthesia* **41**, 589−595.

Kusunoki M., Kimura K., Nakamura M., Isaka Y., Yoneda S. & Abe H. (1981) Effects of hematocrit variations on cerebral blood flow and oxygen transport in ischemic cerebrovascular disease. *Journal of Cerebral Blood Flow and Metabolism* **1**, 413−417.

Laycock J.R.D., Smith C.E., Donati F. & Bevan D.R. (1987) Sensitivity of the adductor pollicis and diaphragm to atracurium in a hemiplegic patient. *Anesthesiology* **67**, 851−853.

Lee C.M. (1975) Train of four quantitation of competitive neuromuscular block. *Anesthesia and Analgesia* **54**, 649−653.

Marx W., Shah N., Long C. *et al.* (1988) Sufentanil, alfentanil and fentanyl: impact on CSF pressure in patients with brain tumors. *Anesthesiology* **69**, A627.

McKeating K., Bali I.M. & Dundee J.W. (1988) The effects of thiopentone and propofol on upper airway integrity. *Anaesthesia* **43**, 638−640.

Mendelow A.D., Teasdale G.M., Russel T., Flood J., Patterson J. & Murray G.D. (1985) Effect of mannitol on cerebral blood flow and cerebral perfusion pressure in human head injury. *Journal of Neurosurgery* **63**, 43−48.

Merckx L., Van Hemelrijck J., Van Aken H., Plets C. & Goffin J. (1988) Total intravenous anesthesia using propofol and alfentanil infusion in neurosurgical patients. *Anesthesiology* **69**, A576.

Michenfelder J.D. (1988) *Anaesthesia and the Brain*, 1st edn, pp. 52−59. Churchill Livingstone, London.

Michenfelder J.D. & Theye R.A. (1968) Hypothermia: effect on canine brain and whole-body metabolism. *Anesthesiology* **29**, 1107−1112.

Moss E. (1992) Alfentanil increases intracranial pressure when intracranial compliance is low. *Anaesthesia* **47**, 134−136.

Moss E., Powell D., Gibson R.M. & McDowall D.G. (1978) Effects of fentanyl on intracranial pressure and cerebral perfusion pressure during hypocapnia. *British Journal of Anaesthesia* **50**, 779−784.

Nakakimura K., Fleischer J.E., Drummond J.C. *et al.* (1990) Glucose administration before cardiac arrest worsens neurologic outcome in cats. *Anesthesiology* **72**, 1005−1011.

Pang D. (1982) Air embolism associated with wounds from a pintype head-holder. *Journal of Neurosurgery* **57**, 710−713.

Pfenninger E. & Himmelseher S. (1991) Perioperative fluid management in neurosurgical anaesthesia. *Current Opinion in Anesthesiology* **4**, 649−652.

Prys-Roberts C., Foex P., Biro G.P. & Roberts J.G. (1973) Studies of anaesthesia in relation to hypertension. V: Adrenergic beta receptor blockade. *British Journal of Anaesthesia* **45**, 671−681.

Puri G.D. & Batra Y.K. (1988) Effect of nifedipine on cardiovascular responses to laryngoscopy and intubation. *British Journal of Anaesthesia* **60**, 579−581.

Ravussin P., Abou-Madi M., Archer D. *et al.* (1988) Changes in CSF pressure after mannitol in patients with and without elevated CSF pressure. *Journal of Neurosurgery* **69**, 869−876.

Richards M.J., Skues M.A., Jarvis A.P.& Prys-Roberts C. (1990) Total I.V. anaesthesia with propofol and alfentanil: dose requirements for propofol and the effect of premedication with clonidine. *British Journal of Anaesthesia* **65**, 157−163.

Risberg J., Lundberg N. & Ingvar D.H. (1969) Regional cerebral blood volume during acute transient rises of the intracranial pressure (plateau waves). *Journal of Neurosurgery* **31**, 303−310.

Risk Factors Consensus Group (1992) *British Medical Journal* **305**, 567−574.

Roberts F.L., Dixon J., Lewis G.T.R., Tackley R.M. & Prys-Roberts C. (1998) Induction and maintenance of propofol anaesthesia. *Anaesthesia* **43** (Suppl.), 14−17.

Rupp S.M., McChristian J.W., Miller R.D., Taboada J.A. & Cronnelly R. (1986) Neostigmine and edrophonium antagonism of varying intensity neuromuscular blockade induced by atracurium, pancuronium or vecuronium. *Anesthesiology* **64**, 711−717.

Scott J.C., Ponganis K.V. & Stanski D.R. (1985) EEG quantitation of narcotic effect: The comparative pharmacodynamics of fentanyl and alfentanil. *Anesthesiology* **62**, 234–241.

Sear J.W. (1989) Drugs by infusion: their use during intravenous anaesthesia and intensive care. In: Atkinson R.S. & Adams A.P. (Eds), *Recent Advances in Anaesthesia and Analgesia*, vol. 16, pp. 43–64. Churchill Livingstone, London.

Sear J.W., Phillips K.C., Andrews C.J.H. & Prys-Roberts C. (1983) Dose–response relationships for infusions of Althesin or methohexitone. *Anaesthesia* **38**, 931–936.

Shapiro H.M., Galindo A., Wyte S.R. & Harris A.B. (1973) Rapid intraoperative reduction of intracranial pressure with thiopentone. *British Journal of Anaesthesia* **45**, 1057–1062.

Sheref S.E. (1985) Pattern of CNS recovery following reversal of neuromuscular blockade: comparison of atropine and glycopyrrolate. *British Journal of Anaesthesia* **57**, 188–191.

Stirt J.A., Grosslight K.R., Bedford R.F. & Vollmer D. (1987) 'Defasciculation' with metocurine prevents succinylcholine-induced increases in intracranial pressure. *Anesthesiology* **67**, 50–53.

Turner D.M., Kassell N.F., Sasaki T., Comair Y.G., Boarini D.J. & Beck D.O. (1984) Effects of naloxone on cerebral blood flow and metabolism in isoflurane/nitrous oxide-anesthetized dogs. *Neurosurgery* **14**, 688–696.

Unni V.K.N., Johnston R.A., Young H.S.A. & McBride R.J. (1984) Prevention of intracranial hypertension during laryngoscopy and endotracheal intubation. Use of a second dose of thiopentone. *British Journal of Anaesthesia* **56**, 1219–1223.

Van Hemelrijck J., Fitch W., Mattheussen M., Van Aken H. & Plets C. (1990) The effect of propofol on the cerebral circulation and autoregulation in the baboon. *Anesthesia and Analgesia* **71**, 49–54.

Van Hemelrijck J., Van Aken H., Merckx L. & Mulier J. (1991) Anesthesia for craniotomy: Total intravenous anesthesia with propofol and alfentanyl compared to anesthesia with thiopental sodium, isoflurane, fentanyl, and nitrous oxide. *Journal of Clinical Anesthesia* **3**, 131–136.

Vandesteene A., Trempont V., Engelman E. *et al.* (1988) Effect of propofol on cerebral blood flow and metabolism in man. *Anaesthesia* **43** (Suppl.), 42–43.

Vucevic M., Purdy G.M. & Ellis F.R. (1992) Esmolol hydrochloride for management of the cardiovascular stress responses to laryngoscopy and tracheal intubation. *British Journal of Anaesthesia* **68**, 529–530.

Wang C.Y., Chee C.P. & Delilkan A.E. (1991) Upward transtentorial herniation of posterior fossa structures. *European Journal of Anaesthesiology* **8**, 469–470.

White M. & Kenny G.N.C. (1990) Intravenous propofol anaesthesia using a computerised infusion system. *Anaesthesia* **45**, 204–209.

Wilson I.G., Meiklejohn B.H. & Smith G. (1991) Intravenous lignocaine and sympathoadrenal responses to laryngoscopy and intubation. The effect of varying time of injection. *Anaesthesia* **46**, 177−180.

Zornow M.H., Todd M.M. & Moore S.S. (1987) The acute cerebral effects of changes in plasma osmolality and oncotic pressure. *Anesthesiology* **67**, 936−941.

Zornow M.H., Scheller M.S., Todd M.M. & Moore S.S. (1988) Acute cerebral effects of isotonic crystalloid and colloid solutions following cryogenic brain injury in the rabbit. *Anesthesiology* **69**, 180−184.

8
Anaesthesia for supratentorial tumour surgery

J.R. DAVID LAYCOCK AND FRANK J.M. WALTERS

Introduction

Tumours within the CNS exert an effect either by local invasion of specific anatomical structures thereby producing specific neurological signs, by non-specific elevation of intracranial pressure, or by production of convulsions. Tumours in the region of the pituitary gland may also produce hormonal effects. Some tumours are amenable to surgical excision, others may be palliated by surgical decompression, insertion of a shunt, or radiotherapy. Marked peritumour oedema is often present in brain tissue surrounding malignant tumours. The larger benign meningiomas are often characterized by high shunt-like blood flows within the tumour. Autoregulation is lost within the tumour itself, and often in the surrounding brain tissue. If by either of these mechanisms there are significant pressure effects and cerebral compression by the tumour, any further increase in intracranial pressure (ICP) may lead to tentorial herniation. The principal consideration for the anaesthetist during tumour surgery is therefore the control of ICP.

Pathology and radiology

The incidence of intracranial tumours is about six per 100 000 population per year. Table 8.1 describes the features of the common primary supratentorial tumours. The plain skull X-ray may show expansion of the sella and erosion of the clinoid in pituitary tumours. Calcification may be present in craniopharyngiomas and oligodendrogliomas. Virtually all supratentorial tumours can be detected with the CT scanner, though occasionally tumours which are isodense with surrounding brain tissue may not be imaged (Wulff *et al.* 1982). In the majority of cases a provisional diagnosis of the nature of the tumour can be arrived at. Figure 8.1 shows examples of glioblastoma and meningioma respectively. A chest X-ray should always be taken if there is a suspicion of a

Table 8.1 Features of common primary supratentorial tumours

Name	Nature	Origin	Percentage
Anaplastic astrocytoma and glioblastoma	Malignant	Astrocytes undifferentiated	45
Meningioma	Benign	Arachnoid granulations	15
Metastasis	Malignant	Breast—lung melanoma	14
Pituitary adenoma	Benign	Adenohypophyseal cells	10
Astrocytoma	Low-grade malignant	Astrocytes	8
Craniopharyngioma	Benign	Buccal epithelium	2
Oligodendroglioma	Low-grade malignant	Oligodendrocytes	2
Colloid cyst	Benign	Embryonic	1
Lymphoma	Malignant	Lymphatic	1
Others			2

secondary; indeed secondary tumours can account for up to 25% of supratentorial tumours. An MRI scan may be useful in further delineating the extent of tumour spread, and is superior to CT scanning in the imaging of posterior fossa tumours. Angiography is used if there is a suspicion that the tumour mass may be a giant aneurysm, for example

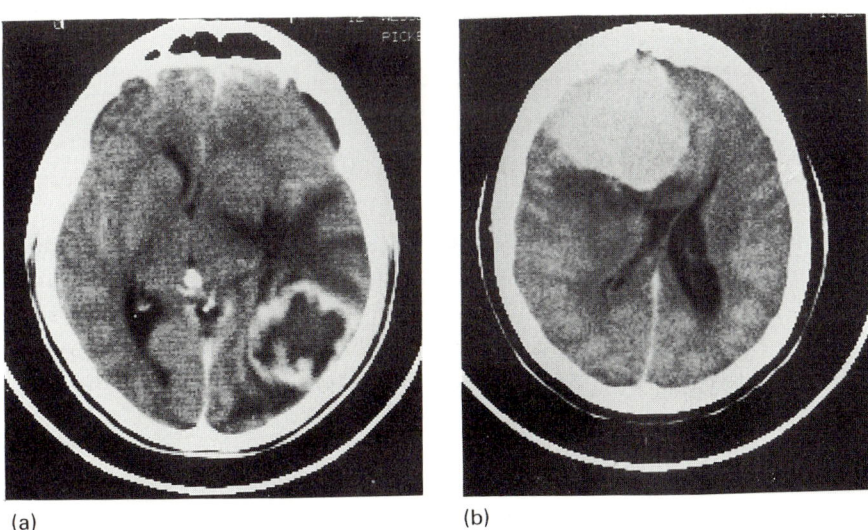

(a)   (b)

Fig. 8.1 CT scan of (a) glioblastoma and (b) meningioma. Note the marked area of oedema surrounding the glioblastoma.

with some pituitary lesions, and to assess the vascularity of some tumours.

Medical management

Once a provisional diagnosis has been made, and a surgical plan formulated, the principal aims of medical management are the control of ICP and treatment of epilepsy. Steroids are effective in reducing the peritumour oedema and increasing brain compliance in most intrinsic malignant tumours, secondaries and the larger meningiomas (French & Galicich 1964, Miller & Leech 1975). The usual dose is dexamethasone 4 mg t.d.s., together with a hydrogen receptor antagonist. In those patients whose level of consciousness is depressed, remarkable improvements are often seen. Care should obviously be taken to exclude an abscess or infective pathology before steroids are administered.

Epilepsy is controlled with phenytoin 100 mg t.d.s. following a loading dose, with estimation of blood levels if necessary. The normal therapeutic range is $40-100\,\mu mol\,l^{-1}$. In a minority of patients, particularly the elderly and those with bulbar problems, nutritional status is poor. If time allows they may benefit from a period of preoperative nasogastric enteral feeding.

Surgery for supratentorial lesions

Burr-hole biopsy

A burr-hole biopsy is performed to establish a tissue diagnosis in malignant brain tumours where resection is not feasible, and to differentiate primary from metastatic brain disease. The procedure itself carries a low mortality (2−4%) (Marshall et al. 1974), principally from haemorrhage into and expansion of the tumour mass, or localized brain swelling. With deep-seated or small lesions a stereotactic biopsy is more appropriate.

Most burr-hole biopsies can be undertaken under local anaesthesia. The scalp, subcutaneous tissues and periosteum are infiltrated with lignocaine and adrenaline, a burr-hole made, and needle aspiration of tissue performed through a cruciate dural incision. The employment of intravenous sedation as an adjunct is not recommended. The occasional patient may be confused and uncooperative, in which case general anaesthesia is indicated. The same considerations will then apply as for craniotomy (Chapter 7).

Shunt procedures

The majority of shunt procedures are performed in paediatric patients. Adult patients with obstructive hydrocephalus associated with an inoperable tumour may benefit from the insertion of a shunt. Similarly, obstructive hydrocephalus can occur following a subarachnoid haemorrhage. Occasionally an emergency shunt is required for a patient with a posterior fossa lesion prior to definitive surgery, though in these circumstances temporary ventricular drainage is often employed. Occasional patients with lesions near the third ventricle require a bilateral shunt.

The ventriculoperitoneal route is favoured for shunt insertion. The ventriculo-atrial is rarely used, generally reserved for those patients in whom for technical reasons it is impossible to site the peritoneal catheter. In patients with benign intracranial hypertension the lumboperitoneal route is often chosen in favour of the ventriculoperitoneal.

The problems of anaesthesia for shunt surgery are discussed in detail in Chapter 13. In adult patients the anaesthetic technique chosen should take into account the nature of the underlying pathology.

Craniotomy

Most benign supratentorial tumours and the less aggressive astrocytomas can be completely excised. Difficulties may occur with some tumours, for example a meningioma en plaque when closely applied to important structures, or base of skull tumours. Most malignant gliomas are so closely associated with normal brain that only partial debulking is possible without causing significant neurological damage. If the lesion is confined to the frontal or temporal lobes then a complete removal may be attempted by lobectomy.

Meningiomas offer a special challenge to both anaesthetist and surgeon, as they are benign and thus curable, but complications from surgery can be devastating. They may reach large sizes before producing clinical signs, and they may be very vascular with the accompanying possibility of large intraoperative blood losses. The following points should be borne in mind. Some convexity meningiomas erode into the vault of the skull as shown in Fig. 8.2. The anaesthetist should be

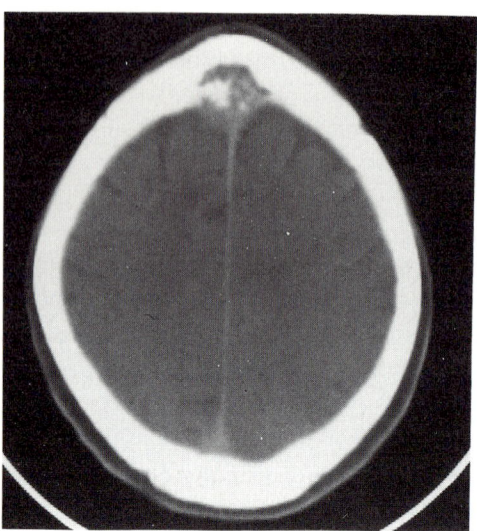

Fig. 8.2 A convexity meningioma eroding into the vault of the skull. Profuse bleeding may occur on elevation of the flap.

prepared for profuse bleeding when the bone flap is raised. This danger is also present with re-do craniotomies for recurrent meningiomas. In these circumstances, and also with tumours of vascular origin, central venous pressure should be monitored. With larger tumours, if pressure gradients exist within the brain, sudden changes in blood pressure and pulse rate may occur on elevation of the flap. With large and vascular tumours hypotension may be employed to reduce bleeding; however, surgical advances have dramatically reduced the blood loss which is experienced with resection of these tumours. Occasional patients show evidence of brain swelling once the resection of the tumour is completed. In this case an intracranial pressure monitor should be inserted and the patient ventilated postoperatively. This ensures that any brain oedema will not be worsened by hypoxia or hypercapnia, nor will the patient be at risk from sudden apnoeic episodes. The presence of an intra-cranial pressure monitor will alert attendant staff to any postoperative haematomas.

In the presence of raised intracranial pressure the principal aim is the avoidance of hypercarbia and hypotension or hypertension. Strategies for achieving this are discussed in Chapter 7. Most patients with cerebral tumours now present much earlier than previously due to the widespread use of the CT scanner, thus many fewer present for anaesthesia obtunded by raised ICP. If the conscious level of the patient is depressed despite treatment with dexamethasone, mannitol may be administered prior to induction. Very rarely, if the patient shows signs of incipient cerebral herniation associated with hydrocephalus, the surgeon can perform a ventricular tap through a burr-hole prior to anaesthesia.

Mannitol may be administered following induction, and will be useful in those patients with large tumours with surrounding oedema. The usual dose is $0.25-1.0\,g\,kg^{-1}$. Frusemide ($0.25-1.0\,mg\,kg^{-1}$) can also be given; this may help to prevent a rebound increase in ICP due to mannitol crossing into areas where the blood−brain barrier is disrupted due to tumour. A urinary catheter is inserted.

Tumours of the orbit and skull base can be exposed through a variety of combined approaches (Anand *et al.* 1991, Uttley *et al.* 1989). Most skull base tumours tend to be benign or of low-grade malignancy. Tumours of the orbit can be exposed with a frontal craniotomy, access achieved by removing the roof of the orbit together with a portion of frontal bone. For tumours of the skull base a variety of approaches are possible. For extended access anteriorly, a transfacial approach is possible. Following a frontal craniotomy the maxilla is split and reflected sideways. If access is required more posteriorly, the nasal septum can be detached from the maxilla, a Le Fort 1 osteotomy performed, and the maxilla down-fractured to give access upwards to the base of the skull. A tracheostomy is recommended for transfacial operations, otherwise prolonged intubation, together with its attendant difficulties, will be required postoperatively.

Some swelling of the brain is inevitable following tumour surgery. Steroids should be continued postoperatively; indeed some centres give an additional bolus of dexamethasone 12−16 mg peroperatively, followed by an increased dose for the first few postoperative days. Areas of ischaemia or trauma at the operation site, as well as blood in the ventricles, will predispose to convulsions. Anticonvulsants may therefore be given, and plasma levels in patients on established therapy should be maintained.

Pituitary surgery

Anatomy

The pituitary sits in the sella turcica, separated by a diaphragm of dura from the optic chiasma. The pituitary stalk traverses the diaphragm to connect the hypothalamus to the pituitary, and contains neurosecretory fibres running from the supraoptic and paraventricular nuclei of the hypothalamus to the posterior pituitary. The carotid arteries lie close to the lateral aspects of the gland, and the third, fourth and sixth cranial nerves run in the cavernous sinus.

Pathophysiology

Tumours can be divided into two broad categories: non-functioning and hypersecreting (Jeffreys 1987).

NON-FUNCTIONING TUMOURS

These account for about 75% of pituitary tumours. They generally become evident when they are large enough to produce a mass effect due to suprasellar extension (Fig. 8.3), or symptoms and signs of hypopituitarism. The mass effects which may be seen include loss of visual fields, ocular nerve palsies from compression of third, fourth or sixth and symptoms and signs of raised intracranial pressure due to obstructive hydrocephalus. Hypopituitarism can manifest itself in a number of ways. Hypothyroidism may occur. Decreased release of gonadotrophic hormones causes amenorrhoea, infertility, impotence and loss of secondary sexual characteristics. Loss of adrenocorticotrophic hormone (ACTH) secretion causes a picture that differs in some respects from Addison's disease. There is no hyperpigmentation because ACTH secretion is reduced, not raised. Sodium and water deficiency does not occur as aldosterone secretion, which is controlled by angiotensin, is normal. Cortisol is, however, necessary for normal water excretion, thus a dilutional hyponatraemia may occur. Lack of normal cortisol secretion also predisposes to hypoglycaemia, hypotension and hypothermia.

HYPERSECRETING TUMOURS

These adenomas, previously classified on their histological properties, are now classified on the basis of hormone produced. Growth hormone (GH), ACTH, prolactin, or thyroid-stimulating hormone TSH are secreted. Occasionally more than one hormone may be produced. Gonadotrophin-secreting tumours are rare. Apart from prolactinomas, patients with hypersecreting tumours usually present before any mass lesion is evident because of endocrine effects.

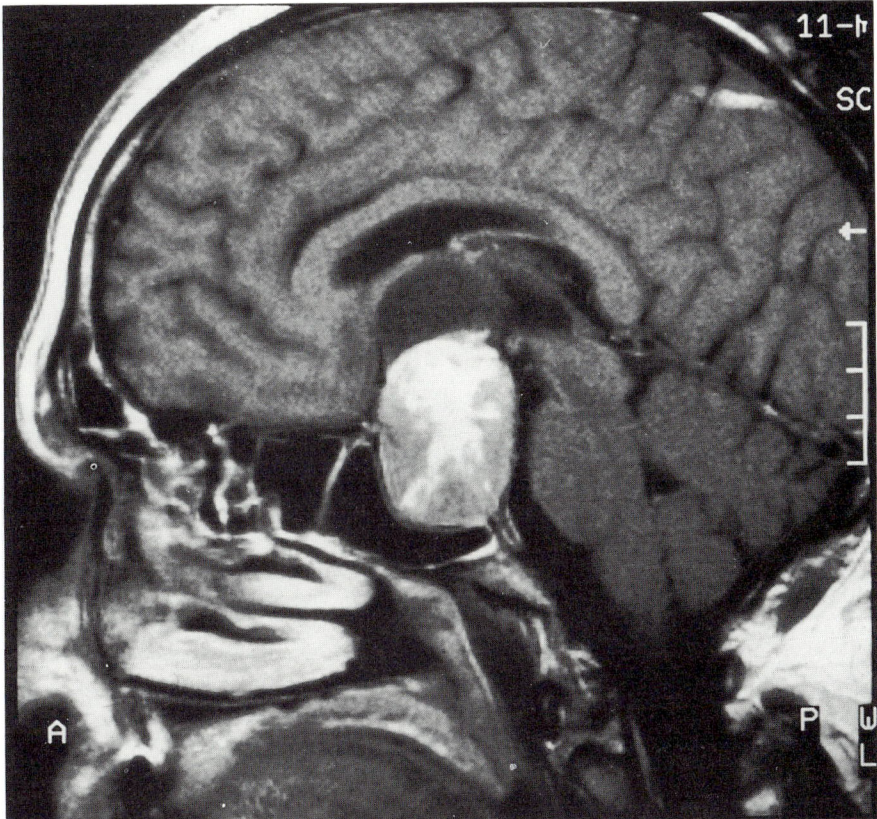

Fig. 8.3 MRI scan of a pituitary tumour with suprasellar extension out of the pituitary fossa.

ACROMEGALY

Apart from the obvious skeletal abnormalities, excess growth hormone secretion can result in hypertension, cardiomyopathy and diabetes mellitus, all of which may require treatment preoperatively and should be considered in planning the anaesthetic management. The features of acromegaly persist when the phase of hypopituitarism has begun. Laryngoscopy and visualization of the cords may be difficult due to overgrowth of the soft tissues in the pharynx, lips and tongue. Intubation may be difficult due to fixation of the vocal cords or hypertrophy and calcification of the laryngeal cartilages resulting in laryngeal stenosis (Edge & Whitwam 1981). The laryngeal aperture may be reduced, and the epiglottis large and fleshy. Some difficulty with intubation using a laryngoscope can be anticipated in approximately 40% of cases (Messick *et al.* 1982). Insurmountable difficulties are fortunately uncommon. Prior to induction, a long-bladed laryngoscope, a selection of bougies, and a selection of different tube sizes should be immediately available.

CUSHING'S DISEASE

Excess ACTH secretion is characterized by hypertension, mild congestive cardiac failure, hirsutes, truncal obesity, insulin-resistant diabetes mellitus, osteoporosis, proximal muscle weakness and hyperaldosteronism with electrolyte disturbances, particularly hypokalaemia and metabolic acidosis. X-rays of the sella are often normal and the microadenoma responsible may be extremely small, of the order of 1–2 mm diameter. These patients are also at increased risk of infection from any invasive procedure. Care is also required when moving or positioning the unconscious patient.

PROLACTINOMAS

In women clinical signs include amenorrhoea, galactorrhoea and hirsutes. In men impotence, galactorrhoea and a female distribution of body fat may occur. These tumours are often large, producing neurological signs. Bromocriptine is used prior to surgery to effect shrinkage of the tumour (Barrow *et al.* 1984). In a proportion of cases it may be possible to control the tumour with bromocriptine alone. It may be unwise to use dopamine antagonists such as the phenothiazines, domperidene and metoclopramide as prolactin secretion can increase resulting in expansion of the tumour mass.

OTHER TUMOURS

Occasionally, other tumours occur in the region of the pituitary gland which may be amenable to a trans-sphenoidal approach. These include craniopharyngiomas, arachnoid cysts, epidermoid tumours, small meningiomas and chordomas.

PITUITARY APOPLEXY

This term signifies sudden enlargement of a tumorous pituitary gland, due either to haemorrhage or haemorrhagic infarction. It usually presents with headache, loss of consciousness and acute visual loss. Once diagnosed it is a neurosurgical emergency, and decompression of the lesion should be undertaken immediately.

BIOCHEMICAL TESTS

Direct assay of pituitary hormones is now possible, and this has to some extent reduced the need for stimulation and suppression tests of pituitary function.

Table 8.2 gives reference values for the four major pituitary hormones. Individual laboratories will vary in their exact figures. Stimulation tests are used to aid in the differential diagnosis of deficient secretion, and suppression tests in the differential diagnosis of excessive secretion. A failure to suppress implies loss of feedback control and an extrapituitary source of effector hormone.

Table 8.2 Reference values for the four major pituitary hormones

Hormone	Blood level
Growth hormone (GH)	$<5\,mU\,l^{-1}$
Thyroid-stimulating hormone (TSH)	$0.8-5.0\,mU\,l^{-1}$
Adrenocorticotrophic hormone (ACTH)	$10-80\,ng\,l^{-1}$
Prolactin	
Male	$<500\,mU\,l^{-1}$
Female	$<1000\,mU\,l^{-1}$

DISTURBANCES OF FLUID BALANCE

Apart from electrolyte disturbances due to hypopituitarism or hypersecreting tumours, the disorders of fluid balance seen in pituitary patients are diabetes insipidus and less commonly inappropriate antidiuretic hormone (ADH) secretion. These usually occur after surgery.

DIABETES INSIPIDUS

This may also occur following cranial trauma. It is characterized by a water diuresis, hypernatraemia and progressive dehydration. Despite a high serum osmolality the urine remains dilute ($50-200\,mosmol\,l^{-1}$) with a low specific gravity (less than 1.005), and outputs in excess of $500\,ml\,h^{-1}$ may occur. As the condition is usually self-limiting, treatment should be aimed at maintaining fluid balance. If urine volumes are not excessive, then sufficient fluid intake should be maintained by either the oral or intravenous routes to replace urinary and insensible losses. Intravenous fluids should consist of 5% dextrose or dextrose saline. If large volumes of dextrose are administered care should be taken that the patient does not become hyperglycaemic. If urinary losses are excessive then DDAVP can be administered ($1-2\,\mu$g subcutaneously 12-hourly). This should then be discontinued after 48 h to assess whether the diabetes insipidus is resolving.

INAPPROPRIATE ADH SECRETION (SIADH)

SIADH causes excessive retention of free water resulting in hyponatraemia and low serum osmolality. The urine osmolality is high relative to the serum osmolality. The patient generally remains normovolaemic. SIADH should be distinguished from other causes of hyponatraemia (Swales 1991), the most common of which in neurosurgical patients is mannitol administration. In patients who have had mannitol the serum osmolality is either normal or raised. The clinical picture of SIADH will depend on the rapidity with which hyponatraemia develops. If the fall in sodium is slow symptoms will be few; however, a rapid fall is characterized by nausea and irritability progressing to seizures and coma.

The treatment of SIADH is water restriction, the patient should be limited to 500 ml per day, and the serum sodium will gradually increase. It should rarely be necessary to administer hypertonic saline solutions with diuretics. These will raise the serum sodium, but should be used with care as the rapid expansion of the intravascular volume can lead to pulmonary oedema.

Preoperative evaluation

In general those patients with deficiency states will be on replacement therapy when presenting for surgery. Very occasionally a patient with hypopituitarism will require urgent surgery. In these circumstances it is important to commence glucocorticoid replacement (hydrocortisone 100 mg 6-hourly) immediately. This should be accompanied by sodium chloride 0.9% infusion under central venous pressure (CVP) control, rarely hypertonic saline is needed if the plasma sodium is less than $115\,\text{mmol}\,l^{-1}$. Glucose should be added to the infusion if indicated by regular blood sugar monitoring. Thyroid replacement is also required, but this must be commenced after glucocorticoid replacement otherwise the increase in metabolic rate will worsen the situation. Tri-iodothyronine (T_3) 10 µg may be given daily by mouth, or if necessary 5−20 µg T_3 may be given intravenously and repeated after 12 h.

In patients with hypersecreting tumours it is important to control any hypertension, diabetes or electrolyte disturbances prior to anaesthesia. The presence of gross obesity in Cushing's disease may necessitate modifications in technique. The airway and cardiac function merit particular attention in acromegalics, as this condition with Cushing's disease may be associated with ischaemic heart disease and congestive cardiac failure.

Surgery of pituitary lesions

The indications for pituitary surgery are given in Table 8.3. This may either be through a craniotomy or via the trans-spenoidal route (Hardy 1971).

CRANIOTOMY FOR PITUITARY LESIONS

Where a pituitary mass is large, sufficient surgical access will be gained only by craniotomy. This is classically by the subfrontal route, though

Table 8.3 Indications for pituitary surgery

Non-functioning tumours
Mass effect
Cranial nerve deficit III, IV and VI
Visual deficits
Hydrocephalus
Neuroendocrine deficits due to hypothalamic dysfunction
Functioning tumours
Cushing's disease
Acromegaly
Prolactinomas
Pituitary apoplexy
Uncertain diagnosis
Sellar and parasellar lesions
Metastatic cancer

more recently the transzygomatic has been used. Anaesthetic consider-ations remain the same as for any craniotomy. Prophylactic antibiotics should be administered as the frontal sinuses are often breached by the former approach, and mini-plates used for repair of the zygoma in the latter.

TRANS-SPHENOIDAL HYPOPHYSECTOMY

In addition to the tumours mentioned above, a trans-sphenoidal approach may be required in the treatment of cerebrospinal fluid (CSF) leaks, or in the treatment of malignant pain from cancers of the breast and prostate. Table 8.4 lists the advantages and disadvantages of the trans-sphenoidal approach.

If intubation difficulties are anticipated in acromegalics then a gaseous induction or an awake fibreoptic intubation should be performed. How-ever, intubation can be achieved in most patients with a long-bladed laryngoscope and good neuromuscular blockade. If there is evidence of raised intracranial pressure, then a suitable neuroanaesthetic technique should be chosen (Chapter 7). In other cases any general anaesthetic technique which allows for rapid emergence is suitable. Direct arterial pressure monitoring is indicated, and will warn of trauma to the hypo-thalamus. Visual evoked responses are measured in some centres to monitor optic nerve function, which can become compromised during surgery near the chiasm.

A preformed RAE tube is ideal for these cases. A pharyngeal pack is inserted after intubation. In order to reduce bleeding from surgical

Table 8.4 Advantages and disadvantages of the trans-sphenoidal approach

Advantages
Morbidity and mortality extremely low
Brain trauma minimized
Well tolerated by the aged and seriously ill
Anaesthetic and convalescent times short
Low incidence of diabetes insipidus
Minimal blood loss

Disadvantages
Neural structures adjacent to large tumour not visualized
Non-sterile approach (meningitis rare)
Suprasellar extension cannot be removed
Cerebrospinal fluid leaks

trauma, the nose is packed with ribbon gauze soaked in 2 ml of 5% cocaine. If 1:200 000 adrenaline is added to this solution this may induce hypertension, which can be treated with beta-blocking drugs, labetalol, or deepening anaesthesia with isoflurane. Some surgeons request prophylactic antibiotics because the surgical route traverses the nose. All patients should receive corticosteroids in the form of hydro-cortisone 100 mg on induction.

The patient is placed supine with a 15° head-up tilt. X-ray screening is used to aid the surgeon in locating the pituitary fossa (Fig. 8.4). A common problem is the occurrence of hypertension during the creation of access through the sphenoid. This is best treated with incremental doses of either labetalol or alfentanil. As the operative time is usually about 1½ h, and rapid emergence is desirable, administration of large doses of fentanyl or volatile agent is not recommended. Sudden brady-cardia or hypertension may also occur as a result of manipulating the dura. Blood loss is usually small, of the order of 500 ml. However, in about 10% of patients haemorrhage is sudden and profuse, and losses of up to 3 l can occur. Air embolism is a potential hazard and will be evidenced by the fall in end-tidal carbon dioxide and blood pressure (Newfield *et al.* 1978).

Fascia lata is used by some surgeons to pack the defect produced by this procedure. Nasal packs are inserted at the end of surgery. After

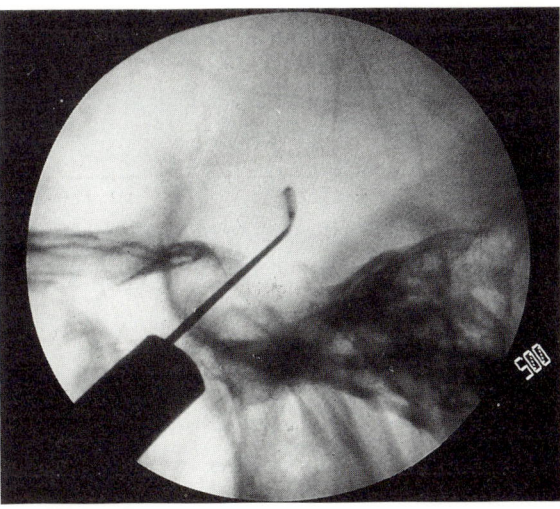

Fig. 8.4 Radiograph of probe in the pituitary fossa during a trans-sphenoidal procedure.

removal of the throat pack and pharyngeal toilet the patient is reversed. In recovery the patient should be sat up as soon as possible in order to reduce any venous bleeding.

Postoperative care

A variety of serious complications may follow trans-sphenoidal surgery. These include haemorrhage, CSF leak, meningitis, blindness, diplopia and perforated nasal septum (Laws & Kern 1975). Parenteral cortico-steroid cover is continued for 48 h (hydrocortisone 100 mg q.d.s.), at which time it may be replaced by oral cortisone acetate. Blood glucose should be measured regularly. Urine output should be closely moni-tored in case diabetes insipidus (DI), which may occur in 10−20% of patients on the first or second postoperative day, develops (Cobb 1980). Urine output may reach 15 l in 24 h and urine osmolality fall to 50−100 mosmol kg^{-1}. Post-hypophysectomy DI usually resolves within 1−2 weeks of operation. A less common complication is inappropriate ADH secretion, which has been reported in the second week post-hypophysectomy (Cusick *et al.* 1984). In addition to disturbances of posterior pituitary function, insufficient steroid replacement may cause hyponatraemia post-hypophysectomy (Whitaker *et al.* 1985).

Patients with acromegaly can develop respiratory difficulties post-operatively. Approximately 40% show signs of sleep apnoea syndrome preoperatively due either to central or peripheral causes (Perks *et al.* 1980). They should therefore be observed for 48 h in a high-dependency unit, and oxygen saturation measured continuously.

CSF rhinorrhoea may occur in the postoperative period. Initially these leaks are treated with a spinal drain. If the patient has to return to theatre, preoxygenation is necessary in order to avoid inflation of the lungs via a face mask. This can otherwise result in intracranial air, and the insufflation of potentially infected material into the brain. When air is known to be present within the skull it is wise to avoid nitrous oxide, as the resultant expansion of the air pocket will worsen the CSF leak during surgery.

References

Anand V.K., Harkey H.L. & Al-Mefti O. (1991) Open-door maxillotomy approach for lesions of the clivus. *Skull Base Surgery* **1**, 217−225.

Barrow D.L., Tindall G.T., Kovacs K., Thorner M.O., Horvath E. & Hoffman J.C. (1984) Clinical and pathological effects of bromocriptine on prolactin secreting and other pituitary tumours. *Journal of Neurosurgery* **60**, 1−7.

Cobb W.E. (1980) Endocrine management after pituitary surgery. In: Post K.D., Jackson I.M.D. & Reichlin S. (Eds), *The Pituitary Adenoma*, pp. 417−435. Plenum Press, New York.

Cusick J.F., Hagen T.C. & Findling J.W. (1984) Inappropriate secretion of antidiuretic hormone after transsphenoidal surgery for pituitary tumours. *New England Journal of Medicine* **311**, 36−38.

Edge W.G. & Whitwam J.G. (1981) Chondro-calcinosis and difficult intubation in acromegaly. *Anaesthesia* **36**, 677−680.

French L.A. & Galicich J.H. (1964) The use of steroids for control of cerebral edema. *Clinical Neurosurgery* **10**, 212−223.

Hardy J. (1971) Transsphenoidal hypophysectomy. *Journal of Neurosurgery* **34**, 582−594.

Jeffreys R.V. (1987) The pituitary adenomas and craniopharyngiomas. In: Miller J.D. (Ed.) *Northfield's Surgery of the Central Nervous System*, 2nd edn, pp. 320−330. Blackwell Scientific Publications, Oxford.

Laws E.R. & Kern E.B. (1975) Complications of trans-sphenoidal surgery. *Clinical Neurosurgery* **23**, 401−416.

Marshall L.F., Jennett B. & Langfitt T.W. (1974) Needle biopsy for the diagnosis of malignant glioma. *Journal of the American Medical Association* **228**, 1417−1418.

Messick J.M., Cucchiara R.F. & Faust R.J. (1982) Airway management in patients with acromegaly. *Anesthesiology* **56**, 157.

Miller J.D. & Leech P. (1975) Effects of mannitol and steroid therapy on intracranial volume−pressure relationships in patients. *Journal of Neurosurgery* **42**, 274−281.

Newfield P., Albin M.S., Chestnut J.S. & Maroon J. (1978) Air embolism during transsphenoidal pituitary operations. *Neurosurgery* **2**, 39−42.

Perks W.H., Horrocks P.M., Cooper R.A. *et al.* (1980) Sleep apnoea in acromegaly. *British Medical Journal* **280**, 894−897.

Swales J.D. (1991) Management of hyponatraemia. *British Journal of Anaesthesia* **67**, 146−153.

Uttley D., Moore A. & Archer D.J. (1989) Surgical management of midline skull-base tumours: a new approach. *Journal of Neurosurgery* **71**, 705−710.

Whitaker S.J., Meanock C.I., Turner J.F. *et al.* (1985) Fluid balance and secretion of antidiuretic hormone following transsphenoidal pituitary surgery. *Journal of Neurosurgery* **63**, 404−412.

Wulff J.D., Proffitt P.Q., Panszi J.G. & Ziegler D.K. (1982) False-negative CTs in astrocytomas: the value of repeat scanning. *Neurology* **32**, 766−769.

9
Anaesthesia for posterior fossa surgery

G. STUART INGRAM AND FRANK J.M. WALTERS

Anatomy and physiology

The posterior fossa is defined as that area bounded by the tentorium cerebelli superiorly, the foramen magnum inferiorly, the occiput posteriorly, and the clivus anteriorly. The clivus supports the pons and is formed from the superior surface of the basilar part of the occiput, and the sloping surface of the sphenoid behind the dorsum sellae. The contents include the midbrain, pons, medulla, and the brainstem, in which the main motor and sensory pathways are situated. The posterior fossa also contains the fourth ventricle, with the respiratory and cardiovascular centres in its floor, the cerebellum, and the lower cranial nerves (Fig. 9.1). A fuller description of the anatomy of the contents of the posterior fossa is given in Chapter 1.

The relatively small size of the posterior fossa, and the presence within it of the major motor and sensory pathways, together with the vital centres controlling the cardiovascular and respiratory systems, means that even localized lesions or small amounts of oedema arising at this site can produce profound neurological changes. It is essential that extensive monitoring is used both during surgery and in the postoperative period. From the third ventricle, cerebrospinal fluid (CSF) passes through the cerebral aqueduct to reach the fourth ventricle before escaping via the two lateral foraminae of Luschka and the medial foramen of Magendie into the subarachnoid space around the brain. Obstruction in the posterior fossa at the level of the aqueduct or fourth ventricle can be caused by a tumour, cyst, oedema or other generalized swelling, which in the presence of continued CSF production from the choroid plexus will then lead to hydrocephalus in the lateral ventricles. The possibility of this happening must be appreciated, particularly in the hours immediately following surgery when brain distension is particularly likely to occur.

Uncontrolled swelling in the posterior fossa will ultimately result in coning. This may take place through the foramen magnum as described

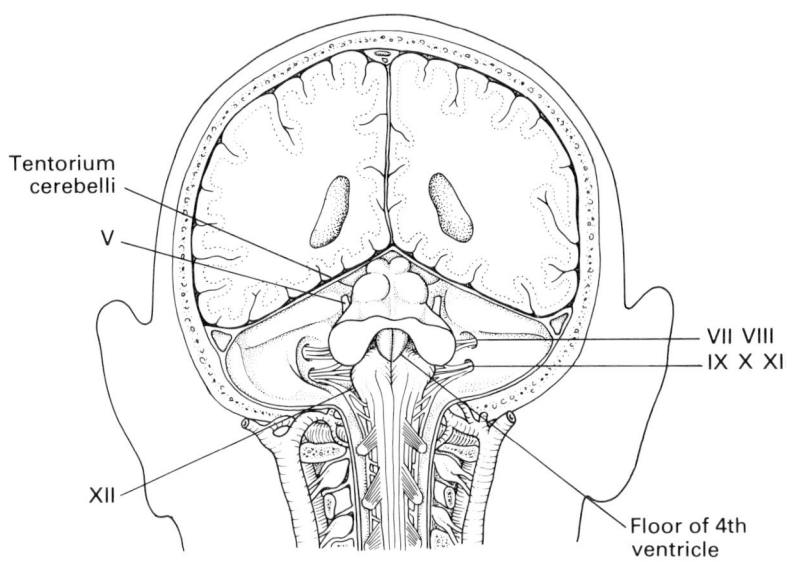

Tentorium
cerebelli

V

VII VIII
IX X XII

XII

Floor of 4th
ventricle

Fig. 9.1 Diagram of the contents of the posterior fossa with the cerebellum removed to reveal the floor of the fourth ventricle and the cranial nerves.

in Chapter 2, or less commonly, as reverse coning where the contents of the posterior fossa are forced upwards into the tentorial hiatus. It can occur in the presence of a large posterior fossa tumour when the lateral ventricles are decompressed, thereby causing a large pressure difference across the tentorium. This may be suspected clinically by the presence of a persistent tachycardia. .

Pathology

In the posterior fossa primary malignant tumours such as astrocytomas are more common in children, whereas secondary tumours in adults frequently metastasize to the cerebellum. Of the benign tumours, meningiomas occur below the tentorium as well as above, and when they arise anteriorly in the midline they present a particularly difficult surgical challenge and may even require an anterior approach transorally or, if high on the clivus, a maxillary split. More commonly meningiomas occur in the cerebellopontine angle, as do acoustic neuromas which are also benign, arising from the eighth nerve. Vascular lesions are uncommon, but angiomas and arteriovenous malformations do occur, as well as aneurysms. The latter generally arise on the posterior inferior cerebellar artery (PICA) and, as this supplies the midbrain, vasospasm can have severe consequences. Compression of the medulla at the foramen magnum may require surgical decompression; this may result from congenital syndromes such as Arnold−Chiari malformations or bony degeneration in the elderly. The cerebellar vermis may reach the cervical vertebrae, obstructing the CSF pathway and producing hydrocephalus in children with the Arnold−Chiari syndrome. Particular care should be taken when moving the head once the patient has been anaesthetized, as any extreme position may interfere with the blood supply to the vital centres in the brainstem which has herniated through the foramen magnum (Meridy *et al.* 1974).

Surgery

The surgical approach to the posterior fossa is through an occipital craniectomy, bone is excised and a defect remains in the skull at the end of the operation. Whilst the anaesthetic management will follow the general principles for intracranial surgery, there are specific additional difficulties. These relate to:

Positioning of the patient;
The risk of air embolism and postural hypotension;
Interference to vital medullary centres;
Damage to cranial nerves;
The potential for hydrocephalus.

In some cases one problem may lead on to another; for instance the choice of sitting position increases the risk of air embolism and postural hypotension.

Prone position (Fig. 9.2)

The patient is positioned with good support under the chest and iliac crests. Care must be taken to ensure free movement of the abdomen and the absence of pressure over the femoral vessels. This allows free venous drainage to reduce the risk of deep-vein thrombosis, and enables the epidural veins and venous sinuses to empty. The prone position gives good surgical access to midline structures, but if heavy bleeding occurs, blood will run down and obscure the surgical field. If head-up tilt is used, a foot support is needed to prevent the patient sliding down

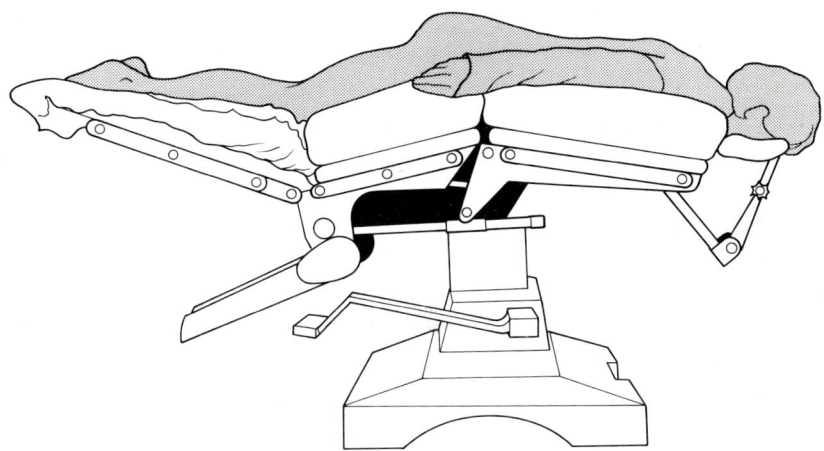

Fig. 9.2 Prone position — the arms are secured to the sides by a sheet folded back under the patient; if more head-up tilt it used a foot piece may be required. From Ingram (1987).

the table. Although air embolism is unlikely to occur, it has been described (Shenkin & Goldfedder 1969).

Lateral position (Fig. 9.3)

In neurosurgical practice this is often referred to as the 'park-bench' position (Gilbert & Brindle 1966) due to its resemblance to a tramp lying on a bench in the park. The patient is placed on the table in a lateral position as described in Chapter 7, but for posterior fossa surgery the body may be slightly rotated towards the prone position, semiprone (Lam 1982). To improve surgical access the upper arm is often pulled down, but care must be taken to avoid injuring the brachial plexus. The neck is flexed and the face rotated towards the floor (Fig. 9.4), ensuring that the jugular veins are not obstructed. The head can be held in a head clamp. If the horseshoe headrest is used, pressure on the lower eye must be avoided. Head-up tilt can be employed to encourage emptying of the venous sinuses.

This position offers a good compromise, especially in older and more frail patients as there is minimal risk of air embolism. It is used for laterally placed lesions, especially those in the cerebellopontine angle, but venous and CSF drainage from the operative field can be poor. However, this position is used successfully in many units where it is

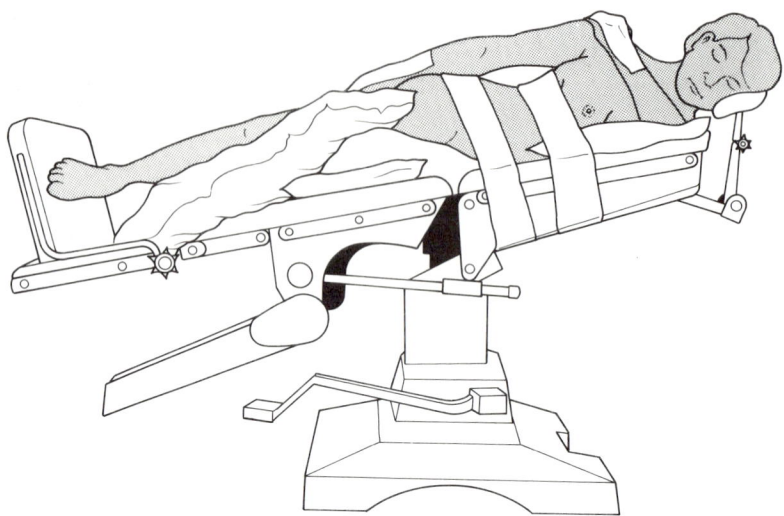

Fig. 9.3 Lateral or 'park bench' position—if strapping is applied around the upper abdomen or lower chest it should not interfere with respiration. The head would ultimately be rotated more towards the floor and secured. From Ingram (1987).

considered that the risks of the sitting position do not justify the surgical advantages.

Sitting position (Fig. 9.5)

The practice of placing patients in the sitting position for posterior fossa surgery originated before World War I, and was popularized by the French neurosurgeon, de Martel (Bingham 1973). At that time, when the techniques of general anaesthesia were limited, it is clear that satisfactory conditions for surgery on the posterior fossa were often lacking when the prone or lateral positions were used. De Martel also advocated the use of local anaesthesia for craniotomy, and influenced Harvey Cushing in changing his own practice from general to local anaesthesia. Cushing did not, however, take up the sitting position, and thus from the outset there were those who felt it to be beneficial despite the additional risks, and others who regarded its use as inherently unsafe.

The advantages of the sitting position are generally stated to be ease of surgical access with good spatial orientation, and free venous and CSF drainage giving a good surgical field. The disadvantages are the problems

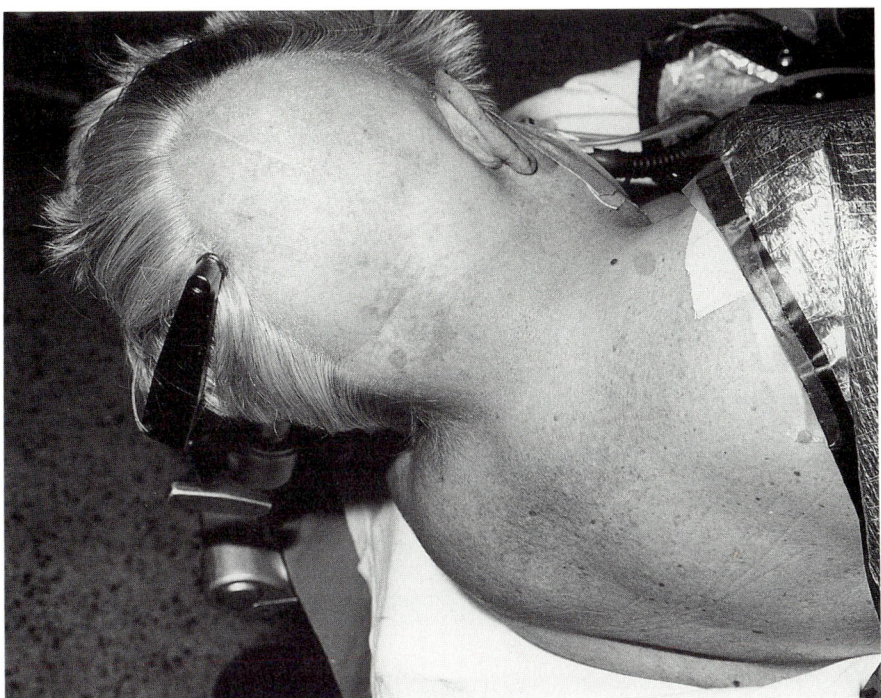

Fig. 9.4 Posterior view of a patient in the lateral position, the head is flexed, rotated and held by a head clamp.

associated with air—embolism and pneumocephalus—and postural hypotension. It is clear that the anaesthetist has to cope with the potential problems, whilst the neurosurgeon reaps the advantages. It is crucial that if the sitting position is used it should only be by mutual agreement, and all involved must fully understand the potential hazards and the measures necessary for their avoidance. In competent and experienced hands the sitting position has a good record of safety (Cuccharia 1984).

In practical terms the sitting position is taken to be any position that allows the surgeon access to the posterior fossa from behind with the head erect. To achieve this the patient may be placed in a range of positions from semirecumbent with extreme head flexion to sitting in a chair with legs dependent. Normally the conventional operating table is arranged so that the body is upright with the head flexed slightly forward to be held in a horseshoe headrest or pinned in a head clamp, and the legs are kept horizontal but slightly flexed (Fig. 9.5). Excluding

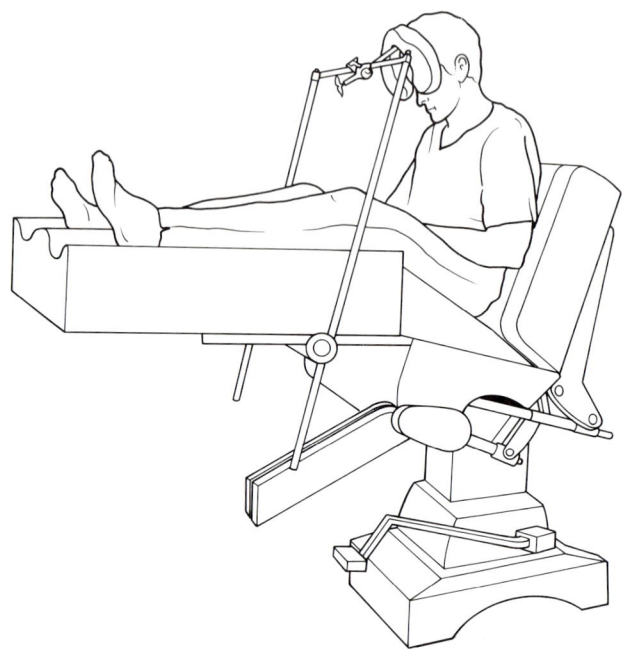

Fig. 9.5 Sitting position—the legs have been elevated and are flexed. Once the head is secured, the operating table can be tilted back if required. From Ingram, 1987.

any preventive measures, the greater the vertical distance between the surgical site and the right atrium, the greater will be the negative pressure in any open vein, and the greater the risk of a significant volume of air being entrained. Figure 9.6 shows the way in which this negative pressure is generated with the upper body fully erect. In practice pressures will be less than this with head flexed. In a series of patients at the National Hospital the mean height between the right atrium and the lower end of the wound was found to be 12.5 cm (Brodrick & Ingram 1988). Similarly with regard to postural hypotension, the more dependent the legs and lower body are placed, the greater the potential will be for it to occur. These problems are not unique to the sitting position; the use of steep head-up tilt for neurosurgery in other positions will expose the patient to the same risks.

Complications: air embolism and postural hypotension

Generally, when a vein is cut during surgery, it collapses, preventing the inflow of air. In the approach to the posterior fossa this is not the case,

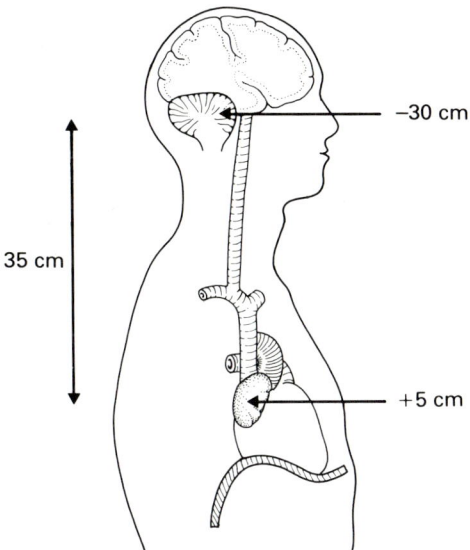

−30 cm

35 cm

+5 cm

Fig. 9.6 Diagrammatic representation of the pressures in the right atrium and intracranial venous system in the erect position.

the venous sinuses do not collapse as they are held open by the surrounding dura, the veins in the skull are held open by their attachment to bone, and outside the skull branches of the sub-occipital plexus may be held open by the fascia of the cervical muscles. The incidence of venous air embolism in the sitting position is variously quoted, usually as between 25% and 40% (Albin *et al.* 1976). However, in the majority of cases the amounts of air will be small and may not be clinically significant, in addition the use of preventive measures, together with the care and skill of the surgeon, can greatly reduce this figure.

MECHANISM AND PHYSIOLOGICAL CHANGES

Entry of air into the venous system occurs either as a large bolus or more insidiously as a slow steady stream of small air bubbles. If a vein is punctured at the operative site and is held open, air will enter the venous system passing through the right atrium and into the pulmonary vascular bed. This will lead to a rise in pulmonary vascular resistance and pulmonary artery pressure, ultimately leading to right ventricular failure with ECG signs of right ventricular strain. There will also be a fall in cardiac output and blood pressure, and an increase in physiological dead space as the bubbles of gas block the pulmonary capillaries, resulting in many alveoli being ventilated but not perfused. There is now a reduction in carbon dioxide exchange causing a sudden fall in the excretion of carbon dioxide (Fig. 9.7).

The mode of respiration can also affect the risk of air embolism. In the past controlled ventilation was held to increase the risks, and spontaneous breathing was recommended (Hunter 1975). Certainly if there is straining on expiration, and an increased intrathoracic pressure, the venous pressure will inevitably be high. But a spontaneously breathing patient in the sitting position who takes a deep inspiration or sigh will generate negative pressures which may well lead to air entry. Now that controlled ventilation is almost always used, the argument is largely academic.

In recent years an awareness of the potential for paradoxical air embolism has raised further concerns about the continued use of the sitting position (Gronert et al. 1979). It is known from post-mortem studies, and has been confirmed intraoperatively using transoesophageal echocardiography (Konstad et al. 1991), that approximately 25% of the general population have a probe patent foramen ovale. The potential therefore exists in these people for air reaching the right atrium to pass directly into the left atrium and enter the systemic circulation. A gradient of 4 mmHg is all that is required to reverse the flow through a shunt, and there is evidence to suggest that pulmonary capillary wedge pressure is lower than the right atrial pressure in patients in the sitting position when air is in the pulmonary vascular bed (Bedford et al. 1981, Perkins-

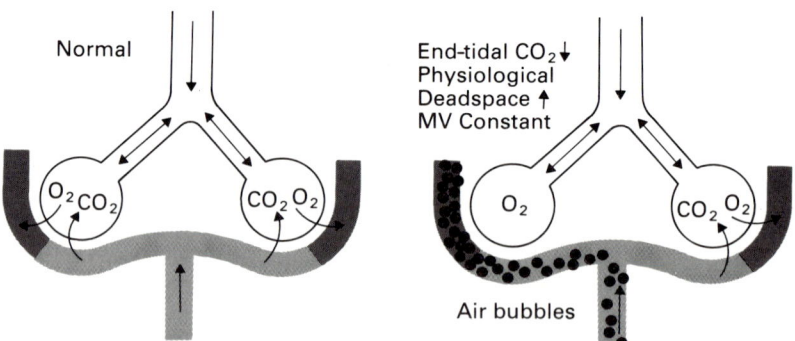

Fig. 9.7 Diagrammatic representation of gaseous exchange in the normal situation on the left. On the right, emboli have obstructed the pulmonary capillary allowing gaseous exchange to take place in only part of the lung, thereby increasing physiological deadspace and decreasing carbon dioxide excretion.

Pearson *et al.* 1982). Furthermore, when there is a significant volume of air in the pulmonary vascular bed there is evidence to suggest that left atrial pressure falls, which will increase the gradient in favour of embolization. It is also possible for paradoxical air embolism to occur in the presence of a normal cardiac anatomy, as the small gas bubbles can cross the pulmonary bed via capillaries or arteriovenous shunts, especially in those patients with raised pulmonary pressure as happens in the presence of air embolism (Clayton *et al.* 1985). If this were to happen in a patient in the sitting position, the air bubbles would form emboli in any organ, but severe complications will arise in the cerebral and coronary circulations. In taking preventive measures against air embolism it is important that this gradient is not reversed.

DETECTION

Precordial Doppler
This device detects the altered reflection of the ultrasonic beams from a blood–gas interface, or bubbles in the blood stream (Michenfelder *et al.* 1972). It is the most sensitive method available, being capable of detecting air bubbles as small as 0.12 ml and hence air entrapment at a rate of 0.2 ml kg^{-1} min^{-1}. The probe, a relatively large flat transducer, is placed over the fourth intercostal space at the right sternal edge; this is the surface marking of the right atrium. Ultrasonic gel is placed on the device, which is then strapped to the chest wall with either tape or a rubber strap. Fixation is important, as any movement will cause the signal to be lost. It has been used successfully with signals focused at a depth of 5–10 cm (Fig. 9.8). Injection of 10 ml of normal saline through a central line has been suggested as a means of checking correct positioning (Tinker *et al.* 1975), but more recently the use of 1 ml of carbon dioxide has been proposed as a more reliable alternative (Schubert *et al.* 1986).

The Doppler technique has two main drawbacks; the first is interference from the diathermy machine. This can be very troublesome as the majority of diathermy occurs when the nuchal muscles are being cut by electrocautery, and this is a period of high risk. Therefore, although machines are available with an automatic cut-out during diathermy, the monitoring cannot be continuous. The second drawback is the familiarity of the observer, who needs to be trained to detect the subtle changes that occur when air passes under the transducer. The normal sounds for

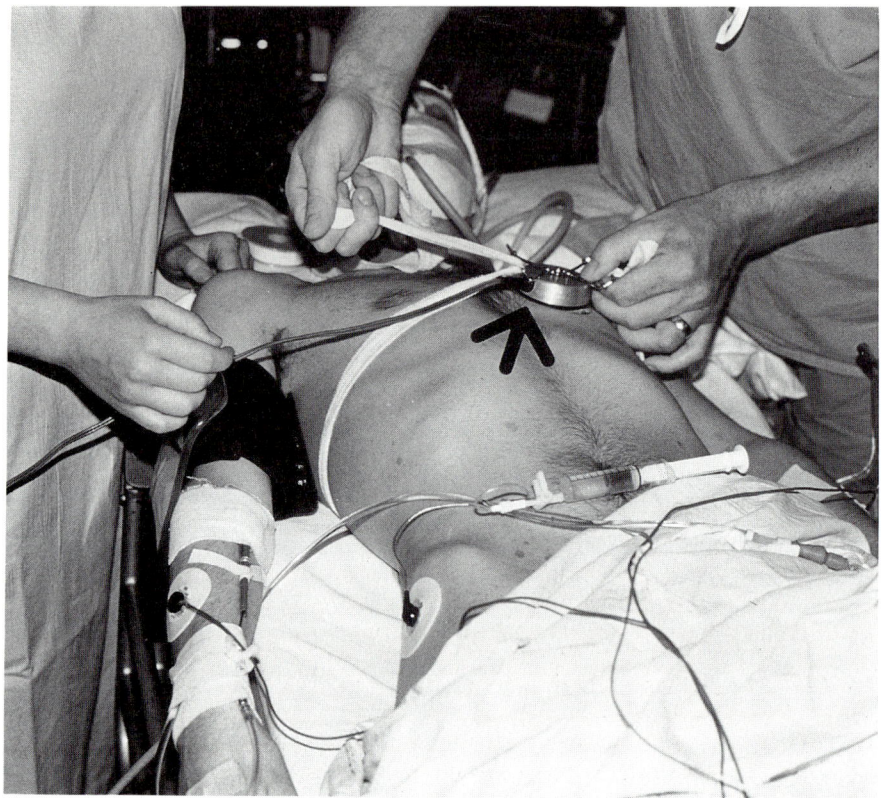

Fig. 9.8 Flat Doppler probe being positioned over the precordium to detect air emboli.

each heart beat, when heard through the Doppler, consist of rough, regular, and low frequency double sound; when air embolism occurs there is a chirping sound superimposed on top of this regular rhythm. Critics of the technique have suggested that the device is oversensitive as it detects air which is clinically insignificant, but with the recognized risk of paradoxical air embolism, this view is difficult to sustain.

Capnograph

When air embolism occurs there is a decrease in excretion of carbon dioxide, which can be detected by continuous monitoring with a capnograph (Bethune & Brechner 1968). Clinically the end-tidal carbon dioxide trace falls as shown in Fig. 9.9; this provides a quantitative indication of the volume of air and the rate of entrainment. The technique is

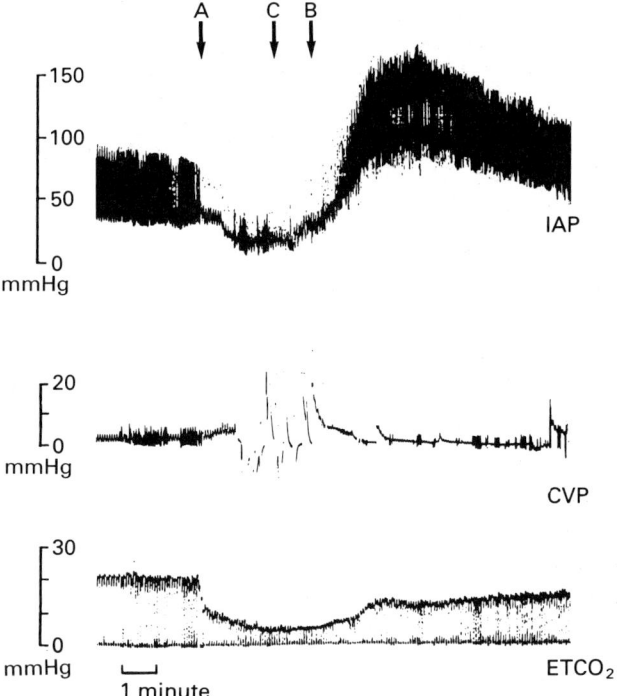

Fig. 9.9 Air embolism — at A: a change in the Doppler signal was noted. At B: an antigravity suit was inflated. At C: air was aspirated from the right atrial catheter, disturbing the CVP trace. From Brodrick (1987).

approximately half as sensitive as the Doppler, detecting air embolism at a rate of $0.4\,\mathrm{ml\,kg^{-1}\,min^{-1}}$ (Gildenberg *et al.* 1981). It has been suggested that this method has an advantage over the Doppler technique as it only detects 'significant air embolism', thereby minimizing delays to the surgery. Confusion can, however, arise when interference with the brainstem by compression, for example, results in an arrhythmia, bradycardia or other response resulting in an abrupt decrease in cardiac output (Fig. 9.10). A decrease in end-tidal carbon dioxide will follow, and this may be falsely interpreted as an air embolism, but in either event the surgeon needs to be warned immediately.

Pulmonary artery pressure
When air enters the pulmonary circulation the pulmonary artery pressure increases, the increase being proportional to the severity of the

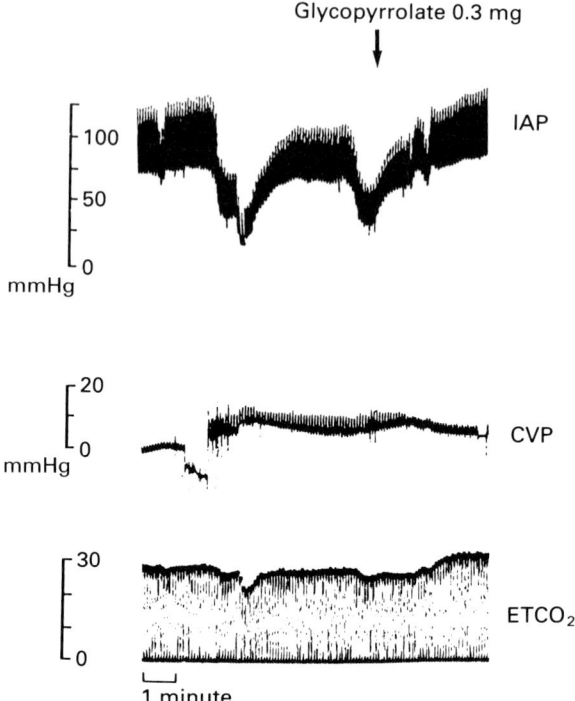

Glycopyrrolate 0.3 mg

Fig. 9.10 Brainstem manipulation—a marked bradycardia has occurred and the end-tidal carbon dioxide has fallen, it would fall further with greater cardiovascular collapse. From Brodrick (1987).

embolism. As an invasive and somewhat difficult technique it is not used in the UK at present, but as it makes possible the identification of patients at risk from paradoxical air embolism by measuring pulmonary capillary wedge pressure and calculating the gradient between right and left atrium, this may change in the future (Marshall & Bedford 1980). The potential for use of Swan–Ganz catheters in neurosurgical practice has been reviewed by Pritz (1986).

Pulse oximetry
As a now widely available, non-invasive method of monitoring, pulse oximetry would be used in any patient undergoing anaesthesia for neurosurgery. Although it does not detect air embolism as early as a capnograph, it is very valuable in the management of an established embolism.

Oesophageal methods
A Doppler with a 360° arc can be positioned in the oesophagus so that the transducer is level with the aortic arch; this has the advantage of overcoming some of the difficulties with precordial placement.

Two-dimensional transoesophageal echocardiography allows the direct visualization, on a screen, of air entering the heart; in addition it can be used to identify patients with probe patent foramen ovale (Rafferty 1992). It is, however, far too expensive for general use and would require someone to watch the screen at all times.

End-tidal nitrogen
An increase in end-tidal nitrogen mirrors the decrease in end-tidal carbon dioxide when air enters the circulation; but nitrogen increase is specific to air embolism and will not result from the circulatory changes that can confuse end-tidal carbon dioxide monitoring. A dedicated mass spectrometer is required, centralized mass spectrometers covering a number of theatres will cause a delay in diagnosis. With small emboli the changes in nitrogen may be difficult to detect, and in general they tend to be of short duration.

Other vascular changes
When there is obstruction to right ventricular outflow a rise in central venous pressure (CVP) will occur, but it would be a relatively late sign. Decrease in blood pressure, right heart strain and dysrhythmias on the ECG, and the presence of a mill-wheel murmur on auscultation, all require large volumes of air.

PREVENTION

Use of nitrous oxide
If air enters the circulation, and the patient is breathing nitrous oxide, then nitrous oxide will diffuse into the embolism and increase its volume. It can be argued that by making the bubbles larger, nitrous oxide aids detection. But equally it must mean that some small air bubbles which would not be clinically significant will enlarge and become so. Clinical studies with 50% nitrous oxide are reassuring (Losasso *et al.* 1992). Certainly if clinically significant air embolism occurs, nitrous oxide should be discontinued.

Volume loading
Patients will often have undergone a degree of voluntary or involuntary fluid restriction preoperatively. In addition to correcting this deficiency, increasing the CVP, provided that the patient's cardiovascular system will tolerate it, will reduce the hydrostatic negative pressure. In addition, if other methods are used such as positive end-expiratory pressure (PEEP) or bandaging, their effect will be more marked if the circulation is well-filled.

PEEP
PEEP, up to a maximum of 10 cm, has been used as a means of decreasing the incidence of air embolism (Lee *et al.* 1981). By raising the pressure in the venous system the negative pressure at an open vein in the posterior fossa will be reduced. But if the patient is fluid-depleted or if cardiovascular reflexes are insufficient the decrease in venous return created by PEEP may lead to a marked decrease in blood pressure. It has been suggested that by increasing right atrial pressure the use of PEEP might increase the risk of paradoxical embolism. Zasslow *et al.* (1988) have shown that 10 cm of PEEP does not change the gradient between left and right atrial pressure, but despite this finding its relevance to clinical safety has been questioned (Drummond 1988).

Compression of the abdomen and/or the lower limbs
Elasticated bandages may be applied to the legs to prevent venous pooling. The medical antishock trousers (MAST), designed for use in trauma and the antigravity suit, as used in aviation, are both used. They can be inflated to a set pressure up to 60 mmHg and compress both the legs and lower abdomen. The MAST may put pressure on the lateral peroneal nerves, whereas the G-suit is designed to avoid this problem. Brodrick and Ingram (1988) demonstrated mean increases in 40 sitting patients of 7 mmHg in CVP using a combination of the G-suit inflated to 60 mmHg and 10 cmH₂O of PEEP.

Central venous catheters
A CVP catheter is valuable as a means of assessing the effectiveness of the methods described above to raise venous pressure; it is also of value in diagnosis, but in addition, if air does enter the circulation, it potentially offers a method of aspiration. For this to be successful the position of the catheter is important; for standard catheters 3 cm above the sinoatrial node close to the point at which the superior vena cava enters the right

atrium appears to be most effective (Bunegin *et al.* 1981). X-ray or intracardiac ECG (Michenfelder *et al.* 1969b) have been used to aid placement. However, the recovery of air is greatly improved when a multiple-orifice catheter is used. A specially designed catheter, the 'Bunegin-Albin', is available commercially.

It has to be recognized that none of the preventive measures described above will guarantee the avoidance of an air embolism, but in combination they can raise venous pressure to a level at which air embolism is very unlikely to occur. Clearly, as in any type of surgery, the anaesthetist wants to keep the venous pressure at the surgical field low to minimize venous bleeding, and to achieve this a combination of good venous drainage and positioning is used. In the sitting position venous drainage is excellent, but the negative pressure created leads to the risk of air embolism. If venous pressure is then increased to a height equivalent to just below the wound, then the situation is similar to any other operation, and if air enters an open vein it will not be immediately drawn into the circulation by a large negative pressure. If attempts to increase venous pressure are excessive, then venous bleeding at the operative site will interfere with surgery.

At the National Hospital the practice is to ensure that the patient is well hydrated prior to induction, and to put a G-suit on the patient once he or she is anaesthetized. The patient is then placed on the operating table in the sitting position with careful monitoring of the blood pressure. If postural hypotension is a problem the patient can be returned to the horizontal and elevated more slowly, or the G-suit can be immediately inflated. Once the G-suit is inflated to 60 mmHg the CVP is measured in relation to the height of the posterior fossa. PEEP can then be applied and further fluid loading with colloid used to achieve a CVP that corresponds to a height close to the lower end of the wound. PEEP is only applied and released once the G-suit is inflated, to minimize blood pressure changes. The G-suit is generally kept inflated for the duration of the operation. Particular care is always taken in removing PEEP or the pressurization of the G-suit, as it is recognized that the sudden reduction of venous pressure is particularly likely to encourage the entry of air.

TREATMENT

Should embolism occur or be suspected:

1 immediately inform the surgeon;

2 the surgeon should flood the field with saline and occlude the wound edges with wet swabs;

3 ventilate the patient with 100% oxygen;

4 raise the venous pressure (squeeze the jugular veins in the neck, Fig. 9.11);

5 aspirate for air from the CVP catheter;

6 if the situation has stabilized the surgeon can look for the open vein—with jugular compression this should now be bleeding;

7 if the situation continues to deteriorate the table must be levelled or placed head-down and general resuscitation measures commenced.

General problems with positioning

Some problems are common to all three positions, although they do not influence the relative merits of each. Pressure on peripheral nerves can result from faulty positioning or lack of adequate padding, and in prolonged surgery peripheral nerve lesions can occur. In the sitting position the arms need to be well supported to avoid traction on the brachial

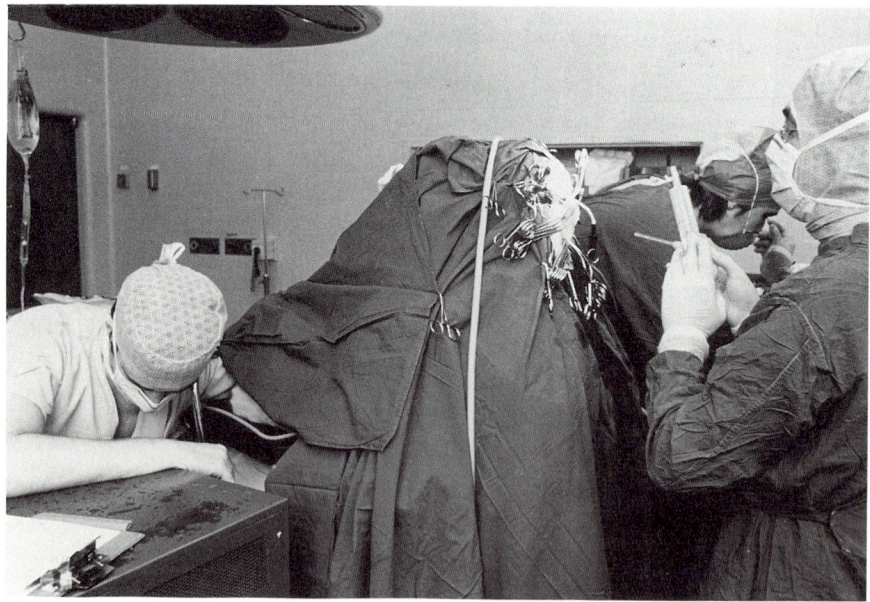

Fig. 9.11 Patient in the sitting position. Air emboli have been detected and the anaesthetist is squeezing the neck to obstruct the jugular veins.

plexus; the ulnar nerve is also vulnerable and the arms are best placed in front of the patient as in Fig. 9.5. The risks to the brachial plexus in the lateral position have been described above.

In the lower limbs, sciatic nerve damage as a result of severe flexion of the hips with the knees straight in the sitting position has been described; the knees should be flexed. The common peroneal nerve in the lower legs should always be well padded in the lateral position, and it is also vulnerable in other positions. When a patient is supported on firm blocks placed over the upper thigh in the prone position the femoral and lateral cutaneous nerves are at risk.

The endotracheal tube should be checked as a matter of routine following final head positioning on the operating table to avoid the possibility of tube migration resulting in one-lung anaesthesia (Conrardy *et al.* 1976). Excessive head flexion can also lead to jugular venous obstruction, and the anaesthetist should ensure that at least the space of two fingers exists between the chin and suprasternal notch. The more horizontally the patient is placed in the sitting position, the more head flexion is needed and the more likely jugular venous obstruction is to occur.

Complications of surgery in the posterior fossa

Some of the problems encountered peroperatively are due to stimulation of the vital centres and retraction of the medulla or midbrain. The cardiovascular centre is in the grey matter in the floor of the fourth ventricle (Fig. 9.12). Hypertension and bradycardia or other dysrhythmias may occur when the periventricular grey area and the medullary reticular formation, ventral to the grey area, are stimulated (Artru *et al.* 1980). The majority of dysrhythmias occur while the surgeon is operating in the vicinity of the pons and roots of the fifth, ninth and tenth nerves. Surgery in this region may be accompanied by a sudden marked rise in blood pressure. Direct stimulation of the vagus will cause severe bradycardia and stimulation of the trigeminal nerve, hypertension. The apneustic centre (APC), which is the normal inspiratory cut-off mechanism, and the dorsal group of neurones (DRG) responsible for the initiation of rhythmic breathing are situated near the cardiovascular centre. If these centres are damaged significantly, the respiratory drive may be seriously disturbed, causing either apnoea or inadequate breathing. The effects may be permanent from direct trauma or temporary due to oedema resulting from injury to adjacent tissues. As the two centres are

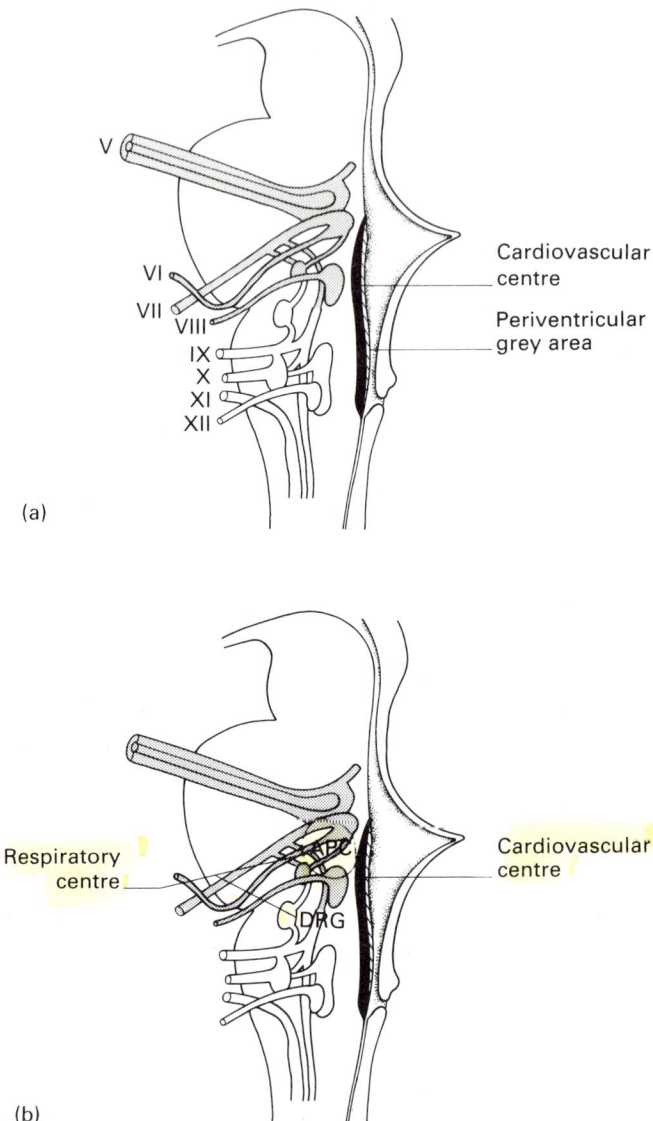

(a)

(b)

Fig. 9.12 Diagram of the pons and medulla containing the fifth to twelfth cranial nerves and nuclei. In the floor of the fourth ventricle is the periventricular grey area, the cardiovascular centre and nearby the respiratory centre represented by the apneustic centre (APC) and the dorsal group of neurones (DRG).

adjacent any injury to one is likely to effect the other (Fig. 9.12). A continuous record of pulse rate, blood pressure and ECG is an effective method of monitoring brainstem retraction, and provides a warning of the brainstem being compromised (Michenfelder *et al.* 1969a). In a paralysed and ventilated patient, therefore, cardiovascular changes may be the only warning the anaesthetist gets that the surgeon is trespassing into the vital centres. Should such changes occur the surgeon should be warned. If further dissection or retraction is unavoidable, the cardiovascular complications can be treated with conventional drugs, remembering that these warning signs have now been obtunded and postoperative respiratory failure may occur.

More recently brainstem auditory evoked potentials (BAEP) monitoring has been used for the detection of untoward surgical dissection near the brainstem, particularly during surgery for acoustic neuromas. Its advocates argue that it is a more sensitive monitor than cardiovascular change during brainstem manipulation. Others argue that the changes are small, and in practice difficult to interpret in a clinical environment.

In some centres spontaneous breathing is maintained during critical periods of surgery so that the breathing pattern can be monitored, using any changes seen as a monitor of surgical transgression into the respiratory centre. This is because changes in respiratory pattern are detectable before any alteration in blood pressure or ECG during manipulation of the vital centre. If, as is usual, controlled ventilation is used for most of the operation, and the patient only allowed to breathe spontaneously during brainstem dissection, this requires great skill from the anaesthetist if the surgical conditions are to remain satisfactory. Carbon dioxide tension will inevitably increase, as will cerebral blood flow, and this may result in poor conditions due to brain swelling. In practice operating conditions are acceptable, probably because of the considerable CSF and venous drainage which takes place. The majority practice in the UK, as elsewhere, is to maintain controlled ventilation and accept the loss of respiration as a monitor of brainstem integrity (Frost 1984).

The sensory nucleus of the trigeminal nerve receiving inputs from the cornea, mandible and anterior two-thirds of the tongue, the motor nucleus for the abducent nerve, the facial nerve and the sensory nucleus for the vestibular component of the eighth nerve are all situated in the dorsal pons and medulla (Fig. 9.12). Therefore they too are at risk from injury during surgery in the posterior fossa. It has been suggested that observation of clinical signs can detect different cranial nerve integrity

Table 9.1 Cranial nerve stimulation in posterior fossa surgery

V	Motor — jaw jerk	
	Sensory — hypertension, bradycardia	
VII	Facial twitch	
X	Hypotension, bradycardia	
XI	Shoulder jerk	

peroperatively (Table 9.1). This is difficult when the patient is prone or in the park-bench position.

During surgery for acoustic neuromas the facial nerve is particularly vulnerable due to the proximity of the nerve to the tumour, especially if it is stretched over it. The nerve can be identified by the surgeon using a pair of dissecting forceps which is also a nerve stimulator. Electromyographic needles placed preoperatively in the face will detect action potentials, and when connected to a loudspeaker will alert the surgeon. This technique precludes the use of full neuromuscular block.

Anaesthetic management

Preoperative assessment

A space-occupying lesion in the posterior fossa can produce the following complications which should be assessed clinically, biochemically and radiologically: (1) raised intracranial pressure is due either to the size of a space-occupying lesion or the production of hydrocephalus by obstruction of CSF flow. Assessment of the intracranial status preoperatively is important; (2) hypovolaemia and electrolyte disturbance are relatively uncommon in adults, but do occur in small children who are severely ill with nausea and vomiting; and (3) cranial nerve involvement may cause a bulbar palsy which will impair both swallowing and the normal glottic protective reflexes, which in turn will lead to a risk of aspiration pneumonia.

Premedication

Patients with lesions in the posterior fossa are particularly sensitive to the respiratory depression caused by opiates and other sedatives, particularly in the presence of raised intracranial pressure and significant brain-stem pathology. In practice premedication consists of a benzodiazepine, diazepam or temazepam, given orally combined with metoclopramide. However, if the patient is drowsy, premedication should be omitted.

Monitoring

The monitoring needs are dictated by the requirements outlined for any neurosurgical operation (Chapter 7), the need to detect the occurrence of air embolism and inadvertent surgical damage to the vital centres in the brainstem. Therefore it is necessary to routinely monitor ECG, arterial pressure continuously with an arterial line, end-tidal carbon dioxide, CVP and temperature as these operations are long and it is easy for the patient to become cold.

Induction and maintenance

INDUCTION

The requirements are the same as for all patients with intracranial pathology: smooth induction with minimal changes in blood pressure (Chapter 7). When surgery involves the brainstem or cerebellopontine angle it is wise to insert a nasogastric tube following induction, to minimize the risk of aspiration in the immediate postoperative period when there is a risk of a temporary bulbar paresis.

MAINTENANCE

In principle, the technique for maintaining anaesthesia is the same as that for any craniotomy. When a patient is not fully paralysed to allow motor nerve monitoring, a propofol infusion can be helpful in preventing sudden movement. Should the patient become light, he or she is less likely to give a sudden cough. In addition, recovery is calmer with no coughing particularly when the head is manipulated while releasing the head fixator (Chapter 7). When the patient is in the sitting position careful monitoring and cautious use of drugs is more important than a particular technique.

Postoperative management and complications

Respiratory complications

Respiratory failure is one of the most important postoperative complications following posterior fossa surgery, presenting as either an abnormal pattern of breathing or apnoea. This can be due to a variety of
pathological changes which can affect the respiratory centre, including
pressure from oedema or acute hydrocephalus and ischaemia following
trauma to the delicate vasculature. Respiratory failure must be treated
by intubation and ventilation (Chapter 15). Patients who are particularly at risk are those where the operation has involved midline structures, in particular the fourth ventricle where, typically, surgery is for
removal of subependymal ependymomas, choroid plexus papillomas
and medulloblastomas.

When medullary herniation is seen at operation there is a high risk
of postoperative apnoea. In these situations the neuromuscular block is
reversed and the patient woken up and observed in an intensive care
unit for 24—48 h. If there is any abnormality in the respiratory pattern
the patient is immediately reintubated and ventilated. For any patient
who may be at risk postoperatively, it is most important to plan admission
to an intensive care unit or high-dependency care unit, and to consider
with the surgeons whether there are indications for elective ventilation.
A decision to ventilate limits the degree of neurological assessment
possible, but with better short-acting sedative drugs this is an area in
which opinion is changing. Whatever the decision, close observation
will allow the early identification and management of complications,
which may be very sudden. Patients particularly at risk would be those
who had undergone major surgical dissection of the brainstem and had
suffered recognized trauma to the vital centres.

Respiratory obstruction, partial or total, may occur as a result of
acute swelling of the tongue or soft tissues in the immediate postoperative period. The exact mechanism is unclear, but it has been suggested
that it may be due to local trauma, venous obstruction, or possibly some
neurogenic mechanism (Moore *et al.* 1988).

Cranial nerve complications

Loss of cranial nerve function can happen with significant clinical effects.
Damage to the sensory portion of the trigeminal nuclei will result in loss

of corneal sensation and the development of corneal drying, which can be prevented by either temporary protective means or tarsorrhaphy. More seriously, loss of the ninth, tenth and twelfth cranial nerves can result in impairment of swallowing, by causing uncoordinated muscle contraction and loss of the protective laryngeal reflexes. As a consequence secretions will tend to accumulate, and repeated aspiration of small volumes of fluid will cause aspiration pneumonia and, if severe enough, respiratory failure. This may on occasions be anticipated, particularly if there have been several episodes of cardiovascular disturbance peroperatively, indicating significant brainstem stress. A nasogastric tube is inserted before extubation, oral fluids withheld, antiemetics such as metoclopramide given electively, and the patient nursed in an intensive care unit. On extubation the gag reflex can be tested and, if impaired, methods to protect the airway should be actively considered. In the short term this can be achieved by an endotracheal tube or a tracheostomy in the immediate postoperative period (Chapter 15). Tracheostomy has the advantage of more easily allowing the patient to breathe spontaneously and be unsedated. Should aspiration occur at all postoperatively, then these measures should be undertaken without further delay. Permanent dysfunction, if unrecognized, will allow chronic aspiration to occur.

Pneumocephalus

This complication involves an intracranial collection of air becoming compressed, and is associated with a rise in intracranial pressure. During surgery CSF is drained out, the combination of steroids, mannitol and hypocapnia reduce brain bulk and thus air is entrained, the volume being greater when patients are sitting up. This problem has been generally reported, therefore, in patients in the sitting position, but it has occurred in the supine position (Miller & Furman 1983). During the recovery phase brain bulk increases due to oedema formation, hypocapnia and reformation of CSF; thus air trapped between the arachnoid and dura mater comes under increasing pressure. Nitrous oxide will diffuse into the air space and may aggravate the situation, but symptoms from pneumocephalus can occur 1½ h after withdrawal of nitrous oxide (Friedman *et al.* 1981).

Pneumocephalus may therefore present some time after the end of the operation. Characteristically there is delayed return of consciousness, with some deterioration in the neurological state, but cardiac arrest due to coning has been described (Thiagarajah *et al.* 1982). Therefore the diagnosis should always be considered in any patient with unexplained postoperative deterioration, especially if the patient has been operated on in the sitting position.

Techniques to prevent the syndrome include attempts to flush out the air with saline via a subdermal catheter as the dura is closed. It has been suggested that nitrous oxide be terminated 15 min before the dura is closed, but more recently it has been shown that when nitrous oxide is continued to the end of the procedure there is no rise in ICP (Pandit *et al.* 1982). A reduction in ventilation towards the end of the operation may, by allowing the arterial carbon dioxide tension to rise, encourage the brain bulk to increase a little, so displacing the air before the dura is closed. The air can linger in the cranial vault for up to 2 weeks, and its presence should be borne in mind if the patient is anaesthetized again during this period.

References

Albin M.S., Babinski M., Maroon J.C. & Jannetta P.J. (1976) Anaesthetic management of posterior fossa surgery in the sitting position. *Acta Anaesthesiologica Scandinavica* **20**, 117–128.

Artru A.A., Cucchiari R.F. & Messick J.M. (1980) Cardiorespiratory and cranial-nerve sequelae of surgical procedures involving the posterior fossa. *Anesthesiology* **52**, 83–86.

Bedford R.F., Marshall W.K., Butler A. & Welsh J.E. (1981) Cardiac catheters for diagnosis and treatment of venous air embolism. A prospective study in man. *Journal of Neurosurgery* **55**, 610–614.

Bethune R.W.M. & Brechner V.L. (1968) Detection of venous air embolism by carbon dioxide monitoring. *Anesthesiology* **29**, 178.

Bingham W.F. (1973) The early history of neurosurgical anaesthesia. *Journal of Neurosurgery* **39**, 568–584.

Brodrick P.M. (1987) The sitting position; monitoring, diagnosis and treatment of air embolism. In: Jewkes D.A. (Ed.), *Anaesthesia for Neurosurgery, Baillière's Clinical Anaesthesiology*, pp. 419–440. Baillière Tindall, London.

Brodrick P.M. & Ingram G.S. (1988) The antigravity suit in neurosurgery. *Anaesthesia* **43**, 762–765.

Bunegin L., Albin M.S., Helsel P.E., Hoffman A. & Hung T.-K. (1981) Positioning the right atrial catheter: a model for reappraisal. *Anesthesiology* **55**, 343–348.

Clayton D.G., Evans P., Williams C. & Thurlow A.C. (1985) Paradoxical air embolism during neurosurgery. *Anaesthesia* **40**, 981–989.

Conrardy P.A., Goodman L.R. & Lainge F. (1976) Alterations in endotracheal tube position. Flexion and extension of the neck. *Critical Care Medicine* **1**, 7–12.

Cuccharia R.F. (1984) Safety of the sitting position. *Anesthesiology* **61**, 790.

Drummond J.C. (1988) The use of PEEP in patients in the sitting position. *Anesthesiology* **69**, 798–799.

Friedman G.A., Norfleet E.A. & Bedford R.F. (1981) Discontinuance of nitrous oxide does not prevent tension pneumocephalus. *Anesthesia and Analgesia* **60**, 57–58.

Frost E.A.M. (1984) Some inquiries in neuroanesthesia and neurological support-ive care. *Journal of Neurosurgery* **60**, 673–686.

Gilbert R.G.B. & Brindle G.F. (1966) Anaesthesia for neurosurgery. *International Anesthesiology Clinics* **4**, 836.

Gildenberg P.L., O'Brien R.P., Britt W.J. & Frost E.A.M. (1981) The efficacy of Doppler monitoring for the detection of venous air embolism. *Journal of Neurosurgery* **54**, 75–78.

Gronert G.A., Messick J.M., Cucchiara R.F. and Michenfelder J.D. (1979) Para-doxical air embolism from a patent foramen ovale. *Anesthesiology* **50**, 548–549.

Hunter A.R. (1975) *Neurosurgical Anaesthesia*, 2nd edn, p. 243. Blackwell Scientific Publications, Oxford.

Ingram S. (1987) Posterior fossa surgery—patient position and mode of venti-lation. In: Jewkes D.A. (Ed.), *Anaesthesia for Neurosurgery, Baillières Clinical Anaesthesiology*, pp. 405–417. Baillières, Tindall, London.

Konstadt S.N., Louie E.K., Black S., Rao T.L.K. & Scanlon P. (1991) Intraoperative dectection of a patent foramen ovale by transoesophageal echocardiography. *Anesthesiology* **74**, 212–216.

Lam A.M. (1982) Proper positioning of the patient. *International Anesthesiology Clinics* **20**, 139–147.

Lee D.S., Lichtmann M.W. & Weintraub H.D. (1981) Effect of PEEP on air embolism during sitting neurosurgical procedures. *Anesthesia and Analgesia* **60**, 262.

Losasso T.J., Muzzi D.A., Dietz N.M. & Cuccharia R.F. (1992) Fifty percent nitrous oxide does not increase the risk of venous air embolism in neuro-surgical patients operated on in the sitting position. *Anesthesiology* **77**, 21–30.

Marshall W.K. & Bedford R.F. (1980) Use of a pulmonary-artery catheter for detection and treatment of venous air embolism: a prospective study in man. *Anesthesiology* **52**, 131–134.

Meridy H.W., Creighton R.E. & Humphreys R.P. (1974) Complications during neurosurgery in the prone position in children. *Canadian Anaesthetist Society Journal* **21**, 445–453.

Michenfelder J.D., Gronert G.A. & Rehder K. (1969a) Neuroanesthesia. *Anes-thesiology* **30**, 65–100.

Michenfelder J.D., Martin J.T. & Altenburg B.M. (1969b) Air embolism during neurosurgery. An evaluation of right-atrial catheters for diagnosis and treatment. *Journal of the American Medical Association* **208**, 1353–1358.

Michenfelder J.D., Miller R.H. and Gronert G.A. (1972) Evaluation of an ultrasonic device (Doppler) for the diagnosis of venous air embolism. *Anesthesiology* **36**, 164–167.

Miller C.F. & Furman W.R. (1983) Symptomatic pneumocephalus after translabyrinthine acoustic neuroma excision and nitrous oxide anesthesia. *Anesthesiology* **58**, 281–283.

Moore J.K., Chaudri S., Moore A.P. & Easton J. (1988) Macroglossia and posterior fossa disease. *Anaesthesia* **43**, 382–385.

Pandit U.A., Mudge B.J., Keller T.S. *et al.* (1982) Pneumocephalus after posterior fossa exploration in the sitting position. *Anaesthesia* **37**, 996–1001.

Perkins-Pearson N.A.K., Marshall W.K. & Bedford R.F. (1982) Atrial pressure in the seated position: implication for paradoxical air embolism. *Anesthesiology* **57**, 493–497.

Pritz M.B. (1986) Swan–Ganz catheter monitoring in neurosurgical patients: Theoretical and practical aspects. *Surgical Neurology* **25**, 67–70.

Rafferty T.D. (1992) Intraoperative transoesophageal saline-contrast imaging of flow-patent foramen ovale. *Anesthesia and Analgesia* **75**, 475–480.

Schubert A., Drummond J.C., Peterson D.G. *et al.* (1986) A comparison of CO_2 and saline injection as tests of adequate Doppler placement in neurosurgery. *Anesthesia and Analgesia* **65** (Suppl.), S135.

Shenkin H.N. & Goldfedder P. (1969) Air embolism from exposure of the posterior cranial fossa in the prone position. *Journal of the American Medical Association* **210**, 726.

Thiagarajah S., Frost E.A.M., Singh T. & Shulmann K. (1982) Cardiac arrest associated with tension pneumocephalus. *Anesthesiology* **56**, 73–75.

Tinker J.H., Gronert G.A., Messick J.M. & Michenfelder J.D. (1975) Detection of air embolism: a test for positioning of right atrial catheter and Doppler probe. *Anesthesiology* **43**, 104–106.

Zasslow M.A., Pearl R.G., Larson C.P., Silverberg G. & Shuer L.F. (1988) PEEP does not affect left atrial–right atrial pressure difference in neurosurgical patients. *Anesthesiology* **68**, 760–763.

10
Anaesthesia for vascular surgery

EDWARD MOSS

Introduction

Patients who present with a cerebrovascular accident may have a lesion which can be treated surgically. Symptoms are due to cerebral ischaemia or haemorrhage into brain tissue or cerebrospinal fluid (CSF). Management includes identification of the lesion by clinical and radiological examination, and either prevention of further haemorrhage or improvement of the circulation to the affected area. Surgical management includes clipping of intracranial aneurysms, excision of arteriovenous malformations (AVM), drainage of haematomata and repair or bypass of stenotic areas in the blood vessels supplying the brain. Over recent years radiological techniques have been developed which allow the occlusion of inaccessible or surgically untreatable aneurysms and AVMs with microspheres, coils and histoacryl glue inserted into the cerebral vessels through intravascular catheters (Halbach *et al.* 1989). Modern anaesthetic techniques have contributed to a reduction in morbidity and mortality from these conditions, largely due to an increased understanding of the pathophysiological processes and the effects of anaesthetic agents and procedures on these processes.

Intracranial aneurysms

Intracranial aneurysms are situated mainly on the circle of Willis and almost always occur at junctions or bifurcations of major vessels; usually where there is a bend changing the axial flow of the blood which maximizes the haemodynamic stress. They occur where there is a weakness or deficiency of the muscular coat which may be congenital. They are frequently associated with Ehlers–Danlos syndrome, coarctation of the aorta and polycystic disease of the kidneys. The most common acquired cause is atherosclerosis and the most common sites are the internal carotid system (41%), the anterior cerebral artery (34%) and

239

the middle cerebral artery (20%). Within the internal carotid system, 61% of aneurysms are on the posterior cerebral artery, and 84% of those on the anterior cerebral system are on the anterior communicating artery. Only 4.5% of aneurysms occur on the basilar and vertebral arteries and its branches (Fig. 10.1) (Shaw 1987). Half of the aneurysms in the vertebrobasilar system occur on the basilar artery, and the remainder are generally on the vertebral or posterior inferior cerebellar arteries. They are most common in the 40–60-year age group, and 60% occur in women; 4% of people have asymptomatic aneurysms and 15–20/100 000 have a subarachnoid haemorrhage from an aneurysm. One-third of those that rupture are on the anterior communicating and middle cerebral arteries. Aneurysms do not generally rupture until they are more than 5 mm in diameter and most commonly present with a subarachnoid haemorrhage or intracerebral haematoma. Sometimes the presenting feature is a focal neurological deficit due to pressure of an enlarging aneurysm on surrounding structures such as the optic nerve.

A subarachnoid haemorrhage presents typically with a sudden head-

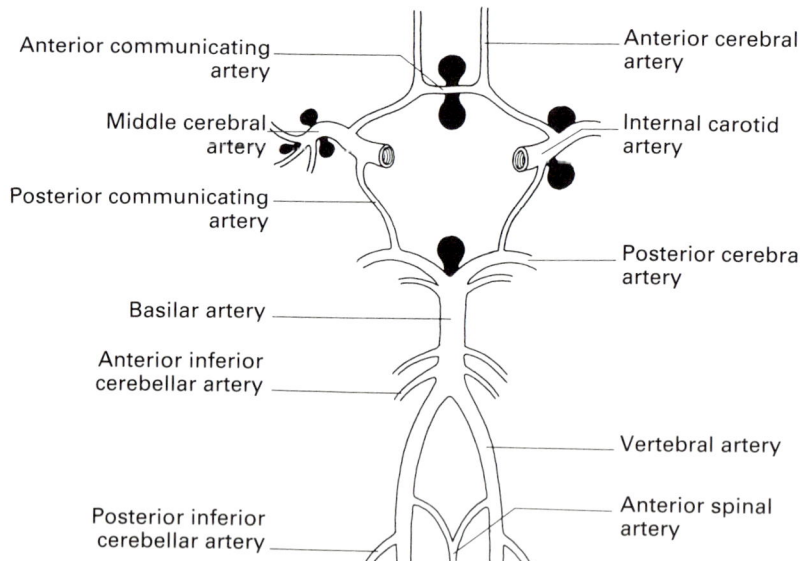

Fig. 10.1 Diagram of the major cerebral arteries with the common sites for the development of aneurysms. Internal Carotid system (41%); posterior communicating artery (61%); anterior cerebral artery (34%); anterior communicating artery (84%); middle cerebral artery (20%).

ache, which is often likened to a blow on the back of the head, and meningism with or without loss of consciousness. Warning leaks days or weeks previously have often been ignored. The intracranial pressure (ICP) increases abruptly to the diastolic arterial pressure and then decreases (Nornes 1973). The patient may die within minutes or hours of the bleed, or have a depressed conscious level for several days, but with less severe bleeds consciousness usually returns rapidly and the patient is orientated, complaining of persistent headache and photophobia. Hypertension, due to intense sympathetic activity, possibly induced by spasm of small vessels supplying the hypothalamus (Doshi & Neil-Dwyer 1977), is common, and arrhythmias and ECG changes may occur.

ECG CHANGES

These are common following subarachnoid haemorrhage and there is a high incidence of peaked P waves, short P−R intervals, long Q−Tc intervals and tall U waves in the ECG of patients who die or develop cerebral arterial spasm. A variety of abnormal cardiac rhythms may also occur (Table 10.1) (Weintraub & McHenry 1974). The presence of a pathological

Table 10.1 Changes in cardiac rhythm and ECG associated with subarachnoid haemorrhage. After Weintraub & McHenry (1974)

Changes in rhythm
Sinus bradycardia
Wandering atrial pacemaker
Paroxysmal atrial tachycardia
Atrial fibrillation
Two-to-one atrioventricular block
Atrioventricular dissociation
Nodal bradycardia
Premature ventricular contractions

General ECG changes
Peaked P waves
Short P−R interval
Prolonged Q−Tc interval
Tall U waves
Pathological Q waves in limb and precordial leads
Raised or depressed ST segments
Inverted T waves
Alteration in shape of T waves (notched, bifid or increased amplitude)

Q wave, raised ST segments or peaking or alteration in shape of the T wave indicates a poor prognosis (Cruickshank *et al.* 1974). These abnormalities may be secondary to increased circulating catecholamine levels (McIntyre *et al.* 1971).

The ECG is not an accurate predictor of myocardial function after subarachnoid haemorrhage, and myocardial dysfunction is related more closely to the patient's neurological state. Delays in treatment of patients with pathological Q waves can be avoided by assessing the cardiac and haemodynamic status using continuous ECG monitoring, isoenzyme determinations and myocardial nuclear scanning to differentiate neurogenic from cardiogenic causes of ECG changes (White *et al.* 1985).

Early focal neurological signs may be due to intracranial haematoma, sudden expansion of an aneurysm or a jet of blood causing pressure effects on cranial nerves (e.g. oculomotor nerve palsy associated with a posterior communicating artery aneurysm). The diagnosis of subarachnoid haemorrhage is confirmed by lumbar puncture, showing xanthochromia of the supernatant after centrifugation, and by CT scan. The cause of the haemorrhage is identified by cerebral angiography.

Hunt and Hess (1968) devised a grading system (Table 10.2) which takes into account the intensity of the meningeal inflammatory reaction, level of consciousness, evidence of focal neurological deficit, presence of

Table 10.2 Classification of patients with intracranial aneurysms according to surgical risk. After Hunt & Hess (1968)

Category*	Criteria
Grade 0	Unruptured aneurysm
Grade I	Asymptomatic, or minimal headache and slight nuchal rigidity
Grade Ia	Stable, residual dysfunction after acute cerebral reaction has settled
Grade II	Moderate to severe headache, nuchal rigidity, no neurological deficit other than cranial nerve palsy
Grade III	Drowsiness, confusion or mild focal deficit
Grade IV	Stupor, moderate to severe hemiparesis, possibly early decerebrate rigidity and vegetative disturbances
Grade V	Deep coma, decerebrate rigidity, moribund appearance

* Serious systemic disease such as hypertension, diabetes, severe arteriosclerosis, chronic pulmonary disease, and severe vasospasm seen on arteriography, result in placement of the patient in the next less favourable category.

severe vasospasm and intercurrent disease. The patient is put into the next less favourable category if he or she has hypertension, diabetes mellitus, severe arteriosclerosis, chronic pulmonary disease or severe vasospasm identified at angiography. The original grading has now been modified to include two further grades, '0' for patients with unruptured aneurysms and 'Ia' for patients with stable, residual dysfunction in whom the acute cerebral reaction has settled. The probability of survival according to the grading on the Hunt and Hess scale has been determined (Alvord *et al.* 1972). Survival rates in any of the clinical grades increase with the interval between the initial haemorrhage and the time that the clinical grade is determined, so that grade I on the first day has a 65% chance of survival whereas the same grade on day 21 has a 95% chance. Chance of survival is reduced as the clinical grade worsens. Deterioration after subarachnoid haemorrhage may be due to cerebral vasospasm causing ischaemia or infarction, rebleeding, development of raised ICP due to hydrocephalus or metabolic disturbances (e.g. hyponatraemia) (Archer *et al.* 1991).

CEREBRAL VASOSPASM

This is a pathological vasoconstriction which may be due to breakdown products of blood constituents in the subarachnoid space. There is a vasculopathy resulting in alterations in the media of vessels or mechanical compression or distortion by the periarterial clot (Archer *et al.* 1991, Kassel *et al.* 1985). Cerebral vasodilators do not reverse vasospasm and may induce an intracerebral steal effect and a reduction in arterial and cerebral perfusion pressures through peripheral vasodilatation. Vasospasm occurs in 70% of patients producing signs of cerebral ischaemia in 20–30% at 3–9 days after the haemorrhage with a peak incidence at 7 days (Archer *et al.* 1991). It may also occur postoperatively. It may be mild or severe, diffuse or local, and causes ischaemia which is worsened by a reduction in arterial pressure and hypoxia. Autoregulation is disrupted in the ischaemic region in patients with vasospasm, and cerebral blood flow (CBF) values may fall in response to only minor changes in arterial pressure. Nimodipine, a calcium antagonist with a greater effect on cerebral vessels, has been shown to improve survival and reduce neurological deficit following subarachnoid haemorrhage (Allen *et al.* 1983). There is no evidence of a reduction in vasospasm following nimodipine, which indicates that the improved survival may be due to an effect of nimodipine at cellular level (Pickard *et al.* 1989). Cerebral metabolism and CBF are reduced by subarachnoid haemorrhage even in the absence of vasospasm. This is apparently due to the presence of blood in the subarachnoid space. A reduction in circulating blood volume and hyponatraemia frequently occurs (Archer *et al.* 1991).

A ruptured aneurysm is very vulnerable to surges in arterial pressure which increase the transmural pressure (the arterial pressure within the aneurysm sac minus the surrounding ICP) (Ferguson 1972) (Fig. 10.2). An increase in arterial pressure or a decrease in ICP will increase the transmural pressure and thus increase the risk of rupture. The risk of rebleeding is maximal during the first 14 days after the initial bleed and then decreases over the next 6 weeks as the blood clot organizes. ICP may be increased by cerebral oedema, haematoma or hydrocephalus due to blood clot blocking the CSF drainage pathways. The preoperative management is aimed at maintaining a normal cerebral perfusion pressure without an increase in arterial pressure, adequate analgesia (codeine phosphate or pethidine) and maintenance of normal fluid balance. Anticonvulsants are administered according to the policy of the neurosurgical unit. The patient should receive 1500 calories per day if possible, and laxatives to prevent straining at stool. The administration of antifibrinolytic agents such as epsilon-aminocaproic acid or tranexamic acid may reduce the risk of rebleeding but cause an increased risk of vasospasm (Adams *et al.* 1987). If rebleeding occurs, ICP should be controlled by the administration of $0.5\,\mathrm{g\,kg^{-1}}$ of 20% mannitol or drainage of CSF from a lateral ventricle. If neurological deterioration occurs the blood volume should be rapidly increased by the infusion of colloid and crystalloid raising the CVP to $10-12\,\mathrm{mmHg}$. If this has no effect the arterial pressure should be raised gradually by infusion of phenylephrine, dopamine or

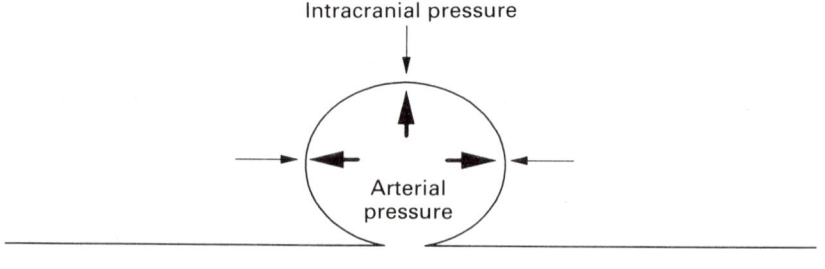

Fig. 10.2 The transmural pressure of an aneurysm is the arterial pressure minus the intracranial pressure. This is the pressure tending to expand the aneurysm. An increase in arterial pressure or a decrease in intracranial pressure will increase the risk of rupture of a cerebral arterial aneurysm.

dobutamine until the deficit is reversed. Complications arising from these measures include rebleeding and circulatory overload. The use of induced hypertension and blood volume expansion in subarachnoid haemorrhage has been reviewed by Archer *et al.* (1991).

Surgical management

The aim of surgery is to prevent rebleeding, and its timing is controversial. Some neurosurgeons believe in operating early, before vasospasm develops, to prevent the risk of early rebleeding and to reduce the incidence of pneumonia, thromboembolism and fluid and electrolyte abnormalities. Removal of blood from the subarachnoid space may reduce the incidence of vasospasm (Kassell *et al.* 1985) and, when the aneurysm has been clipped, volume expansion and measures to increase arterial pressure and reduce vasospasm can be started without the risk of rupture of the aneurysm. Others delay surgery until the tenth to fourteenth day, to avoid operating when the incidence of vasospasm is highest and allow any brain swelling to settle, but 10–20% will have recurrent haemorrhage during this period (Shaw 1987). If there is evidence of severe vasospasm the operation is postponed until the neurological condition improves.

Surgical procedures

Aneurysms on the anterior part of the circle of Willis and basilar artery are approached through a frontal or frontoparietal craniotomy, and those on the vertebral system and posterior inferior cerebellar artery require a posterior fossa craniectomy. The procedure of choice is to place a clip across the base of the aneurysm isolating the sac from the circulation whilst maintaining flow through the feeding artery. Modern microsurgical techniques involve sharp dissection round the base of the aneurysm, and identification of any small perforating arteries or branches nearby. A removable spring clip can be placed across the neck of the aneurysm as close to the feeder artery as possible without narrowing it (Fig. 10.3). If the clip is too distal a new aneurysm can develop, and if too proximal flow through the feeding artery will be impaired. The mortality is less than 5% in the hands of an experienced surgeon, and even less if the aneurysm has not bled. As the size of the aneurysm increases the morbidity and mortality increase.

If clipping proves to be technically impossible the aneurysm may be trapped by occluding the vessels proximal and distal to the aneurysm, provided that collateral flow to the brain normally supplied by the

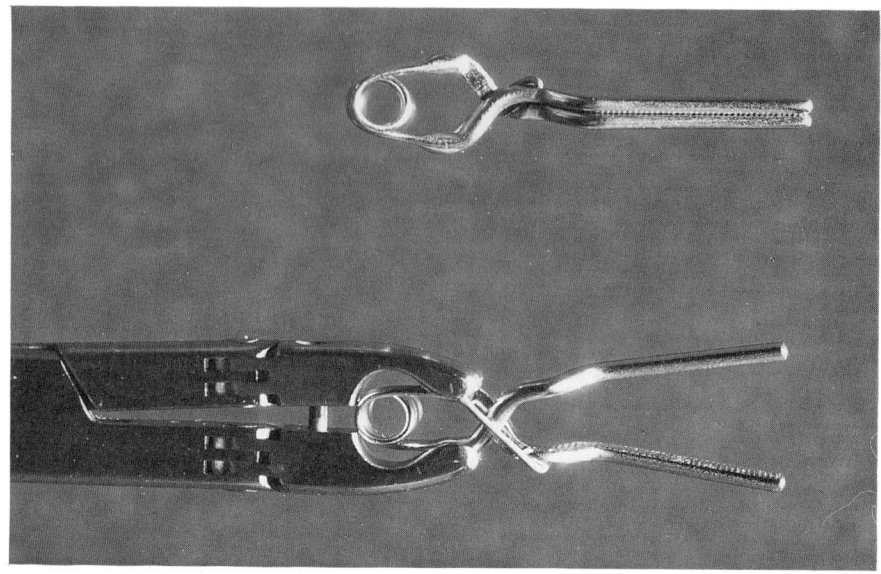

(a)

(b)

Fig. 10.3 (a) A spring loaded aneurysm clip closed, and held open in a clip applicator. (b) A cerebral artery aneurysm before and after clip application.

occluded vessels is sufficient. Carotid ligation can be used to reduce the pressure inside some large or otherwise inoperable aneurysms, reducing the chance of rupture and encouraging thrombosis in the sac. The clamp can be applied under general anaesthesia and then gradually closed over several days. If complete occlusion does not cause any neurological deficit the artery is permanently ligated at a second operation. Alternatively, a trial occlusion of the artery can be performed under local anaesthesia with permanent ligation if there is no deficit. It is possible to ligate other vessels after the collateral circulation has been improved by extracranial to intracranial bypass. Postoperative hypotension should be avoided after arterial ligation. If all these techniques prove impossible, the aneurysm can be reinforced by wrapping with gauze, gelfoam or plastic materials in an attempt to promote fibrosis and prevent further enlargement and rupture. Wrapping does not eradicate the aneurysm sac completely, or reduce the size of large aneurysms which may be causing pressure effects on adjacent structures. Fibrosis takes time to develop, so the aneurysm is still likely to rupture if hypertension occurs during emergence and recovery. As a last resort thrombotic material has been introduced into the aneurysm at surgery.

Multiple aneurysms occur fairly frequently (in about 20% of patients presenting with subarachnoid haemorrhage) and, if on the same side as the one that has bled, can be clipped at the same operation. Giant aneurysms are technically difficult, but have been successfully ligated during circulatory arrest under profound hypothermia with cardio-pulmonary bypass (Silverberg *et al.* 1981).

Interventional neuroradiology

Advances in angiography technology have made it possible to cannulate feeder arteries of aneurysms and AVMs and insert balloon catheters, glue, coils or microspheres in order to occlude the vessels or aneurysms. These are particularly useful in inaccessible aneurysms and AVMs. Iron has been inserted into aneurysms by stereotactic methods to encourage thrombosis.

AVMs and angiomas

These are dilated arteries and veins with no intervening capillaries. They may present clinically with subarachnoid or intracerebral haemorrhage, epilepsy or headaches. The high flow may steal blood from the adjacent brain and cause ischaemia. The morbidity following leakage is lower than following rupture of an aneurysm, and they are either surgically excised or devascularized using interventional neuroradiological techniques. The latter technique may be used to reduce vascularity before surgery.

VEIN OF GALEN ANEURYSMS

These are AVMs which consist of a direct communication between the great cerebral vein of Galen and one or more branches of the carotid or vertebral circulation (Gold *et al.* 1964, Wilkins 1985). They may present in neonates with hydrocephalus and an enlarging head. The mortality is high because the AVM is large and the considerable shunt through the lesion causes high-output congestive cardiac failure which is frequently the cause of death. Infants present with hydrocephalus or convulsions, and postoperative cerebral hyperperfusion is likely. In later childhood and adult life the lesions are smaller, the symptoms usually result from subarachnoid haemorrhage, mass effect causing headaches or cerebral steal causing neurological signs, and the operative mortality is lower than in younger patients.

Preoperative assessment

In addition to the history, physical examination and investigations appropriate for any patient undergoing intracranial surgery, the clinical grade should be assessed (Hunt & Hess 1968) and a 12-lead ECG should be obtained. The neurological observation chart should be scrutinized for any neurological deterioration which coincides with episodes of arterial hypotension, because the arterial pressure should not be allowed to fall below this threshold level during the operation. It is useful to determine the patient's normal arterial pressure and maintain this level during surgery. Patients who have been nursed recumbent for several days may be dehydrated with disturbance of electrolytes and may have reduced sympathetic tone. Both these factors will contribute to hypotension during induction and maintenance of anaesthesia. Deep venous thrombosis and pulmonary embolism are rare despite prolonged immobility. The body temperature may be raised and should be restored to normal, if possible, before surgery to reduce cerebral oxygen requirements. Aneurysms of the anterior part of the circle of Willis may affect the hypothalamus leading to endocrine disturbances, notably inappropriate antidiuretic hormone (ADH) secretion. Anticonvulsants and antihypertensive therapy should be continued throughout the perioperative period. It is normal practice for these patients to receive oral nimodipine to reduce the incidence of neurological deficits and possibly vasospasm. The half-life of nimodipine is short, so it should be given by infusion during the perioperative period when oral administration is not possible. The CT scan should be assessed for signs of increased ICP, haematoma or oedema, and arteriography will reveal the site of the aneurysm or AVM. The vascularity of AVMs can be assessed by arteriography, allowing anticipation of haemorrhage and the need for induced hypotension.

Anaesthesia for intracranial aneurysms

PREMEDICATION

Ideally, the patient should be relaxed and comfortable on arrival in the anaesthetic room so that tachycardia and hypertension are avoided. An oral benzodiazepine such as diazepam 10−15 mg or temazepam 20−30 mg with metoclopramide 10 mg is usually effective. If the conscious level is depressed reduced doses are given, or premedication is omitted. If the patient is taking beta-adrenergic blocking drugs or other antihypertensive agents these are given with the premedication, and anticonvulsant medication should be continued throughout the perioperative period. Beta-blockers attenuate the hypertensive response to intubation and reflex tachycardia during induced hypotension. They also reduce rebound hypertension during recovery. They can be given orally with the premedication or, alternatively, the short-acting beta-blocking agent, esmolol, which has a half-life of 9 min, can be given intravenously before induction of anaesthesia (Miller *et al.* 1991).

MONITORING

The usual monitoring for intracranial surgery including ECG, pulse oximetry, end-tidal carbon dioxide tension, fractional inspiratory oxygen concentration (FIO_2), ventilator disconnection alarm, nasopharyngeal and peripheral temperatures, direct arterial and central venous pressure measurement is employed, and has been discussed in Chapter 7. It is important to control the arterial pressure within relatively narrow limits during induction, so it must be measured repeatedly during this time.

Continuous recording of the arterial pressure is useful. The arterial line can be inserted under local anaesthesia before induction of anaesthesia. However, this can cause pain and hypertension, and many centres use an automated NIBP machine until anaesthesia is induced. Internal jugular vein cannulation is best avoided because of the danger of trauma to the internal carotid artery. However, fibreoptic oximetry probes have been developed which, if inserted into the jugular bulb by retrograde catheterization of the internal jugular vein, allow continuous monitoring of jugular venous oxygen saturation (SjO_2) and blood sampling for lactate measurement. These may be useful for providing early warning of cerebral ischaemia.

INDUCTION OF ANAESTHESIA

The anaesthetist aims to avoid increases in arterial pressure which increase the transmural pressure of the aneurysm and the potential for rupture. Marked reduction in arterial pressure should also be avoided, and may require infusion of fluid before and during induction to avoid a significant fall in cerebral perfusion pressure (CPP) and cerebral ischaemia.

The induction of anaesthesia and intubation should be smooth, using an intravenous hypnotic such as thiopentone $4-7\,\text{mg}\,\text{kg}^{-1}$ or propofol $2-3\,\text{mg}\,\text{kg}^{-1}$ titrated to effect and atracurium $0.75\,\text{mg}\,\text{kg}^{-1}$ or vecuronium $0.15\,\text{mg}\,\text{kg}^{-1}$. Pancuronium is best avoided because of its potential to increase arterial pressure (Kelman & Kennedy 1971) and tubocurarine can cause a dramatic reduction in arterial pressure (Moss *et al.* 1978). The use of fentanyl $5\,\mu\text{g}\,\text{kg}^{-1}$ given just before the induction agent, so that at least 3 min elapse before intubation, reduces the hypertensive response to intubation (Helfman *et al.* 1991). Alfentanil will also reduce the cardiovascular response to intubation, but when given as a bolus dose can cause marked increases in ICP and reductions in CPP (Chapter 4). Esmolol, which has a short half-life, may be the beta-blocking agent of choice (Cucchiara *et al.* 1986, Miller *et al.* 1991, Vucevic *et al.* 1992). Other agents used to reduce the cardiovascular response to intubation include nicardipine (Omote *et al.* 1992). If a difficult intubation is anticipated suxamethonium is the relaxant of choice.

MAINTENANCE

Anaesthesia can be maintained with nitrous oxide supplemented with an opioid analgesic and a volatile anaesthetic (enflurane 0.6—1.5% or isoflurane 0.5−1%) or an infusion of intravenous anaesthetic (propofol $6-12\,mg\,kg^{-1}h^{-1}$). Many neuroanaesthetists prefer to avoid nitrous oxide because it increases CBF. This requires the use of oxygen-enriched air and maintenance of anaesthesia with higher concentrations of volatile anaesthetic or larger doses of intravenous agent. Larger doses of opioid are also required because the analgesic effect of nitrous oxide is lost. Fentanyl is the opioid of choice because it has no effect on CBF and ICP (Moss *et al.* 1978). Infusion of alfentanil is a suitable alternative but bolus doses should be used with care because they can cause increase in ICP (Jung *et al.* 1990, Moss 1992). The surgeon can reduce the pressor response to skin incision, and therefore the requirement for analgesia, by infiltrating the scalp with bupivacaine 0.25% (Engberg *et al.* 1990).

Neuromuscular blockade is maintained with a non-depolarizing muscle relaxant such as atracurium $0.5\,mg\,kg^{-1}h^{-1}$. Ventilation is controlled to maintain a $PaCO_2$ of 30−38 mmHg until the dura is incised to avoid a significant reduction in ICP and maintain a satisfactory trans-mural pressure. Thereafter, the $PaCO_2$ is reduced to 26−30 mmHg to induce cerebral vasoconstriction and reduce brain bulk and retraction pressures on the brain. The role of hyperventilation in patients with subarachnoid haemorrhage remains unresolved in the presence of severe vasospasm, because hypocapnia may reduce collateral circulation and worsen ischaemia, whereas the reduction in ICP may improve CPP in grade III and IV patients. It is advisable to maintain normocapnia during induced hypotension (Archer *et al.* 1991). The administration of mannitol $0.5\,g\,kg^{-1}$ followed after 15 min by frusemide 0.5 $g\,kg^{-1}$ further reduces brain bulk and retraction pressures (Roberts *et al.* 1987). The diuresis induced requires an indwelling bladder catheter, and leads to a loss of sodium and potassium (Schettini *et al.* 1982), so serum potassium levels should be monitored and potassium administered if necessary. It also causes hypovolaemia so it is the author's practice to administer up to 1 litre of hetastarch to restore the central venous pressure (CVP) to its previous level. This maintains the cerebral circulation without the risk of increasing brain water content and restores some of the sodium lost during the diuresis. Intravenous fluids should be warmed unless moderate hypothermia is intended, and glucose-containing fluids should be avoided. Blood should be given if blood loss exceeds 20% of blood volume. Operating conditions can be further improved by drainage of CSF either by ventricular drainage at craniotomy or by spinal CSF drainage. CSF should not be removed until the dura has been incised to avoid an increase in transmural pressure.

INDUCED HYPOTENSION

This has been in common use during anaesthesia for clipping of intra-cranial aneurysms because it reduces the risk of rupture during the dissection by reducing the intraluminal pressure and making the aneurysm sac less tense. Improved surgical techniques using the operating micro-scope and sharp dissection have reduced the need for hypotension, and there is evidence that induced hypotension may increase that incidence of ischaemic deficits in some patients (Pickard *et al.* 1980, Farrar *et al.* 1981), particularly those with vasospasm and impaired autoregulation. It is now generally accepted that it is better to maintain a normal arterial pressure during aneurysm surgery, and that hypotension should be employed only if the surgery cannot be performed without it. Hypotension should not be used if vasospasm has been demonstrated at angiography or is suspected on clinical grounds. Some authorities advocate raising the arterial pressure to improve perfusion to ischaemic brain beyond areas of vasospasm. The place of induced hypertension and volume expansion in the management of subarachnoid haemorrhage has been reviewed by Archer and colleagues (1991). It is usually necessary to infuse fluids to maintain intravascular volume and normotension. Large volumes of crystalloid will increase cerebral oedema, so colloid solutions such as hetastarch or human albumin solution are more suitable and should be given until the CVP has returned to the preoperative level.

One situation where induced hypotension may be life-saving is when the aneurysm ruptures during dissection and the haemorrhage is so brisk that the surgeon cannot see to apply a clip to the base of the aneurysm or a temporary clip to a feeding vessel. Under these circum-stances the systolic arterial pressure can be reduced to 60−80 mmHg, or less if absolutely essential, for as short a period as is necessary for the surgeon to arrest the haemorrhage. This can be achieved by infusing a mixture of trimetaphan and sodium nitroprusside (Chapter 4). Usually, when an aneurysm ruptures during dissection the surgeon can control the bleeding sufficiently with tamponade and suction to allow isolation with temporary clips prior to application of the clip to the neck of the aneurysm. If feeding vessels are temporarily occluded the arterial pressure should be returned to, or maintained at, normal levels to minimize the risk of ischaemia and, if possible, thiopentone $3−5\,\mathrm{mg\,kg^{-1}}$ should be given before application of the clip, to give some cerebral protection. There is no point in administering barbiturates while the circulation is arrested because if the collateral circulation is sufficient to deliver the drugs to the ischaemic brain the barbiturates are probably not necessary, and if the collateral circulation is inadequate the drugs will not reach the ischaemic tissues. Post-operative ventilation should be considered if temporary clips have been applied for an extended period.

Anaesthesia for AVMs

Surgery for AVMs is not urgent unless there is a haematoma causing pressure effects. The patient can be allowed to stabilize and recover after the haemorrhage. The operative procedure can be associated with considerable blood loss, and intraoperative use of cell-savers and autotransfusion may be considered. Two large-bore venous cannulas should be inserted and all intravenous fluids should be warmed to body temperature. There is no risk of cerebral vasospasm so induced hypotension can be used to reduce blood loss with relative safety. CVP measurement is useful in assessing the efficacy of fluid replacement and a pulmonary artery catheter is useful if myocardial function is impaired. Children often have high-output cardiac failure due to the intracerebral shunt, and congestive cardiac failure may be precipitated by excision of the lesion.

Intraoperative EEG monitoring may be necessary if feeding arteries are ligated extracranially, but care should be taken in using this technique during anaesthesia, particularly with isoflurane, because tolerance to ischaemia is increased (Messick *et al.* 1987). The low cerebral blood flow tolerated during anaesthesia may not be tolerated when the patient is awake. Temporary balloon occlusion during angiography while the patient is conscious is more reliable in assessing the effect of occlusion on neurological function.

Anaesthesia can be managed in the same way as for clipping of aneurysms, but concentrating more on reducing brain bulk and reducing arterial pressure rather than maintaining normotension. Measures should be taken to reduce the haemodynamic response to laryngoscopy, intubation and application of skull fixation. Hyperventilation with humidified gases to a $PaCO_2$ of 26−30 mmHg is instituted as soon as anaesthesia is induced because a reduction in ICP is desirable and there is no risk of haemorrhage from an aneurysm.

FLUID BALANCE

As during aneurysm surgery crystalloid should be used sparingly because excessive use may cause increased cerebral oedema, and glucose-containing fluids should be avoided intraoperatively to avoid worsening the effects of cerebral ischaemia. Colloid solutions maintain the intravascular volume without increasing brain water. In fact artificial colloid solutions, through their greater osmolality, tend to draw fluid into the vascular space and will help to combat cerebral oedema and reduce brain bulk. Blood should be replaced when the blood loss exceeds 20% of the blood volume in adults.

POSTOPERATIVE HYPERPERFUSION

Some regions of the brain near the AVM may have been chronically ischaemic due to shunting of blood through the AVM which leads to arteriolar dilatation and loss of autoregulation. Following excision of the AVM the sudden increase in perfusion pressure to these regions causes an increase in CBF and ICP, and may cause intracerebral haemorrhage. The transmission of the increased pressure directly to the capillaries leads to filtration of more fluid into the brain interstitial fluid, causing cerebral oedema and a further increase in ICP. This is more likely to occur with large AVM and in patients who had symptoms of cerebral steal and ischaemia preoperatively, or showed poor flow through normal arteries surrounding the AVM at angiography. Preoperative embolization, in addition to reducing the vascularity and operative haemorrhage, may increase flow in arteries surrounding the AVM allowing the restoration of autoregulation preoperatively. In patients at risk from cerebral hyperperfusion maintenance of moderate hypotension and hyperventilation postoperatively will help to restore autoregulation and control cerebral oedema.

Recovery from anaesthesia following aneurysm and AVM surgery

Ideally the patient should regain consciousness as soon as possible after the completion of surgery for cerebral aneurysms or AVM, to allow early recognition and treatment of operative complications. However, for rapid awakening light levels of anaesthesia are required during surgical closure, which may cause hypertension with an increased risk of intracranial haematoma, hyperperfusion and cerebral oedema. Lignocaine 1.5 mg kg^{-1} can be given intravenously before reversal to attenuate the cardiovascular response associated with extubation. Respiratory depression due to opioid analgesics can be reversed with naloxone. This should be carefully titrated to effect because excessive doses can cause hypertension.

Following aneurysm surgery the arterial pressure is maintained within or slightly above the normal range, by infusion of fluids and vasopressors if necessary (Brown *et al.* 1978), and following AVM surgery within or slightly below the normal range using hypotensive agents if necessary. The patients are best nursed on a high-dependency unit with continuous monitoring of ECG, arterial pressure, CVP and haemoglobin saturation, and regular neurological observations.

Weak opioids with little effect on respiration such as codeine phosphate 30–60 mg intramuscularly or orally can be used to control pain. These may be supplemented with nonsteroidal anti-inflammatory drugs such as intramuscular ketorolac 30 mg 6-hourly, but there is some concern that these drugs may increase the risk of postoperative intracranial haematoma; 100 ml h^{-1} of glucose 4%/saline 0.18% is given to maintain fluid balance, and colloid solutions or blood can be given if necessary to maintain a normal CVP. If neurological deficits and a deterioration of level of consciousness occur in the postoperative period, a CT scan should be performed and consideration should be given to improving cerebral blood flow by volume expansion and raising the arterial pressure using inotropes or vasopressors (Levy *et al.* 1982, Archer *et al.* 1991).

Vein of Galen aneurysms

The anaesthetic management in older patients is the same as for the more common forms of AVM, using induced hypotension to reduce blood loss and treat hyperperfusion after obliteration. In neonates and infants it is advisable to monitor cardiac filling pressures. Hyperperfusion and cerebral oedema, should they occur, are treated by hyperventilation, control of arterial pressure and diuretics to control ICP.

Extracranial and intracranial occlusive and ulcerative arterial disease

Occlusive and ulcerative arterial lesions develop at the branches of both the extracranial and intracranial vessels, most commonly at the carotid bifurcations, origins of the internal carotid arteries and origins and course of the vertebral arteries. Stenosis is considered haemodynamically significant when the internal diameter of the artery is reduced by 75%. Cerebral ischaemic events in the carotid circulation are most likely to be due to embolism, while in the vertebrobasilar circulation they are commonly due to haemodynamic factors. The vast majority of new cerebrovascular accidents are caused by thromboembolism (Sherman & Hart 1992). Transient ischaemic attacks (TIA) last for less than 24 h and resolve completely. Reversible ischaemic neurological deficits (RIND) persist for more than 24 h but less than 3 weeks. Progressing stroke (PS) is a situation where over minutes or hours there is worsening of the deficit because of expansion of an area of ischaemia, and in completed stroke (CS) the ischaemic deficit has persisted for more than 24 h and is not clearly worsening or improving at that point. If the vertebrobasilar circulation is involved the presenting symptoms include vertigo, tinnitus and ataxia. Untreated TIA carry a risk of subsequent stroke of about 5% per year for the first 3 years and 3% per annum thereafter (Sherman & Hart 1992).

INVESTIGATION

Investigation includes plain skull and cervical radiography, CT scan with contrast to determine the size of the infarct, Doppler ultrasound measurement of blood flow through the cerebral vessels, digital vascular imaging and/or cerebral arteriography.

MEDICAL TREATMENT

This includes the use of anticoagulant and antiplatelet agents.

SURGERY

Surgery should be reserved for those with more severe disease (Winslow *et al.* 1988), because the mortality from surgery in experienced hands is 1.5% and the morbidity due to perioperative stroke is about 5% (Wong 1991). Myocardial ischaemia is the major cause of death in the follow-up period in this group of patients (Allcutt *et al.* 1991). The most suitable patients for surgery are those who present with TIA, amaurosis fugax, ischaemic neurological deficits or minor stroke with good functional recovery, and also have an appropriate internal carotid artery plaque demonstrated angiographically (Wong 1991). Severe stenosis or ulcerative plaques near the carotid bifurcation are best treated by carotid end-arterectomy to remove the source of emboli and improve the cerebral circulation. Complete occlusion or inaccessible stenosis of the internal carotid or middle cerebral arteries have been treated by extracranial to intracranial anastomosis, but this procedure was not proven to be effective in an international randomized controlled trial (Barnett *et al.* 1985). This conclusion is supported by the results of 13 series of extracranial to intracranial bypass surgery reviewed by Holohan (1991). However, case selection in the international trial has been criticized, and it is possible that this operation may prove useful in suitably selected patients with symptomatic atherosclerotic disease of the internal carotid artery (Relman 1987).

Surgery for ischaemic cerebrovascular disease

Patients with ischaemic cerebrovascular disease frequently have multi-system disease. They may be hypertensive, have ischaemic heart disease or diabetes mellitus and many are heavy smokers with associated chronic obstructive airways disease. All these conditions must be appropriately investigated and treated before surgery. Recent myocardial infarction and unstable angina are definite contraindications to surgery. Poorly controlled hypertension is a relative contraindication, systolic pressures of more than 100 mmHg being associated with an adverse surgical outcome (Brown & Humphrey 1992). These patients may be taking a variety of drugs including digoxin, diuretics, antihypertensives, antiarrhythmics, anticoagulants, insulin, bronchodilators and corticosteroids. Most of these drugs should be continued throughout the perioperative period but anticoagulants and aspirin should be discontinued for up to 1-week before surgery to allow clotting to return to normal for intracranial surgery. If it is not considered safe to discontinue the anticoagulants the oral anticoagulants should be stopped and heparin substituted.

A grading system has been devised at the Mayo Clinic to assess the risk of perioperative morbidity and mortality in patients undergoing initial surgery for carotid stenosis (Messick & Sundt 1990).

Grade 1 is neurologically stable; no major medical or angiographically defined risk factors.

Grade 2 is neurologically stable; no major medical risk factors; significant angiographically defined risk factors (extensive atheromatous plaque, soft thrombus, occlusion of contralateral carotid artery).

Grade 3 is neurologically stable; major medical risks; with or without significant angiographically defined risk factors.

Grade 4 is neurologically unstable; with or without major medical or angiographically defined risks.

Grade 5 are patients with known symptomatic acute internal carotid artery occlusion, who have a progressing neurological deficit or who have sustained a major neurological deficit within 4 h before examination.

The morbidity and mortality ranges from less than 1% in grade 1 to 8.5% in grade 4.

Anaesthesia for carotid endarterectomy

The aim of anaesthetic management for carotid endarterectomy is the avoidance of drugs or techniques that could cause or increase cerebral ischaemia or have detrimental effects on the myocardium. Anaesthetic techniques should optimize CPP, CBF and the ratio of cerebral metabolic rate for oxygen ($CMRO_2$) to CBF. Consideration should be given to the provision of cerebral protection, and the brain should be monitored to detect cerebral ischaemia. Arterial pressure is usually maintained in the normotensive range during the operation because impairment of auto-regulation and dependence on collaterals make oxygen delivery to the brain very sensitive to changes in perfusion pressure. Increases in arterial pressure should be avoided in the postoperative period because they may cause cerebral oedema.

PREMEDICATION

The same considerations apply as for aneurysm surgery, with the relief of anxiety as the main aim. Diazepam, lorazepam or temazepam are suitable agents given in doses appropriate to the patient's age and physical status. Regular medication for intercurrent illness should normally be continued throughout the perioperative period. A glyceryl trinitrate patch can be prescribed with the premedication if there is evidence of ischaemic heart disease.

LOCAL ANAESTHESIA

Carotid endarterectomy can be successfully performed under deep cervical plexus block with general sedation (Rainer *et al.* 1966). The advantages of this method are the avoidance of a general anaesthetic in patients of ASA grade III or higher, and the ability of the anaesthetist and surgeon to monitor the neurological state. The disadvantages are that an inadequate block causes pain and stress for the patient, which can lead to restlessness, hypertension and tachycardia; certain drugs which provide cerebral protection cannot be given; the $Paco_2$ and arterial pressure are not easily controlled, and an unexpected deficit may develop after an uneventful test period.

The technique involves a paravertebral nerve block of C2, C3 and C4 spinal nerves as they emerge from the foramina in the cervical vertebrae. The patient lies supine with the head turned away from the side to be blocked. Three needles are inserted, the first at the level of C2, one finger's-breadth caudal to the mastoid process on a line from the tip of the mastoid process to Chassaignac's tubercle on C6. Two further needles are inserted at the level of C3, one finger's-breadth below the first needle on the same line, and C4, one finger's-breadth below the second needle. Three 22 gauge needles 5 cm in length are directed medially and caudally until contact is made with the transverse processes and paraesthesia is obtained. All three needles should be inserted to the same depth, and if they are at different depths the most superficial is the correctly placed one. Too-deep insertion can cause epidural or spinal block. After aspiration testing, injection of 3−4 ml 1% lignocaine or its equivalent for each nerve are usually adequate for anaesthesia (Murphy 1987). Infiltration of local anaesthetic in the area of the nerves to the carotid body and sinus helps to prevent arrhythmias and fluctuations in arterial pressure during surgery under local and general anaesthesia.

GENERAL ANAESTHESIA

General anaesthesia is more comfortable for the patient, allows control of arterial pressure, $Paco_2$ and Pao_2 and the use of agents which decrease cerebral metabolic rate (Wong 1991). Surgery is technically easier and less hurried. However, these patients have arterial disease affecting both cerebral and coronary vessels, and are at increased risk from general anaesthesia. The anaesthetic agents which have beneficial effects on the brain may have the opposite effect on the heart, and maintenance of an adequate CPP may increase myocardial work load.

Most anaesthetists prefer a balanced anaesthetic technique using a combination of nitrous oxide, opioid analgesic, volatile anaesthetic agent and muscle relaxant. Induction of anaesthesia should be carried out with the agents with which the anaesthetist is most familiar, with the aim of maintaining cardiovascular stability. Hypertension and tachycardia associated with laryngoscopy and intubation should be avoided, but so should hypotension during induction and maintenance of anaesthesia. Normocapnia is maintained, avoiding hypocapnia, because of the decrease in CBF and the shift of the oxyhaemoglobin dissociation curve to the left impairing oxygen delivery, and hypercapnia which may cause cerebral steal and arrhythmias. Nitrous oxide, supplemented by an opioid analgesic and isoflurane, are frequently used because isoflurane may protect against cerebral ischaemia (Michenfelder *et al.* 1987). Coronary steal is not a problem with the low concentrations of isoflurane employed during balanced anaesthesia, but there is evidence that nitrous oxide may abolish the depressant effects of isoflurane on cerebral metabolic rate (Baughman *et al.* 1989). So nitrous oxide may be best avoided in these patients, particularly as it will increase the size of air emboli occurring during positioning of the shunt. Propofol may prove useful for maintenance of anaesthesia as it is a free radical scavenger (Murphy *et al.* 1992) and may have cerebral protective effects (Kochs *et al.* 1992).

FLUID THERAPY

The aim is to maintain a normal intravascular volume and CPP. Some haemodilution will improve flow for the same perfusion pressure but adequate oxygen-carrying capacity should be ensured. Glucose-containing fluids are avoided unless there is a danger of hypoglycaemia.

MONITORING

This should include routine ECG, direct arterial pressure, respiratory gases, pulse oximetry, temperature, neuromuscular function, fluid balance and arterial blood gases. In patients with significant myocardial dysfunction monitoring CVP, pulmonary arterial wedge pressure (PAWP) and cardiac output may be indicated. A monitor which allows the clinician to switch between lead II and either V_4 or V_5 gives good detection of atrial arrhythmias and myocardial ischaemia (London *et al.* 1988).

Monitoring adequacy of cerebral perfusion

Preoperative tests available for predicting the haemodynamic consequences of cross-clamping during carotid endarterectomy include angiography, transcranial Doppler ultrasonography and EEG during compression of the common carotid artery (Wong 1991). Various techniques have been used to assess adequacy of CBF during carotid endarterectomy. These include neurological examination during regional anaesthesia, assessment of neuronal function, measurement of carotid artery stump pressure, measurement of CBF and measurement of jugular venous oxygen saturation.

ASSESSMENT OF NEURONAL FUNCTION

EEG remains the most effective method of detection of cerebral ischaemia affecting cortical function, and various monitors are available which display a processed EEG signal. The cerebral function monitor is not as good as the standard 16-channel EEG for detecting cerebral ischaemia, but the sensitivity is better when both electrodes are placed over the hemisphere at risk than when the electrodes are placed on opposite sides of the head (Cucchiara *et al.* 1979). Somatosensory evoked potentials (SEP) have also been used successfully to monitor cerebral function during carotid endarterectomy (Markand *et al.* 1984, Lam *et al.* 1991) but SEP monitors only a small part of the CNS pathway. Electrophysiological monitoring is discussed in more detail in Chapter 5.

STUMP PRESSURE

This is the pressure in the carotid artery distal to the clamp and is easily measured. Its use was based on the belief that cerebral perfusion was inadequate when the stump pressure was less than 50 mmHg. However, the stump pressure does not correlate well with CBF (McKay *et al.* 1976) and EEG changes indicative of ischaemia with critical levels of regional CBF have occurred when the stump pressure was greater than 50 mmHg. Conversely, there was no evidence of ischaemia in some patients with stump pressures less than 50 mmHg. Stump pressure measures the pressure in the collateral vascular bed and is influenced by vascular resistance as well as flow. Therefore, anaesthetics can influence stump pressure by altering cerebrovascular resistance.

CEREBRAL BLOOD FLOW

CBF can be measured using rapid intracarotid injection of xenon-133 just before temporary occlusion of the internal carotid artery and a single collimated scintillation detector positioned perpendicular to the scalp overlying the distribution of the middle cerebral artery (Sundt *et al.* 1974). During carotid endarterectomy flows greater than 24 ml $100\,g^{-1}\,min^{-1}$ are adequate whereas flows less than 18 ml $100\,g^{-1}$

min^{-1} are inadequate (McKay *et al.* 1976). However, the measurements are intermittent and may not detect complications caused by embolization, hypotension or ischaemia at all times during the operation, and thus may not correlate well with neurological outcome (Wong 1991).

JUGULAR VENOUS OXYGEN SATURATION

Fibreoptic probes are now available for continuous monitoring of SjO_2 (Andrews *et al.* 1991). A fall in the ipsilateral SjO_2 indicates cerebral ischaemia, but the critical level is not known and the measurement is global and may not detect regional cerebral ischaemia. The measurement of jugular venous lactate concentration may make the technique more sensitive. The place of SjO_2 measurement in monitoring during carotid artery surgery is still uncertain.

DOPPLER ULTRASONOGRAPHY

Transcranial Doppler ultrasonography gives a measure of flow velocity in the middle cerebral artery, but a change may be due to a change in diameter of the vessel or a change in flow, therefore, a decrease in velocity may not indicate a reduction in CBF. However, it may be useful in detecting middle cerebral artery emboli during carotid endarterectomy (Spencer *et al.* 1990).

OTHER METHODS

Transconjunctival oxygen tension should reflect internal carotid artery oxygen tension because the capillary network on the palpebral conjunctiva is supplied by the internal carotid artery (Shoemaker & Lawner 1983), but Gibson and colleagues (1986) found no correlation between transconjunctival Po_2 and regional CBF or EEG evidence of cerebral ischaemia. *Supraorbital photoplethysmography* and *oculoplethysmographic monitoring* have been investigated as a continuous and noninvasive method of measuring carotid artery blood flow (Pearce *et al.* 1979, 1980). They are particularly useful in the detection of haemodynamically significant reductions in shunt flow due to retractors or shunt displacement during carotid endarterectomy. *Nasal plethysmography* using a light-emitting diode to indicate nasal blood flow showed no correlation between pulse amplitude and CBF during carotid artery occlusion (Cucchiara & Messick 1981).

No single monitoring technique is absolutely reliable in detecting cerebral ischaemia and predicting postoperative neurological complications in all patients, because these complications may be due to embolization and not carotid occlusion.

TEMPORARY SHUNTING

The advantages of a temporary shunt include the maintenance of flow and avoidance of hypoperfusion during occlusion of the artery, it permits unhurried surgery and provides a stent for closure of the arteriotomy. However, the shunt does not guarantee adequate perfusion because of the potential for thrombus or kinking of the shunt, dissection of the intima or particulate or air emboli. In addition, the shunt may impede surgical exposure. The use of a shunt is still controversial and practices include routine insertion, insertion when indicated by detection of inadequate flow and never shunting (Wong 1991). The combined mortality and minor and major morbidity associated with shunting is approximately 3%, whereas the risk of a major neurological deficit without the use of shunting when indicated is about 12% (Sundt *et al.* 1986).

Complications of carotid endarterectomy

Myocardial infarction is a major cause of death. Intraoperative embolization and postoperative occlusion of the internal carotid artery may cause major strokes. If embolization of a major artery occurs intraoperatively the patient should be heparinized and thiopentone should be given to produce burst suppression on the EEG. If, on completion of the endarterectomy, the EEG appearances do not improve, angiography and middle cerebral embolectomy through a craniotomy should be performed. Ipsilateral hyperperfusion syndrome may occur several days after the operation and presents with vascular headache, migraine variants, seizures and intracerebral haemorrhage. In view of these serious potential complications it is accepted that carotid endarterectomy should only be performed for appropriate indications (Winslow *et al.* 1988).

Anaesthesia for extracranial–intracranial anastomosis

The pathological features and anaesthetic considerations and techniques are very similar to those for carotid endarterectomy. Surgery involves anastomosis of small arteries to vessels on the surface of the cortex, and excessive movements of the brain due to respiration will make surgery very difficult. Increasing the frequency of ventilation and reducing tidal volume will reduce brain movement, as will high-frequency ventilation. The brain should not fall away from the cranial defect when the dura is incised so brain bulk should not be reduced. Normocapnia will maintain a normal CBV as well as normal physiological levels of CBF. At the end of the procedure coughing and straining should be avoided because this will increase venous pressure and put a strain on the anastomosis.

A multicentre study demonstrated that extracranial–intracranial anastomosis was no better than medical management in reducing the risk of ischaemic stroke in patients with occlusive disease of cerebral vessels (Barnett *et al.* 1985). Consequently the popularity of this procedure has declined, but the methodology of this study has been criticized (Relman 1987) and there may be a resurgence of interest in this procedure for specific indications.

Special techniques

Induced hypotension

Induced hypotension is used much less frequently during intracranial surgery than previously, particularly, during aneurysm surgery. There are significant risks from induced hypotension which may impair blood flow through diseased vessels in the brain and other organs. Ischaemia under the brain retractor is increased when mean arterial pressure is reduced (Rosenorn & Diemer 1982). It is important to determine the level to which the arterial pressure can be safely reduced. It is accepted that there is no major depression of the EEG when mean arterial pressure (MAP) is greater than 60 mmHg (Prior 1985). In patients with normal cerebral circulation MAP values of 50–60 mmHg are associated with a normal CBF and the EEG, at 30–50 mmHg CBF is reduced by up to 50% and there may be EEG changes, at 25–30 mmHg the CBF is borderline to inadequate and the EEG shows slow waves or burst suppression, and below 25 mmHg the CBF is inadequate and the EEG shows burst suppression or is isoelectric (Spaerel 1982). Brain damage is unlikely at MAP values of greater than 30 mmHg, but below that brain damage is likely if hypotension is prolonged and below 25 mmHg brain damage is likely after very short periods (<5 min) of hypotension. These figures assume uniform blood flow throughout the brain, but there is always a danger that flow in the boundary zones, or regions supplied by narrowed vessels, will be reduced to critical levels at higher arterial pressures than in normal brain. When MAP is reduced to less than 60 mmHg cerebral activity should be monitored and MAP increased if there is any depression of activity on the EEG.

Moderate hypotension (MAP 70−80 mmHg) is used during excision of vascular tumours or AVMs and more profound hypotension (MAP 50−70 mmHg) is sometimes induced for short periods during aneurysm surgery. In order to allow close control of arterial pressure drugs with a rapid onset and short duration of action are infused, using a volumetric infusion controller or syringe pump. Ideally the drugs should be given through a central line because peripheral pooling can occur with delay in action if a peripheral line is used. The drugs should be diluted in saline rather than glucose because hyperglycaemia will worsen the effects of any cerebral ischaemia.

The agents used to induce hypotension are discussed in detail in Chapter 4. Posture, controlled ventilation and anaesthesia with volatile agents may be sufficient to provide satisfactory control of arterial pressure. Halothane and enflurane may be used but isoflurane is the agent of choice because it reduces MAP mainly by peripheral vasodilatation, it reduces cerebral metabolic rate and has a minimal effect on the cerebral vasculature (Chapter 4). Labetalol may be effective in supplementing the hypotension if tachycardia develops and esmolol has been used as the sole hypotensive agent during surgery for intracranial arteriovenous malformations (Ornstein *et al.* 1991).

More profound hypotension requires the infusion of a short-acting vasodilator such as sodium nitroprusside, trimetaphan or glyceryl trinitrate. If the MAP is to be reduced to 60 mmHg or less sodium nitroprusside is recommended because it allows better maintenance of cerebral perfusion at lower arterial pressures. The author has found the 10:1 mixture of trimetaphan and nitroprusside described by Macrae and colleagues (1981) very useful during intracranial vascular surgery. Trimetaphan 125 mg and sodium nitroprusside 12.5 mg in 500 ml 0.9% saline titrated to effect allows rapid adjustment of arterial pressure without the wide swings seen when sodium nitroprusside alone is used. The use of a volatile agent smoothes the blood pressure control and reduces the dose of hypotensive agent required. Isoflurane may provide some cerebral protection because when used to reduce mean arterial pressure to 40−50 mmHg in dogs there was no anaerobic metabolism (Newberg *et al.* 1983, 1984).

During induced hypotension the anaesthetic technique should be meticulous, ensuring good oxygenation which is monitored by oximetry and arterial blood gases. At the end of the procedure the arterial pressure should be increased gradually, over 10–20 min, to reduce the hyperaemic response and reduce the likelihood of oedema formation as the cerebral capillaries are exposed to sudden increases in pressure. Autoregulation is impaired for up to 2 h after induced hypotension with sodium nitroprusside, halothane and probably other cerebral vasodilators. In order to reduce the risk of reactionary haemorrhage and postoperative intra-cranial haematoma, the dura should not be closed until the arterial pressure has returned to normal levels (a systolic pressure of more than 100 mmHg).

Induced hypothermia

The rationale behind the use of induced hypothermia is the reduction in metabolism and consumption of energy-rich compounds as temperature falls. Unlike the barbiturates, which only reduce the cerebral metabolism associated with cerebral electrical activity (activation metabolism) (Steen *et al.* 1983), hypothermia continues to reduce cerebral metabolic rate even after the EEG is isoelectric (residual metabolism) (Astrup *et al.* 1981, Steen *et al.* 1983). There is some evidence that smaller decreases in brain temperature from 36°C to 34°C may have some cerebral protective effect (Sano *et al.* 1992). The metabolic rate is reduced by 50% at 30°C, 66% at 25°C and 75% at 20°C, giving approximate safe ischaemic times of 6 min at 30°C and 10–12 min at 25°C (Gordon 1981), although these times are also influenced by the anaesthetic technique and presenting disease. Hypothermia offers the additional advantage of reducing brain bulk.

There has been a significant decline in the use of hypothermia since the early 1960s (McDowall 1971) due to better anaesthetic and surgical techniques and understanding of pathophysiology. Mild to moderate hypothermia (30°C) tends to be used only if temporary arrest of the circulation to part of the brain is anticipated during, for instance, surgical treatment of difficult aneurysms (Belopavlovic & Buchtal 1980).

Profound hypothermia (10–25°C) using cardiopulmonary bypass and total arrest of the circulation may be required for surgery to giant aneurysms. Cerebral metabolic rate is linearly related to body temperature so that the lower the temperature the longer the safe ischaemic time, but the complication rate increases at lower temperatures. Hypothermia may be used during resection of extensive highly vascular tumours or AVM if it is anticipated that temporary clipping of a major vessel will be required (Silverberg *et al.* 1981).

Anaesthetic technique

Cooling should be even and controlled, and shivering and vasoconstriction should be avoided.

MILD TO MODERATE HYPOTHERMIA

Chlorpromazine should be included in the premedication to inhibit shivering and produce peripheral vasodilatation. Anaesthesia is induced, maintained and monitored as for intracranial vascular surgery. Use of a non-depolarizing muscle relaxant will prevent shivering and a volatile agent with increments of chlorpromazine 10−25 mg will help to maintain peripheral vasodilatation. Ideally, temperature should be recorded from skin, subcutaneous tissue, muscle, oesophagus and rectum (Gordon 1981), but nasopharyngeal or tympanic membrane temperature are often used to monitor core temperature because of their close correlation with brain temperature. Arterial blood gases should be measured at regular intervals to detect abnormalities of $Pa\text{CO}_2$, to allow adjustment of ventilation and to detect the development of metabolic acidosis due to severe vasoconstriction. The aim is to keep the pH as near the normal value as possible. Cooling is usually performed with a water blanket connected to a heat exchanger or with air at 10°C. These methods have superseded immersion in a bath of cold water and the use of ice. Active cooling should be stopped when the central temperature is between 2°C and 3°C above the desired temperature, because there is a further 'after-drop' in body temperature after cooling is stopped. Bradycardia is a normal accompaniment of hypothermia and treatment of arrhythmias should be confined to runs of ventricular extrasystoles. Blood volume should be maintained with fluids warmed to the patient's temperature.

Rewarming should be gradual with warm air or water circulated around or under the patient. The temperature of the warming blanket should be monitored and should not exceed 40°C. As the temperature rises the blood pressure may fall due to vasodilatation, and intravenous fluids will be required. Anaesthesia should be maintained until the central temperature is greater than 34°C to avoid shivering which may lead to ventricular fibrillation or asystole due to the extra load placed on the hypothermic heart. Elective postoperative controlled ventilation has been suggested with the use of droperidol or chlorpromazine to prevent shivering and the associated increase in oxygen consumption (Gordon 1981).

PROFOUND HYPOTHERMIA

Profound hypothermia requires the use of cardiopulmonary bypass and the use of a heat exchanger. This technique has been used successfully to induce profound hypothermia (17–20°C) with femoro-femoral bypass and an arrest time of 7–15 min for the surgical management of eight giant aneurysms and one haemangioblastoma (Silverberg *et al.* 1981). Intracranial bleeding is a potentially lethal complication so potential clotting factor deficiencies were prevented by giving protamine sulphate, platelets, fresh-frozen plasma, calcium chloride, the patient's own unchilled blood and factor IX complex to all patients. The technique is not without problems and should be used only in selected cases.

References

Adams H.P., Kassell N.F., Turner J.C. & Haley E.C. (1987) Predicting cerebral ischaemia after aneurysmal subarachnoid haemorrhage: influences of clinical condition, CT results, and antifibrinolytic therapy. *Neurology* **37**, 1586–1591.

Allcutt D.A., Chakraborty M. & Sengupta R.P. (1991) Neurosurgical experience with carotid endarterectomy: a 12-year study. *British Journal of Neurosurgery* **5**, 257–264.

Allen G.S., Ahn M.S., Preziosi T.G. *et al.* (1983) Cerebral arterial spasm—a controlled trial of nimodipine in patients with subarachnoid haemorrhage. *New England Journal of Medicine* **308**, 619–624.

Alvord E.C., Loeser J.D., Bailey W.L. & Copass M.K. (1972) Subarachnoid hemorrhage due to ruptured aneurysms. A simple method of estimating prognosis. *Archives of Neurology* **27**, 273–284.

Andrews P.J.D., Dearden N.M. & Miller J.D. (1991) Jugular bulb cannulation: description of a cannulation technique and validation of a new continuous monitor. *British Journal of Anaesthesia* **67**, 553–558.

Archer D.P., Shaw D.A., Leblanc R.L. & Tranmer B.I. (1991) Haemodynamic considerations in the management of patients with subarachnoid haemorrhage. *Canadian Journal of Anaesthesia* **38**, 454–470.

Astrup J., Sorensen P.M. & Soresen H.R. (1981) Inhibition of cerebral oxygen and glucose consumption in the dog by hypothermia, pentobarbitial, and lidocaine. *Anesthesiology* **55**, 263–268.

Barnett H.J.M., Sackett D.L., Taylors S.J. *et al.* (1985) Failure of extracranial-intracranial arterial bypass to reduce the risk of ischemic stroke. Results of an international randomised trial. *New England Journal of Medicine* **313**, 1191–1200.

Baughman V.L., Hoffman W.E., Thomas C., Albrecht R.F. & Miletich D.J. (1989) The interaction of nitrous oxide and isoflurane with incomplete cerebral ischemia in the rat. *Anesthesiology* **70**, 767–774.

Belopavlovic M. & Buchtal A. (1980) Cardiac arrest during moderate hypothermia for cerebrovascular surgery. *Anaesthesia* **35**, 368–371.

Brown F.D., Hanlon K. & Mullan S. (1978) Treatment of aneurysmal hemiplegia with dopamine and mannitol. *Journal of Neurosurgery* **49**, 525–529.

Brown M.M. & Humphrey P.R.D. (1992) Carotid endarterectomy: recommendations for management of transient ischaemic attack and ischaemic stroke. *British Medical Journal* **305**, 1017–1074.

Cruickshank J.M., Neil-Dwyer G. & Brice J. (1974) Electrocardiographic changes and their prognostic significance in subarachnoid haemorrhage. *Journal of Neurology, Neurosurgery and Psychiatry* **37**, 755–759.

Cucchiara R.F. & Messick J.M. (1981) The failure of nasal plethysmography to estimate cerebral blood flow during carotid occlusion. *Anesthesiology* **55**, 585–586.

Cucchiara R.F., Sharbrough F.W., Messick J.M. & Tinker J.H. (1979) An electro-encephalographic filter-processor as an indicator of cerebral ischemia during carotid endarterectomy. *Anesthesiology* **51**, 77–79.

Cucchiara R.F., Benefiel D.J., Matteo R.S., Dewood M. & Albin M.S. (1986) Evaluation of esmolol in controlling increases in heart rate and blood pressure during endotracheal intubation in patients undergoing carotid endarterectomy. *Anesthesiology* **65**, 528–531.

Doshi R. & Neil-Dwyer G. (1977) Hypothalamic and myocardial lesions after subarachnoid haemorrhage. *Journal of Neurology, Neurosurgery and Psychiatry* **40**, 821–826.

Engberg M., Melsen N.C., Herlevsen P., Haraldsted V. & Cold G.E. (1990) Changes of blood pressure and cerebral arterio-venous oxygen content differences ($AVDO_2$) with and without bupivacaine scalp infiltration during craniotomy. *Acta Anaesthesiologica Scandinavica* **34**, 346–349.

Farrar J.K., Gamache F.W., Ferguson G.G., Barker J., Varkey G.P. & Drake C.G. (1981) Effects of profound hypotension on cerebral blood flow during surgery for intracranial aneurysms. *Journal of Neurosurgery* **55**, 857–864.

Ferguson G. (1972) Physical factors in the initiation, growth and rupture of human intracranial aneurysms. *Journal of Neurosurgery* **37**, 666–677.

Gibson B.E., McMichan J.C. & Cucchiara R.F. (1986) Lack of correlation between transconjunctival O_2 and cerebral blood flow during carotid artery occlusion. *Anesthesiology* **64**, 277–279.

Gold A.P., Ransohoff J. & Carter S. (1964) Vein of Galen malformation. *Acta Neurologica Scandinavica* **40** (Suppl. 11), 1–31.

Gordon E. (1981) Induced hypothermia. In: Gordon E. (Ed.), *A Basis and Practice of Neuroanaesthesia*, pp. 331–343. Excerpta Medica, Amsterdam.

Halbach V.V., Higashida R.T. & Hieshima G.B. (1989) Interventional neuro-radiology. *American Journal of Roentgenology* **153**, 467–476.

Helfman S.M., Gold M.I., De Lisser E.A. & Herrington C.A. (1991) Which drug prevents tachycardia and hypertension associated with tracheal intubation: lidocaine, fentanyl or esmolol? *Anesthesia and Analgesia* **72**, 482–486.

Holohan T.V. (1991) Extracranial-intracranial bypass to reduce the risk of ischaemic stroke. *Canadian Medical Association Journal* **1**: 144(11), 1457–1465.

Hunt W.E. & Hess R.M. (1968) Surgical risk as related to time of intervention in the repair of intracranial aneurysms. *Journal of Neurosurgery* **28**, 14–20.

Jung R., Shah N., Reinsel R. *et al.* (1990) Cerebrospinal fluid pressure in patients with brain tumors: impact of fentanyl versus alfentanil during nitrous oxide–oxygen anesthesia. *Anesthesia and Analgesia* **71**, 419–422.

Kassell N.F., Sasaki T., Colohan A.R.T. & Nazar G. (1985) Cerebral vasospasm following aneurysmal subarachnoid hemorrhage. *Stroke* **16**, 562–572.

Kelman G.R. & Kennedy B.R. (1971) Cardiovascular effects of pancuronium in man. *British Journal of Anaesthesia* **43**, 335–338.

Kochs E., Hoffman W.E., Werner C., Thomas C., Albrecht R.F. & Schulte Am Esch J. (1992) The effects of propofol on brain electrical activity, neurologic outcome, and neuronal damage following incomplete ischemia in rats. *Anesthesiology* **76**, 245–252.

Lam A.M., Manninen P.H., Ferguson G.G. & Nantau W. (1991) Monitoring electrophysiologic function during carotid endarterectomy: a comparison of somatosensory evoked potentials and conventional electroencephalogram. *Anesthesiology* **75**, 15–21.

Levy W.J., Bay J.W., Sawhny B. & Tank T. (1982) Aminophylline plus nitro-prusside and dopamine for treatment of cerebral vasospasm. A preliminary report. *Journal of Neurosurgery* **56**, 646–649.

London M.J., Hollenberg M., Wong M.G. *et al.* (1988) Intraoperative myocardial ischemia: localization by continuous 12-lead electrocardiography. *Anesthesiology* **69**, 232–241.

McDowall D.G. (1971) The current use of hypothermia in British neurosurgery. *British Journal of Anaesthesia* **43**, 1084–1087.

McIntyre J.W.R., Dobson D., Weir B.K.A., West R. & Overton T.R. (1971) Monitoring under anaesthesia, with reference to subarachnoid haemorrhage, and the T-wave as an electrocardiographic manifestation. *Canadian Anaesthetists Society Journal* **18**, 293–297.

McKay R.D., Sundt T.M., Michenfelder J.D. *et al.* (1976) Internal carotid artery stump pressure and cerebral blood flow during carotid endarterectomy: modification by halothane, enflurane, and Innovar. *Anesthesiology* **45**, 390–399.

Macrae W.R., Wildsmith J.A.W. & Dale B.A.B. (1981) Induced hypotension with a mixture of sodium nitroprusside and trimetaphan camsylate. *Anaesthesia* **36**, 312−315.

Markand O.N., Dilley R.S., Moorthy S.S. & Warren C. (1984) Monitoring of somatosensory evoked responses during carotid endarterectomy. *Archives of Neurology* **41**, 375−378.

Messick J.M. & Sundt T.M. (1990) Ischemic cerebral vascular disease. In: Cucchiara R.F. & Michenfelder J.D. (Eds), *Clinical Neuroanesthesia*, p. 269. Churchill Livingstone, New York.

Messick J.M., Casement B., Sharbrough F.W., Milde L.N., Michenfelder J.D. & Sundt T.M. (1987) Correlation of regional cerebral blood flow (rCBF) with EEG changes during isoflurane anesthesia for carotid endarterectomy: critical rCBF. *Anesthesiology* **66**, 344−349.

Michenfelder J.D., Sundt T.M., Fode N. & Sharbrough F.W. (1987) Isoflurane when compared to enflurane and halothane decreases frequency of cerebral ischemia during carotid endarterectomy. *Anesthesiology* **67**, 336−340.

Miller D.R., Martineau R.J., Wynands J.E. & Hill J. (1991) Bolus administration of esmolol for controlling the haemodynamic response to tracheal intubation: the Canadian Multicentre Trial. *Canadian Journal of Anaesthesia* **38**, 849−858.

Moss E. (1992) Alfentanil increases intracranial pressure when intracranial compliance is low. *Anaesthesia* **47**, 134−136.

Moss E., Powell D., Gibson R.M. & McDowall D.G. (1978) Effects of fentanyl on intracranial pressure and cerebral perfusion pressure during normocapnia. *British Journal of Anaesthesia* **50**, 779−784.

Murphy T.M. (1987) Somatic blockade of head and neck. In: Cousins M.J. & Bridenbaugh P.O. (Eds), *Neural Blockade in Clinical Anesthesia and Management of Pain*, pp. 551−554. J. B. Lippincott, Philadelphia.

Murphy P.G., Myers D.S., Davies M.J., Webster N.R. & Jones J.G. (1992) The antioxidant potential of propofol (2,6-diisopropylphenol). *British Journal of Anaesthesia* **68**, 613−618.

Newberg L.A., Milde J.H. & Michenfelder J.D. (1983) The cerebral metabolic effects of isoflurane at and above concentrations that suppress cortical activity. *Anesthesiology* **59**, 23−28.

Newberg L.A., Milde J.H. & Michenfelder J.D. (1984) Systemic and cerebral effects of isoflurane-induced hypotension in dogs. *Anesthesiology* **60**, 541−546.

Nornes H. (1973) The role of intracranial pressure in the arrest of hemorrhage in patients with ruptured intracranial aneurysm. *Journal of Neurosurgery* **39**, 226−234.

Omote K., Kirita A., Namiki A. & Iwasaki H. (1992) Effects of nicardipine on the circulatory responses to tracheal intubation in normotensive and hypertensive patients. *Anaesthesia* **47**, 24−27.

Ornstein E., Young W.L., Ostapkovich N., Matteo R.S. & Diaz J. (1991) Deliberate hypotension in patients with intracranial arteriovenous malformations:

esmolol compared with isoflurane and sodium nitroprusside. *Anesthesia and Analgesia* **72**, 639–644.

Pearce H.J., Becchetti J.J. & Brown H.J. (1980) Supraorbital photoplethysmographic monitoring during carotid endarterectomy with the use of an internal shunt: an added dimension of safety. *Surgery* **87**, 339–342.

Pearce H.J., Lowell J., Tubb D.W. & Brown H.J. (1979) Continuous oculoplethysmographic monitoring during carotid endarterectomy. *American Journal of Surgery* **138**, 733–735.

Pickard J.D., Matheson M., Patterson J. & Wyper D. (1980) Prediction of late ischemic complications after cerebral aneurysm surgery by the intraoperative measurement of cerebral blood flow. *Journal of Neurosurgery* **53**, 305–308.

Pickard J.D., Murray G.D., Illingworth R. *et al.* (1989) Effect of oral nimodipine on cerebral infarction and outcome after subarachnoid haemorrhage. British aneurysm nimodipine trial. *British Medical Journal* **298**, 636–642.

Prior P.F. (1985) EEG monitoring and evoked potentials in brain ischaemia. *British Journal of Anaesthesia* **57**, 63–81.

Rainer W.G., McCrory C.B. & Feiler E.M. (1966) Surgery on the carotid artery with cervical block anaesthesia. Technical considerations. *American Journal of Surgery* **112**, 703–705.

Relman A.S. (1987) The extracranial–intracranial arterial bypass study. What have we learned? *New England Journal of Medicine* **316**, 809–810.

Roberts P.A., Pollay M., Engles C., Pendleton B., Reynolds E. & Stevens F.A. (1987) Effect on intracranial pressure of furosemide combined with varying doses and administration rates of mannitol. *Journal of Neurosurgery* **66**, 440–446.

Rosenorn J. & Diemer N.H. (1982) Reduction of regional cerebral blood flow during brain retraction pressure in the rat. *Journal of Neurosurgery* **56**, 826–829.

Sano T., Drummond J.C., Patel P.M., Grafe M.J., Watson J.C. & Cole D.J. (1992) A comparison of the cerebral protective effects of isoflurane and mild hypothermia in a model of incomplete forebrain ischemia in the rat. *Anesthesiology* **76**, 221–228.

Schettini A., Stahurski B. & Young H.F. (1982) Osmotic and osmotic-loop diuresis in brain surgery. Effects on plasma and CSF electrolytes and ion excretion. *Journal of Neurosurgery* **56**, 679–684.

Shaw M.D.M. (1987) Aneurysms. In: Miller J.D. (Ed.), *Northfield's Surgery of the Central Nervous System*, p. 380. Blackwell Scientific Publications, Oxford.

Sherman D.G. & Hart R.G. (1992) Stroke and transient ischemic attack: thromboembolism and antithrombotic therapy. In: Fuster V. & Verstraete W.B. (Eds), *Thrombosis in Cardiovascular Disorders*, pp. 409–422. W.B. Saunders, Philadelphia.

Shoemaker W.C. & Lawner P.M. (1983) Method for continuous conjunctival oxygen monitoring during carotid artery surgery. *Critical Care Medicine* **11**, 946–947.

Silverberg G.D., Reitz B.A. & Ream A.K. (1981) Hypothermia and cardiac arrest in the treatment of giant aneurysms of the cerebral circulation and haemangioblastoma of the medulla. *Journal of Neurosurgery* **55**, 337–346.

Spaerel W.E. (1982) Monitoring the safe levels of hypotension. 1. General considerations. *International Anesthesiology Clinics* **20**, 111–119.

Spencer M.P., Thomas G.I., Nicholls S.C. & Sauvage L.R. (1990) Detection of middle cerebral artery emboli during carotid endarterectomy using transcranial Doppler ultrasonography. *Stroke* **21**, 415–423.

Steen P.A., Newberg L., Milde J.H. & Michenfelder J.D. (1983) Hypothermia and barbiturates: individual and combined effects on canine cerebral oxygen consumption. *Anesthesiology* **58**, 527–532.

Sundt T.M., Sharbrough F.W., Anderson R.E. & Michenfelder J.D. (1974) Cerebral blood flow measurements and electroencephalograms during carotid endarterectomy. *Journal of Neurosurgery* **41**, 310–320.

Sundt T.M., Sharbrough F.W., Marsh W.R., Ebersold M.J., Piepgras D.G. & Messick J.M. (1986) The risk–benefit ratio of intraoperative shunting during carotid endarterectomy. Relevancy to operative and postoperative results and complications. *Annals of Surgery* **203**, 196–204.

Vucevic M., Purdy G.M. & Ellis F.R. (1992) Esmolol hydrochloride for management of the cardiovascular stress responses to laryngoscopy and tracheal intubation. *British Journal of Anaesthesia* **68**, 529–530.

Weintraub B.M. & McHenry L.C. (1974) Cardiac abnormalities in subarachnoid hemorrhage: a resume. *Stroke* **5**, 384–392.

White J.C., Parker S.D. & Rogers M.C. (1985) Preanesthetic evaluation of a patient with pathologic Q waves following subarachnoid hemorrhage. *Anesthesiology* **62**, 351–354.

Wilkins R.H. (1985) Natural history of intracranial vascular malformations: a review. *Neurosurgery* **16**, 421–430.

Winslow C.M., Solomon D.H., Chassin M.R., Kosecoff J., Merrick N.J. & Brook R.H. (1988) The appropriateness of carotid endarterectomy. *New England Journal of Medicine* **318**, 721–727.

Wong D.H.W. (1991) Perioperative stroke. Part 1: General surgery, carotid artery disease and carotid endarterectomy. *Canadian Journal of Anaesthesia* **38**, 347–373.

11
Anaesthesia for spinal surgery

IAN CALDER

Introduction

Surgical treatment of spinal pathology is a relatively recent phenomenon. For instance, lumbar disc protrusion was not recognized as a clinical entity until 1934 (Mixter & Barr, 1934). The revolution in diagnostic radiology produced by the invention of CT and MRI has led to increasingly complex surgery. Both orthopaedic and neurosurgical specialists have regarded the spine as falling within their sphere of interest. There has been a call for a separate superspecialty of 'spinal surgery', which would have a training programme drawing upon orthopaedic and neurosurgical areas of expertise (Crockard 1992). The greatest advances have occurred in the treatment of lesions in the cervical spine, and most attention will be given to that region in this chapter.

Symptoms and signs in spinal disease

The symptoms and signs encountered in patients with spinal disease are principally due to damage to nerve roots (radiculopathy) or the spinal cord (myelopathy).

RADICULOPATHY

Sensory fibre damage causes pain and/or paraesthesiae in the appropriate distribution.
Motor damage causes lower motor neurone type weakness, wasting, and fasciculation of the muscles, with diminished reflexes.

MYELOPATHY

Sensory damage may cause loss of joint position sense and a sensory 'level'. Special patterns such as Brown–Sequard syndrome may

274

occur. 'L'Hermitte's phenomenon' is an 'electric shock' sensation in the arms/legs/trunk, provoked by movement of the neck.

Motor damage causes limb weakness of upper motor neurone type, with spasticity and increased reflexes. The muscles are flaccid during the acute phase of cord injury.

Sympathetic damage in acute cord injury may result in hypotension, bradycardia and postural hypotension. Hypotension is more likely with high lesions.

Bladder and bowel control may be lost, due to a combination of sensory, motor, and autonomic palsy in either myelopathy or lumbar radiculopathy.

Cervical disease can present with brachalgia and weakness of arm muscles (radiculopathy), or weakness of the legs with a sensory level (myelopathy). Both radiculopathy and myelopathy may be present. *Thoracic* disease commonly presents with a myelopathy, whereas *lumbar* disease presents as a radiculopathy (the spinal cord ends about L1/L2).

Cervical spine

ANATOMY OF THE CERVICAL SPINE

There are seven cervical vertebrae. C1 (atlas) and C2 (axis) are specialized in structure and function, forming the cervical component of the *cranio-cervical junction.* The atlas is a ring perforated by the odontoid peg or 'dens' (dens = tooth), which projects upwards from the body of the axis. The dens fuses from three elements in the first 9 months of life. Failures of fusion occur (classically in Down's syndrome), leading to malformed, short or separated pegs — 'os odontoideum'. The dens is restrained by the transverse and apical ligaments. The transverse ligament, which is as strong as the lateral ligament of the knee, runs across the atlas and is the principal structure preventing atlanto-axial subluxation. The apical ligaments run from the tip of the dens to the base of the skull.

BLOOD SUPPLY OF THE CERVICAL CORD

The blood supply of the cervical cord comes from the carotid and vertebral arteries. There are named vessels (anterior and posterior spinal arteries), but much of the cord's blood supply comes from vessels reaching the cord along the dentate ligaments. A communicating plexus of vessels surrounds the cord, so that it is usually unscathed by carotid or vertebral occlusion. The vasculature of the cord appears to behave in the same way as the cerebral vessels. Autoregulation of cord blood flow may be abolished by disease, so that hypotension and hypertension may produce oligaemia or hyperaemia of the cord.

RADIOLOGY OF THE CERVICAL SPINE

Identification of the cervical vertebrae on a lateral radiograph is facilitated by first finding the axis vertebra; *the spine of the axis is large and square,* and the 'lateral masses' (the transverse processes) create a characteristic oval shadow (Fig. 11.1). The other vertebrae can then be identified. The

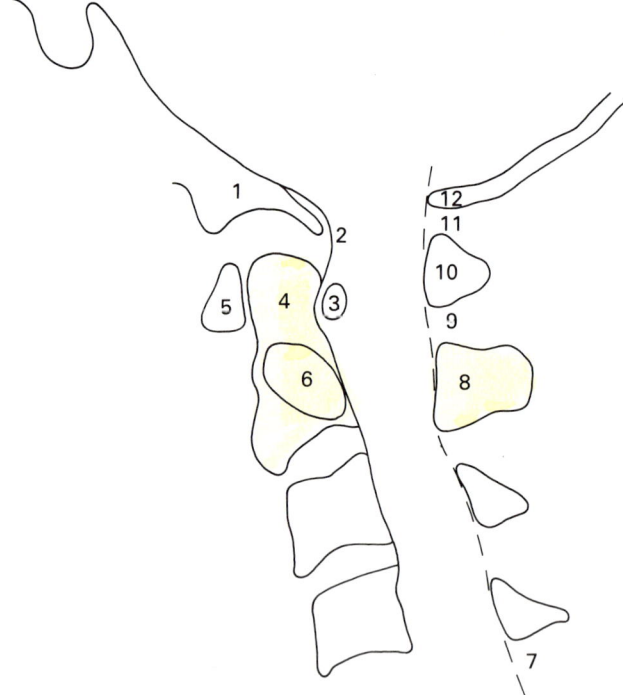

Fig. 11.1 The craniocervical junction. This diagram should be compared with a lateral cervical X-ray to assist in identifying the bony structures. 1, clivus; 2, tectorial membrane; 3, transverse ligament; 4, odonoid peg; 5, anterior arch of atlas; 6, lateral mass of axis; 7, subspinous line; 8, spine of axis; 9, atlanto-axial gap; 10, posterior arch of atlas; 11, atlanto-occipital gap; 12, occiput.

alignment of the vertebrae is best assessed by drawing an imaginary subspinous line.

MRI is currently the premier investigation, since soft tissue can be visualized. CT, often combined with myelography, may be preferred for the study of bony abnormalities.

MOVEMENTS OF THE CERVICAL SPINE

The movements at the craniocervical junction are of paramount importance to the anaesthetist. Flexion/extension amounts to about 25°, shared equally between the atlanto-occipital and atlanto-axial joints. It has been suggested that the first two vertebrae and their joints should be considered as a unit — 'the occipito-atlanto-axial (OAA) complex' (White & Panjabi 1978). The range of movement at the OAA complex is limited (in health) by the tectorial membrane, which is the prolongation of the posterior longitudinal ligament, inserted on to the clivus. Flexion/ extension movements betweeen the other cervical vertebrae are limited, but add up to an impressive 66°, being maximal at C4/5/6 (White & Panjabi 1978). The range of movement decreases with increasing age (Hayashi *et al.* 1987). Rotatory movements occur principally at the atlanto-axial joint.

STABILITY OF THE CERVICAL SPINE

The thoracic and lumbar spines rarely become unstable. The intervertebral joints in the lumbar and thoracic regions are made for stability rather than movement, but the cervical spine is required to be both mobile and stable. The magnitude of this undertaking can be appreciated when one considers that the head weighs about 6 kg and may move 600 times per hour (Konttinen *et al.* 1991).

The atlanto-axial joint is particularly prone to instability. The joint is inherently less stable, because of its rotatory function. It relies heavily on the integrity of the transverse and apical ligaments.

The cervical spine can be considered in terms of two or three 'columns'. In the two-column description the anterior column is composed of the anterior longitudinal ligament, the disc and the posterior longitudinal ligament, with the posterior column composed of the facet joints, neural arch (pedicles and laminae), interspinous and supraspinous ligaments. Instability is more likely when the posterior column is disrupted (McCrae 1981). Some authors have separated the posterior column into two, so that the middle column comprises the facet joints and neural arch. Adherents of the three-column model suggest that instability is unlikely if only one column is damaged (Hirschfeld 1990). The musculature of the neck also contributes to stability.

CAUSES OF CERVICAL INSTABILITY

Trauma causes the most severe grades of instability at all levels of the cervical spine. Instability can also result, at any level, from tumours, tuberculosis and rheumatoid arthritis. Congenital atlanto-axial instability is seen in Down's syndrome, Morquio's syndrome, Sprengel's syndrome, sporadic agenesis of the odontoid peg, Marfan's syndrome, Hurler's syndrome, and the fetal warfarin syndrome (Van Gilder *et al*. 1987a).

DIAGNOSIS OF INSTABILITY

Instability of the cervical spine is not necessarily associated with symptoms and signs. Chronic instability in rheumatoid arthritis and Down's syndrome may be symptomless and the onset of signs insidious (Collins *et al*. 1911, Hreidarsson *et al*. 1982). In a study by Bohlman (1979) one-third of fractures were missed at the time of presentation. Secondary neurological deterioration occurred more frequently in the patients whose fractures had been missed. A high index of suspicion is required (Fig. 11.2).

A lateral radiograph of the cervical spine cannot exclude instability. Flexion/extension views are required, and preferably flexion/extension CT or MRI scans.

STABILIZATION OF THE UNSTABLE NECK

It is surprisingly difficult to immobilize the cervical spine. Up to 25% of total cord injury has been blamed on poor immobilization after trauma (Podolsky *et al*. 1983).

Cervical collars, whether hard or soft, are mostly unable to prevent movements. Hard collars allow about 70% of normal flexion and extension. A combination of hard collar, bilateral sandbags and tape is much more effective (Podolsky *et al*. 1983). This effectively prevents flexion and limits extension to 35% of normal.

Short-board technique: splinting both head and torso to a rigid board has been shown to prevent movements in all planes (Cline *et al*. 1985). Sophisticated, MRI-compatible, boards are available.

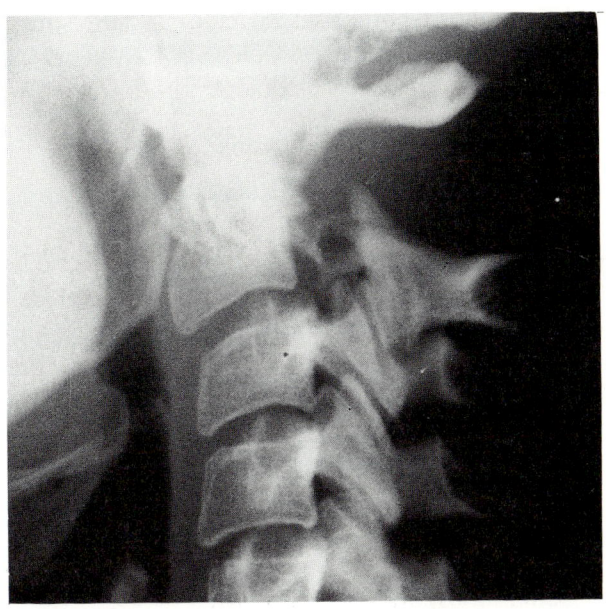

Fig. 11.2 Fracture of the axis vertebra (often known as the 'Hangman's fracture' — apparently inappropriately, since James and Nasmyth-Jones (1992) found that only three of 34 executions in Britain produced this fracture). This patient attended work for 2 weeks after hitting the windscreen. The radiograph was taken because of persistent neck pain. (Courtesy of Mr A. Crockard).

In-line traction can be applied manually by an assistant, or more formally with varying weights after the application of skull tongs. Traction is a traditional method of discouraging movement. The danger of causing distraction of the cord by longitudinal traction is increasingly appreciated (Kaufman *et al.* 1982, Marshall *et al.* 1987, Bivins *et al.* 1988). Traction should be applied with caution. Distraction is particularly likely when traction is applied to ankylosing spondylitis patients with fractured cervical spines. Traction should not be used in such patients (Rowed 1992).

Halo body frames: prolonged effective immobilization can be achieved with external rigid fixators. Airway obstruction has been reported during (Meakam *et al.* 1990) and after (Kainuma & Yamada 1985) application of halo body frames under general anaesthesia. The possibility that the head and neck may be fixed in a position that encourages airway obstruction must be borne in mind.

Internal fixators: an ever-increasing range of screws, plates, rectangles and loops, as well as bone and other materials, such as coral, are used in stabilization procedures.

GENERAL ANAESTHESIA AND THE UNSTABLE CERVICAL SPINE

The fearful possibility is that an unstable patient might be rendered quadriplegic by an anaesthetic manoeuvre. This has not been reported, although publication might not be sought after such an event. An enquiry of the members of the British Cervical Spine Society failed to elicit any knowledge of such a case (Calder 1990). The only contribution was of a patient with Klippel–Feil syndrome whose neck had been broken in a road traffic accident. This patient became quadriplegic after being subjected to rigid bronchoscopy.

Anaesthetic technique
In addition to the overriding requisite of adequate oxygenation at all times there are two objectives.
1 Minimal movement at the unstable site.
2 Cardiovascular stability, so that perfusion of the cord is maintained.
Most attention has been given to techniques of tracheal intubation.

Awake fibreoptic intubation
The fibreoptic endoscope allows tracheal tubes to be placed under topical anaesthesia. Keeping the patient conscious might have some benefits. First, the conscious patient might be able to prevent dangerous movements by voluntary and reflex muscular activity. Secondly, continuous examination of the neurological state is possible, so that any manoeuvre causing deterioration can be reversed at once. This is a particularly attractive feature during positioning for surgery (see below), indeed for surgery itself. A series of surgical stabilizations performed under local anaesthesia has been reported (Zigler *et al.* 1987).

It has been pointed out that coughing can be severe during awake fibreoptic intubation (Wells & Tredrea 1987). Ovassapian *et al.* (1983) reported a 16% incidence of 'severe' coughing. However, in skilled hands coughing is usually minimal and a large series of uncomplicated awake fibreoptic intubations in unstable patients has been reported (Meschino *et al.* 1992). The intubations were mostly performed by residents.

A major argument in favour of awake intubation is the impressive cardiovascular stability that can be achieved (Ovassapian *et al.* 1983).

Awake intubation is obviously impossible in unconscious and uncooperative patients. Fibreoptic intubation can be carried out under general anaesthesia, but most methods require the presence of a skilled assistant and are associated with cardiovascular instability (Smith 1988, Smith *et al.* 1992).

Tracheal intubation under general anaesthesia

Cadaver studies on airway interventions have shown that all the usual manoeuvres (jaw lift, head extension, airway insertion, cricoid pressure, direct laryngoscopy, oral and nasal intubation) produce movement at unstable sites (Bivins *et al.* 1988, Aprahamian *et al.* 1984). Cadaver studies cannot, of course, tell us what movements might occur during awake fibreoptic intubation. These studies have not been backed up by clinical reports of neurological damage. On the contrary, large numbers of patients have been treated using conventional orotracheal intubation after muscle paralysis, mask ventilation and cricoid pressure (Doolan & O'Brien 1985, Stellin *et al.* 1989, Grande *et al.* 1988, Suderman *et al.* 1991). The cadaver finding, that blind nasal intubation produced slightly less movement at the unstable site than oral intubation (Aprahamian *et al.* 1984), led to the recommendation in the Advanced Trauma Life Support protocols of the American College of Surgeons, that blind nasal intubation should be performed when cervical instability is suspected (American College of Surgeons 1990). Other than the cadaver findings there appears to be no basis for this recommendation, while evidence that blind nasal intubation is more difficult and traumatic than oral intubation exists (Dronen *et al.* 1987). It is interesting to note that direct laryngoscopy has been reported to have little effect on the disposition of the lower cervical vertebrae (Horton *et al.* 1989), which are the most often injured (Bohlman 1979). The arguments have been reviewed by Wood & Lawler (1992).

The paradox of the unstable cervical spine

Ironically, the unstable patient is often quite the reverse when presented for anaesthesia. Fixation devices have usually been applied, so that the practical problem becomes more one of difficult direct laryngoscopy. It is principally for this reason that fibreoptic skills are extremely useful.

If direct laryngoscopy is undertaken, a 'gum elastic bougie' should be to hand, since less exposure of the glottis is required when this aid is used (Nolan & Wilson 1992). The laryngeal mask has a place in establishing an emergency airway (Logan 1991, Pennant *et al.* 1992).

The laryngeal mask allows fibreoptic intubation under general anaesthesia without a skilled assistant (Silk *et al.* 1991).

Conclusion

There is no evidence to support the 'therapeutic legend' (Rosen & Wolfe 1989), that orotracheal intubation is neurologically more dangerous than blind nasal or awake fibreoptic intubation. Some 'unstable' patients are difficult direct laryngoscopies unless their stabilizing devices are removed; fibreoptic techniques are useful. Awake fibreoptic intubation is associated with cardiovascular stability.

Difficult intubation in cervical spine disease

It has long been recognized that cervical disease can cause difficult intubation (Brechner 1968). The overall incidence of difficult direct laryngoscopy in patients having cervical surgery at the National Hospital is 19% (Cormack and Lehane grades 3 or 4 at direct laryngscopy). The incidence in the general population is only 1–3% (Benumof 1991).

It must be understood that it is currently not possible to identify the difficult patients without a high incidence of false-positives. Even if we had a test, or combination of tests, giving a specificity (negativity in health) of 99% and a sensitivity (positivity in disease) of 95%, with an incidence of 1%, half the positive predictions would be false (Calder 1992a). We have no test, or combination of tests, that approaches such levels of sensitivity and specificity. It has therefore to be appreciated that, although we can hope to identify the easy patients with some confidence, it must be accepted that our predictions of difficulty will often be false.

CAUSES OF DIFFICULT INTUBATION

There are three causes of difficult intubation: poor mouth opening, poor cervical movements and narrowed airway.

POOR MOUTH OPENING

This is often a feature in cervical disease, since temporomandibular joint dysfunction is common. Loss of protrusion is more important than the absolute measurement of interdental distance. When protrusion is lost, the line of vision obtained at direct laryngoscopy may be *worse* with increasing interdental distance. Shortening of the neck (loss of joint spaces or vertebral collapse) can mean that the mandible's movements are restricted by the manubrium. Limitation of mouth opening can be iatrogenic. Patients with facial fractures are presented with interdental wiring, or the application of a stiff collar can restrict mouth opening.

The function of the temporomandibular joint should be tested by asking the patient to protrude the mandible so that the lower incisors (or dentures) lie in front of the upper incisors (position A); if this can be achieved difficult direct laryngoscopy is very unlikely, provided that the jaw can hinge without obstruction. Restriction of protrusion to position B (upper and lower incisors touching) or C (lower incisors cannot be brought forward to touch the upper incisors) indicates difficulty. Difficult direct laryngoscopy is invariable if protrusion is grade C.

The Mallampati examination (Mallampati *et al.* 1985) is a useful test in patients with cervical disease. A Mallampati class 3 (hard palate only) has a high positive predictive value in this group (>70% in rheumatoid patients — I. Calder unpublished observations), although the test is not as sensitive as mandibular protrusion. The high positive predictive value (percentage of patients predicted to be difficult, who actually are difficult) in cervical disease, contrasts with the low values (4.2% and 6.6%) quoted for general surgical (Oates *et al.* 1991) and obstetric patients (Rocke *et al.* 1992).

POOR CERVICAL MOVEMENTS

Poor movement at the top end of the cervical spine is much more likely to produce difficulty than restricted movement at the lower end. Thus rheumatoid is a frequent cause, and spondylosis an infrequent cause, of difficult intubation.

Testing cervical movements is not easy. An impression can be formed as to whether the head extends satisfactorily on the neck by restraining the flexed neck with one hand and extending the head with the other. However, diminution of movement has to be considerable before it can be reliably diagnosed. The Patil examination, which measures the thyromental distance with the head extended, is simple and quick to do (Patil *et al.* 1983), but the author has found it to be insensitive with a poor predictive value in cervical disease.

If available, radiographic evidence of diminished top end movement should be studied. Absence of a gap between the posterior elements of the atlas and occiput or axis on a flexion lateral radiograph has predictive significance. Approximately half the patients with an absent atlanto-occipital gap are difficult, whilst 80% of those with an absent atlanto-axial gap are difficult (Calder *et al.* 1991). An 'absent gap' can also be diagnosed if the gap is small and fixed on flexion and extension (Fig. 11.3a, b).

NARROWED AIRWAY

This is an unusual cause of difficulty in cervical disease. Tumour or abscesses occasionally deform the airway. MRI can provide useful information (Schneider *et al.* 1989). Preoperative examination with a fibre-optic laryngoscope can be used to evaluate the situation.

OVERALL ASSESSMENT

As well as the examinations already mentioned, one should consider other factors.

Disease
Difficulty is so common in cervical rheumatoid (except reducible atlanto-axial subluxation) that it should be considered a powerful predictor.

Presence of fixation device
Any metal device such as a halo body frame or an internal fixator such

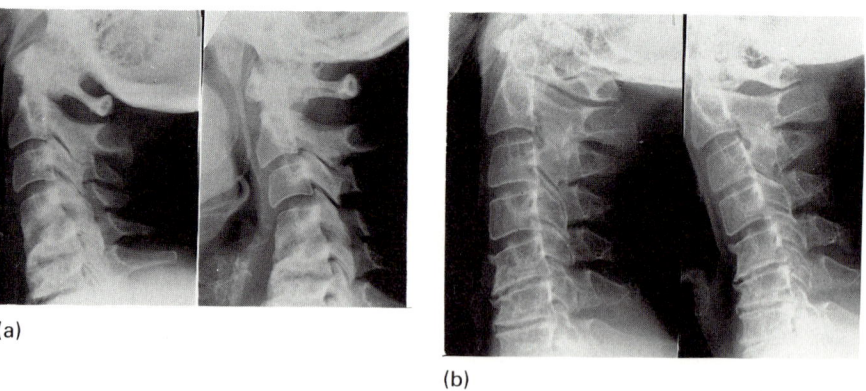

(a)

(b)

Fig. 11.3 (a) Cervical spondylosis: flexion/extension lateral radiographs. Posterior atlanto-occipital and atlanto-axial gaps present. (b) Cervical spondylosis: gaps absent.

as a Ransford loop or Hartshill rectangle will almost always mean difficulty, but skull traction is less likely to be associated with problems.

Dental condition
The presence of precarious teeth or expensive dental restorations must be taken into account.

When making a preoperative assessment of these factors it is helpful to collect all the information onto a single form (Fig. 11.4).

MANAGEMENT OF EXPECTED DIFFICULT INTUBATION

Awake fibreoptic intubation is the most satisfactory technique. The first report of fibreoptic-assisted intubation was by Murphy (1967), who was then a registrar at the National Hospital. A detailed description of a suitable technique for fibreoptic intubation is given at the end of this chapter.

Extubation following cervical spine surgery

Whilst fibreoptic intubation now allows safe intubation in nearly every patient, extubation has become the major problem for the anaesthetist. Awake extubation although generally the safest technique, may not always be advisable (as in cervical spondylosis, described below). If it is

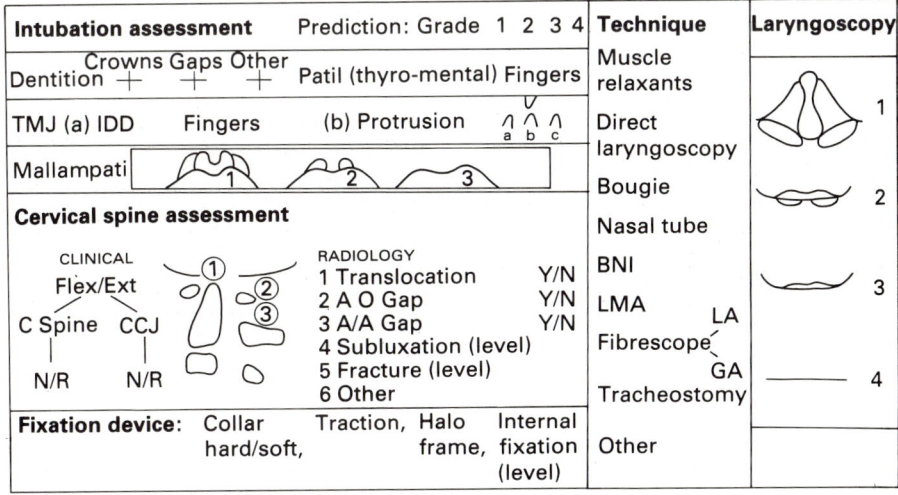

Fig. 11.4 Tracheal intubation assessment form in use at the National Hospital.

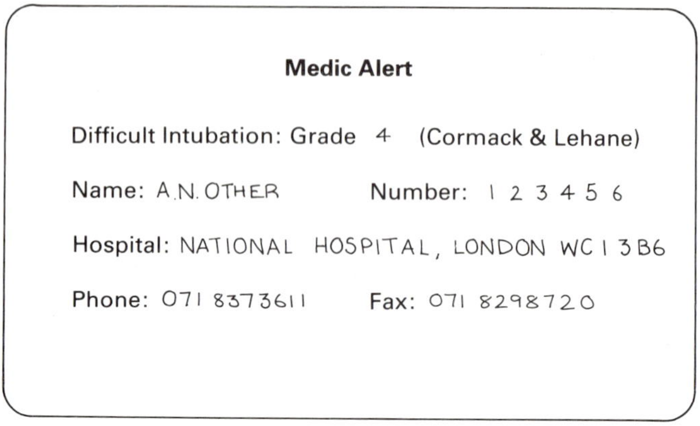

```
┌─────────────────────────────────────────────────┐
│                                                   │
│               **Medic Alert**                     │
│                                                   │
│   Difficult Intubation: Grade  4   (Cormack & Lehane) │
│                                                   │
│   Name: A.N. OTHER        Number: 1 2 3 4 5 6     │
│                                                   │
│   Hospital: NATIONAL  HOSPITAL, LONDON WC 1 3 B6  │
│                                                   │
│   Phone: O71 8373611    Fax: O71 8298720          │
│                                                   │
└─────────────────────────────────────────────────┘
```

Fig. 11.5 Medic-Alert card.

used, a propofol/alfentanyl infusion can be recommended to aid smooth extubation.

Prior to extubation the anaesthetist should consider the following.

1 *Was the patient quadraparetic before surgery, or may have become so during surgery?* If myelopathy was severe enough to cause weakness of all four limbs, the anaesthetist should establish that the neurological findings are at least as good as the preoperative state before extubation. Extubation during a period of neurological deterioration is unwise.

2 *Is the patient likely to be difficult to re-intubate?* Direct laryngoscopy should be performed at the conclusion of the procedure. Patients who will be difficult to re-intubate, should not be extubated if experienced staff are not going to be close at hand.

Stannard and Goat (1990) have suggested the insertion of a 13-gauge cricothyroid cannula (VBM Medezintecnik, West Germany) to provide a conduit for oxygen in the event of postoperative respiratory problems in patients, who have been difficult to intubate. However, Benumof and Scheller (1989) consider that the morbidity of cricothyroid cannulation and transtracheal jet ventilation to be such that the procedure 'should only be undertaken in desperate emergencies or in carefully thought out elective situations'. Unfortunately, most patients who are difficult to intubate because of cervical disease are also difficult to cannulate.

The grade of laryngoscopy should be recorded and if the grade is 3 or 4 the patient given a Medic Alert card (Fig. 11.5).

3 *Was the surgery prolonged and/or bloody?* Hypothermia and hypovolaemia are relative contraindications to extubation. Surgery on major cases often finishes late in the day, and it is safer to allow the temperature and circulation to approach normality by sedating, ventilating and re-suscitating the patient with intravenous fluids overnight.

4 *Do all staff understand the limitations of pulse oximetry and the significance of stridor?* Tissue oxygen saturation readings may generate a false sense of security in the recovery period, when the patient is receiving additional oxygen. This is because desaturation due to hypoventilation is effectively corrected by increasing the percentage of inspired oxygen. Serious hypo-ventilation with respiratory acidosis and reduced Pao_2 may occur, whilst the oximeter readings remain normal (John & Peacock 1993). Stridor is a very serious sign and requires urgent assessment by experienced staff.

Cervical spine pathology

INDICATIONS FOR SURGERY

In one year the indications for cervical surgery at the National Hospital were:

Cervical spondylosis	43.6%
Rheumatoid arthritis	27.0%
Congenital abnormality	11.0%
Disc protrusion	6.8%
Osteoarthritis	5.1%
Tumour	4.3%
Fracture	4.3%
Infection	0.9%

These are the conditions likely to be encountered. It can be seen that ankylosing spondylitis is not mentioned; spinal surgery is rarely required. Ossification of the posterior longitudinal ligament (OPLL) did not present for surgery in the year quoted, although it is a common indication in the Far East. At other units the proportions would be different, reflecting different areas of interest and expertise.

Cervical spondylosis

It is difficult to be sure of the difference between cervical 'spondylosis' and cervical osteoarthritis. The pathological findings are the same, but the term spondylosis is generally used when only one or two joints are

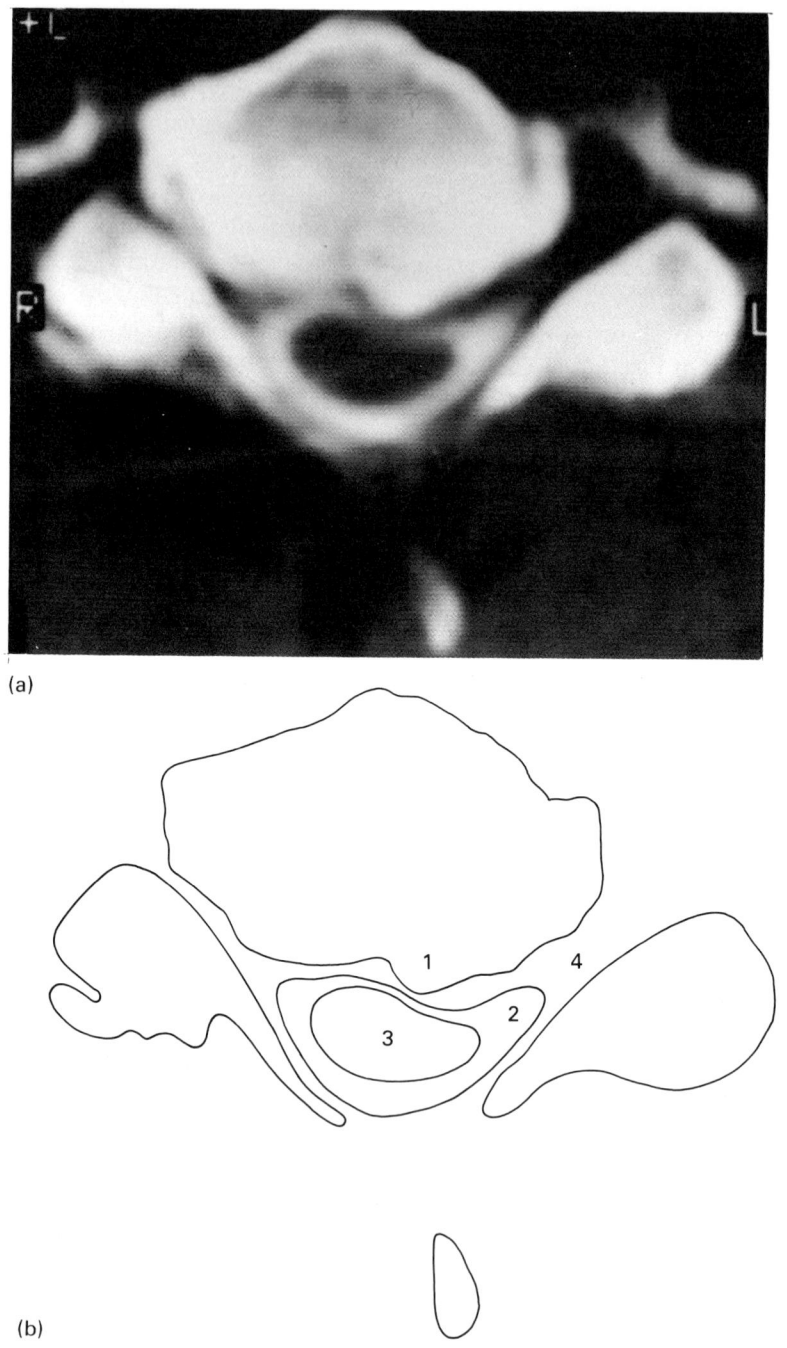

(a)

(b)

Fig. 11.6 Cervical spondylosis. (a) CT myelogram. (b) Explanatory diagram. 1, Osteophyte; 2, dye in dura; 3, deformed spinal cord; 4, root canal.

affected. The lower part of the cervical spine (C4/5, 5/6, 6/7) is most often involved. The disease is characterized by osteophytic projections or disc protrusions, which compress the nerve roots producing a radiculo-pathy, or the spinal cord producing a myelopathy or both. Diagnosis involves CT myelography or MRI scan (Fig. 11.6).

SURGERY

Variations of anterior discectomy and removal of osteophytes, followed by bony fusion of the joint, are popular (Robinson & Smith 1955, Cloward 1958). Internal fixation of the bone grafts by anterior cervical plating is becoming popular when multiple-level surgery is performed. Decompression of the cord by posterior laminectomy is now unusual.

ANAESTHESIA

Difficult direct laryngoscopy occurs in about 7% of cases (I. Calder, unpublished observations), i.e. only two or three times normal. This low incidence reflects the facts that the disease occurs at the lower end of the cervical spine and the temporomandibular joint is not usually affected. Induced hypotension is not required. Damage to the vagus or recurrent laryngeal nerve occasionally occurs (Heeneman 1973); the risk increases with surgery at multiple levels. It is usually difficult to obtain a clear view of the cords at the end of surgery, except with a fibreoptic laryngo-scope. At the National Hospital we do not check cord movement as a routine. The diagnosis is obvious when the patient complains of a weak voice and has a 'lowing' cough. Recovery may take 6 months.

Coughing on extubation must carry a risk of bone graft displacement and should be avoided (cervical dislocation due to coughing during an ether induction has been reported — Schurno 1967). The author's practice is to extubate whilst the patient is still deeply anaesthetized. Swallowing may be difficult for some days if several levels have been treated and plated. A nasogastric tube should be placed at induction in patients having anterior cervical plating. This can be removed as soon as the patient can swallow. Perforation of the oesophagus, pharynx, trachea and most of the major vessels has been reported (Ehni 1984).

Wound haematomas have the same dire implications as in thyroid surgery. The formation of a haematoma may go unobserved, since it is customary to place the patient in a cervical collar at the end of the operation (Tew & Mayfield 1976). If any hint of airway obstruction occurs postoperatively, urgent consideration should be given to guaranteeing the airway by intubating the trachea. The author knows of several cases of severe airway obstruction from this cause, with one fatality. In every case intubation was easily performed after direct laryngoscopy. It is interesting to speculate as to why this should be. Presumably the oedematous obstruction is easily compressed as the tube is passed. If the airway obstruction is so severe as to have caused loss of consciousness then either direct laryngoscopy and intubation with a small tube, or cannulation of the trachea, percutaneously or surgically, will be required. In less acute circumstances inhalational induction with halothane, or awake fibreoptic intubation, are appropriate techniques. Airway obstruction can also follow wound infection (Gwinnutt *et al.* 1992).

The posterior approach to spondylitic lesions is now a rarity. It may be required for decompression of OPLL. Posterior surgery carries a greater risk of damage to the cord. Invasive blood pressure monitoring is required, so that sudden falls due to neurotrauma can be detected. Some surgeons like to operate with the patient sitting.

Rheumatoid arthritis

Rheumatoid arthritis can affect any joint. Cervical involvement is common, 44–88% of rheumatoid patients have been found to have clinically affected cervical spines (Van Gilder *et al.* 1987b). Cervical disease usually presents late; patients have commonly undergone surgery for the replacement of other joints. Collins *et al.* (1991) found that 60% of rheumatoid patients undergoing surgery for hip or knee replacement had radiological evidence of cervical instability, but less than half of these had cervical symptoms. Any cervical joint can be affected by rheumatoid arthritis but, in contrast to spondylosis, the upper end of the cervical spine is most often attacked. Headache, at the back of the head, is a common symptom. The onset of muscle weakness due to cord damage is usually insidious and easily confused with myopathy or general debility.

PATHOLOGICAL FEATURES IN CERVICAL RHEUMATOID DISEASE

1 Osteoporosis.
2 Subluxation—particularly atlanto-axial subluxation.
3 'Settling'—loss of joint spaces.
4 Pannus formation—spinal cord compression is occasionally partially due to pannus pseudotumour.

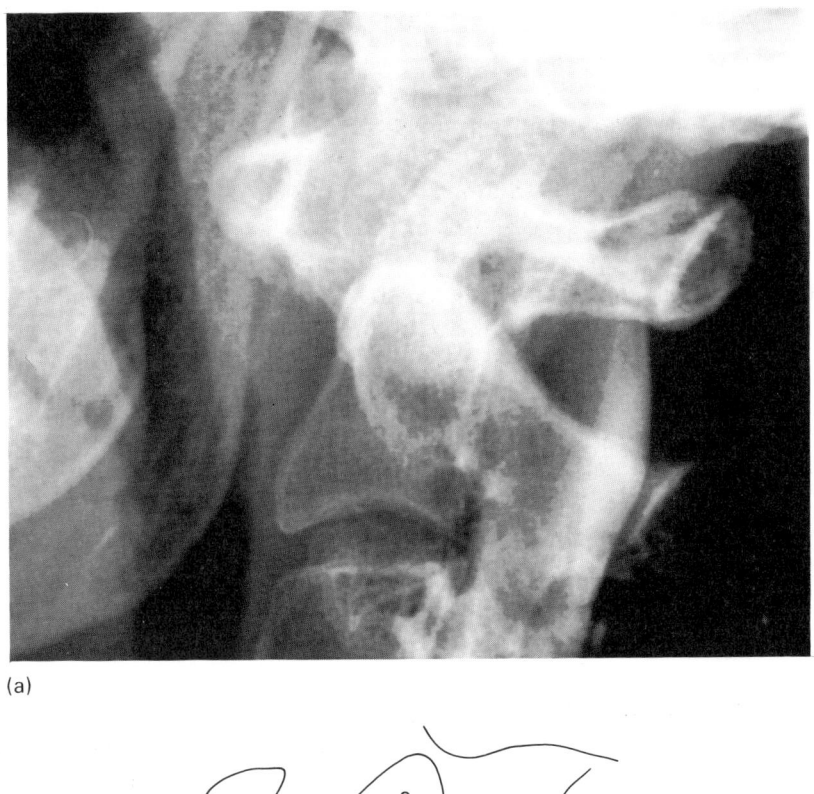

(a)

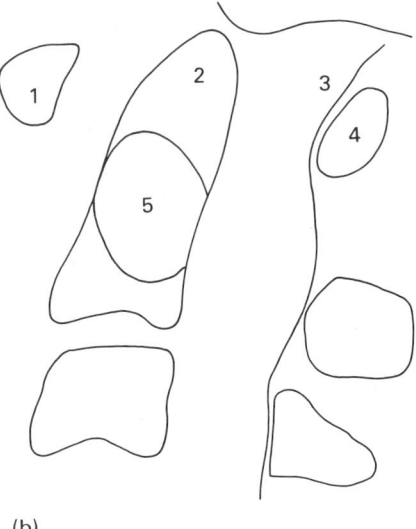

(b)

Fig. 11.7 (a) Cervical rheumatoid arthritis. Cervical myelogram (flexion film), showing atlanto-axial subluxation. (b) Explanatory diagram. 1, Anterior arch of atlas; 2, odontoid peg; 3, indented dura; 4, posterior arch of atlas; 5, lateral mass of axis.

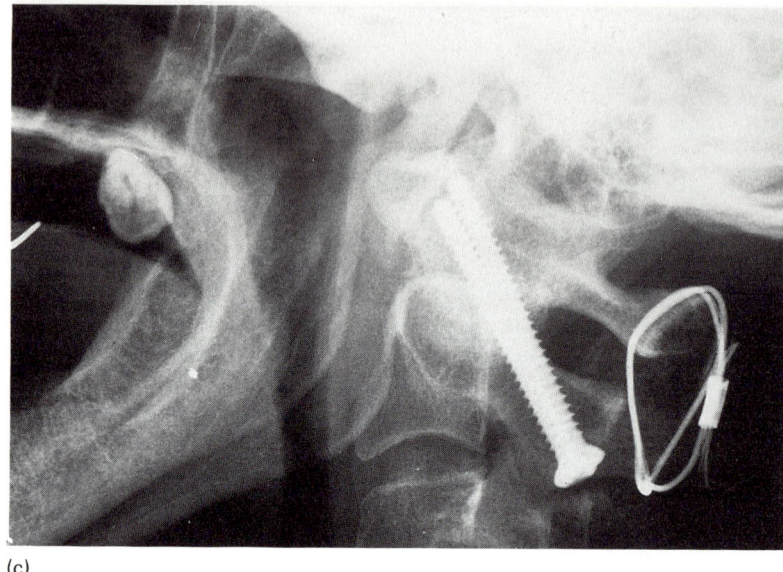

(c)

Fig. 11.7 (c) Atlanto-axial subluxation reduced in extension and fixed with screws and sublaminar wires.

5 Gross disorganization of the cervical spine — due to a combination of the previous features.

ATLANTO-AXIAL SUBLUXATION
IN CERVICAL RHEUMATOID DISEASE

Damage to the transverse and apical ligaments allows the atlas to slip forward on flexion. The subluxation is initially reducible in extension, but becomes fixed when settling occurs (Fig. 11.7). Correlation between symptoms, physical signs and the degree of subluxation seen on lateral radiographs of the neck is poor. Neurological damage is unusual if subluxation is less than 9 mm (Weissman *et al.* 1982).

The subluxation is nearly always anterior; the altas slides forward on the axis. Flexion of the neck is thus the precipitating factor and such patients are at risk if this occurs in the anaesthetized state. Very rarely the subluxation is posterior, in which case extension should be avoided. Subaxial subluxation is a late feature, sometimes resulting in a 'staircase spine'.

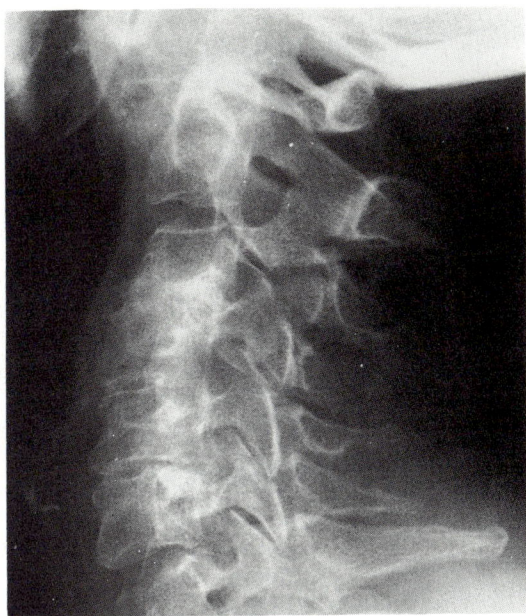

Fig. 11.8 Cervical rheumatoid arthritis. Lateral radiograph in extension, showing fixed atlantoaxial subluxation and 'settling'.

'SETTLING' IN RHEUMATOID CERVICAL SPINE DISEASE

As the disease progresses, the intervertebral spaces disappear. The term 'settling' was coined by Menezes (1984) to describe the radiological appearances (Fig. 11.8). The dens can enter the foramen magnum (translocation of the dens), causing cervical myelopathy or even brainstem signs. Translocation is referred to as vertical subluxation in some texts. Gross deformity of the cervical spine can result from collapse of osteoporotic vertebrae plus joint incompetence. It is sometimes difficult to believe that the radiological appearances are compatible with life (Fig. 11.9).

TEMPOROMANDIBULAR JOINT DISEASE
IN RHEUMATOID CERVICAL SPINE DISEASE

Temporomandibular joint disease is common in patients with cervical rheumatoid disease. The sliding component of the joint's function is lost so that the patient cannot protrude his jaw. It is the combination of temporomandibular joint and occipito-atlanto-axial complex disease that

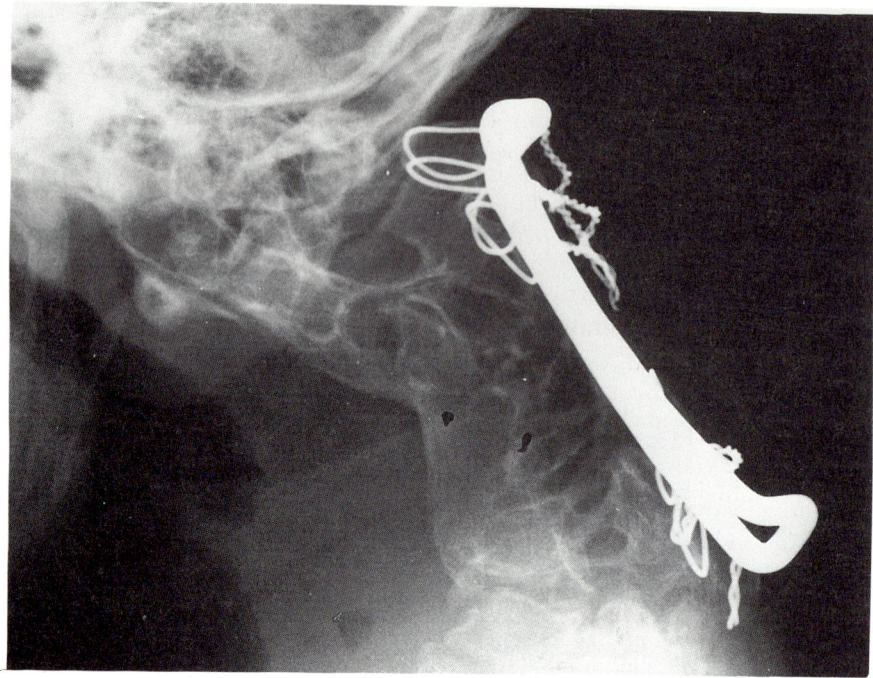

Fig. 11.9 Cervical rheumatoid arthritis. A Hartshill rectangle has been inserted to try to prevent collapse.

causes the very high incidence of difficult intubation in cervical rheumatoid arthritis. Details of the structure of the temporomandibular joint have been described by Aiello and Metcalf (1992).

PULMONARY AND OTHER PROBLEMS
IN RHEUMATOID CERVICAL SPINE DISEASE

Rheumatoid arthritis can affect the lungs. Diffusion defects are uncommon but restrictive abnormalities, due to muscle weakness, rib cage stiffness and cervical myelopathy, are common. This reduces the patient's ability to cough and clear secretions. Pulmonary function tests are often abnormal and values of forced vital capacity (FVC) of less than 50% of predicted are common; if this is the case arterial blood gases should be measured. Patients with respiratory failure are rarely improved by surgery and, once on a ventilator, they can be very difficult to wean. An intuitive estimation of muscular strength is probably the most useful guide to postoperative course. Arthritis of the arytenoid joints can occur in up to 25% of cases (Lofgren & Montgomery 1962) and may cause intermittent hoarseness and stridor. Serious airway obstruction is unusual, but has been reported following difficult intubation in a patient with a history of intermittent stridor (Funk & Raymon 1975).

Advanced cervical rheumatoid disease could be regarded as a malignant condition. Most patients with untreated rheumatoid cervical myelopathy die within 1 year; those who have been bedridden for more than a very few weeks do particularly badly. Rheumatoid arthritis is a generalized disease; other organs such as the kidneys and heart can be involved, also drug therapy with steroids, non-steroidal anti-inflammatory drugs (NSAID) and other drugs may pose additional problems for anaesthesia.

SURGERY

Reducible atlanto-axial subluxation can be treated with a procedure designed to fix the atlas to the axis. Several operations, prostheses and screw fixations have been described. Some involve passing wires under the lamina of C1, which can produce severe falls in blood pressure. Myelopathy due to non-reducible subluxation or translocation is not so easy to treat. Transoral excision of the dens and posterior occipito-cervical fusion is the treatment in the author's unit (Crockard *et al.* 1990).

ANAESTHESIA

Most patients with reducible atlanto-axial subluxation are in fairly good condition. Direct laryngoscopy and tracheal intubation is rarely difficult, provided that temporomandibular joint function is normal. The hazards of flexing the neck, for instance in lifting the head to place a pillow, must be remembered.

Fixed subluxation or settling causes craniocervical junction stiffness, and involvement of the temporomandibular joint usually guarantees difficult intubation. An awake fibreoptic intubation is the easiest method (Marks *et al.* 1986, Calder 1987) and the nasal route is usually the most straightforward in these patients, because of their short necks and poor temporomandibular joint function. The procedure should be covered with antibiotics.

Patients having posterior fixations alone can usually be extubated at the end of the procedure, but those undergoing transoral surgery usually require 12–48 h of postoperative ventilation. The occasional patient, in a better physical condition than most, can be extubated at the end of the procedure. The neurological status should be checked before extubation, a deterioration in neurological findings being a contraindication to extubation. Transoral excision of the dens is not associated with postoperative swelling in the author's experience (>100 cases). However, there have been three cases of postextubation respiratory obstruction. One developed stridor about 8 h after extubation, which settled with adrenaline nebulizer treatment. Another developed stridor after a similar interval, which appeared to settle with adrenaline nebulization, but total obstruction suddenly occurred and the patient died. The third developed pulmonary oedema 2 days after extubation; this probably resulted from airway obstruction. The airway was secured with a laryngeal mask and a tracheostomy performed (Calder *et al.* 1990).

The high incidence of crico-arytenoid joint arthritis should be borne in mind. It is advisable to establish a tracheal airway in patients who develop stridor after extubation. One patient presented with stridor preoperatively. Fibreoptic laryngoscopy revealed adducted immobile cords; an elective tracheostomy was performed.

Most severe rheumatoid patients have very fragile skin and extensive damage can be caused if great care is not taken to pad and protect vulnerable areas. If there is significant renal impairment and the creatinine is increased, renal dopamine should be given. Every effort must be made to avoid hypoxia and hypotension as transient periods, insignificant in normal patients, can result in further complications in a patient with severe rheumatoid arthritis.

CERVICAL RADIOLOGY BEFORE NON-CERVICAL SURGERY IN RHEUMATOID PATIENTS

Should patients with rheumatoid disease have flexion/extension lateral radiographs before anaesthesia for other conditions? The rationale for this practice is that unsuspected atlanto-axial subluxation may be recognized. Admission for surgery is a convenient time to arrange this investigation. Elective surgery need not be delayed in a symptomless patient, in order to obtain the films, provided that the patient is treated as a potential subluxer. Flexion of the neck should be avoided; all staff should be made aware of the potential hazard. Current opinion suggests that symptomless subluxers need not have fixations performed, but should be closely followed up (Agarwal *et al.* 1993). Patients with suggestive symptoms or signs (headache, paraesthesiae, L'Hermitte's phenomenon, spasticity, weakness), should be investigated before being submitted to general anaesthesia.

Congenital abnormality

The commonest problem is Down's syndrome. Children with this syndrome suffer atlanto-axial subluxation or dislocation due to a combination of lax ligaments and unfused dens (os odontoideum). Atlanto-axial instability in Down's syndrome is similar to that caused by rheumatoid arthritis, in that it is often asymptomatic and neurological deterioration is usually insidious, rather than acute. Semine *et al.* (1978) found that 12% of Down's syndrome patients had an abnormal atlantodental interval on flexion (greater than 4.5 mm) and 6% had abnormal odontoid pegs. None of the abnormal group had evidence of myelopathy, and only one developed signs on follow-up. Myelopathy may be difficult to diagnose in children, presenting as 'regressive ambulatory skills' (a child that has walked reverts to crawling), clumsiness and fatigue (Moore *et al.* 1987, Hreidarsson *et al.* 1982). Acute neurological deterioration is unusual, but has been reported following anaesthesia (Moore *et al.* 1987). Staff should therefore be alerted to the danger of excess cervical movements whilst the child's conscious level is reduced. A combination of craniocervical flexion and rotation is thought to be the most dangerous manoeuvre (Sherk & Nicholson 1969). Placing Down's syndrome patients in a soft cervical collar as a method of warning staff has been suggested (Calder 1988). Morquio's syndrome (MPS-IV) is also associated with atlanto-axial instability for the same reasons. A complete list of causes has already been given. Other diseases such as Klippel–Feil syndrome or various dwarfisms occasionally need surgery, to relieve cord or root compression.

Disc protrusion

Protrusions are often found at surgery for spondylosis but isolated disc problems are relatively rare, and are usually associated with a history of trauma. Discectomy is performed using an anterior approach, as for spondylosis.

Tumours

Tumours are discussed in relation to the thoracic and lumbar spine, but when they arise at the cervical level instability can occur. Vertebrectomy and metal stabilization may be necessary.

Fracture/dislocation

The majority of cervical fracture/dislocations occur in young males (80% less than 40 years, M : F 2.4 : 1), and are associated with road traffic accidents, sports injuries and alcohol (Green *et al.* 1981). Twenty per cent of fractures occur at C7, which is notoriously difficult to see on lateral X-rays. The traditional treatment has been conservative. Many patients do well, but Cheshire (1969) found that 42% of patients treated conservatively remained clinically or radiologically unstable after 3 months. Conservative treatment is not free from morbidity and mortality, due to pulmonary emboli, pressure sores and infections. Surgical intervention is becoming more common, both to relieve cord compression and to perform stabilizing procedures.

ANAESTHESIA

The two major imperatives, minimal movement at unstable sites and maintenance of cord perfusion, have already been mentioned. It must be remembered that any form of manipulation of spinal injuries can result in neurological deterioration. Marshall *et al.* (1987) found that 3% of patients undergoing operative treatment deteriorated neurologically as a result. In addition 5% of patients deteriorated as a result of the application of skull traction. Anaesthetic record-keeping should be meticulous. It may be necessary to show that blood pressure or respiratory changes were the result rather than the cause of neurological deterioration.

ACUTE SPINAL CORD INJURY (ASCI)

There are about 1000 new cases of ASCI annually in Britain (Swain *et al.* 1985). The majority of cases are associated with fracture/dislocation of the spine, but cord damage can be sustained without evidence of structural damage. Acute neurological deterioration occasionally occurs days or weeks after injury without obvious precipitating cause.

Emergency room and intensive care
Patients with ASCI frequently have polytrauma and other problems such as inhalation of vomit or water. The initial treatment is directed towards establishing satisfactory 'ABCs' (Hirschfeld 1990). As with head-injured

patients, the aim of treatment is to prevent 'second injury'. The functional spinal level makes a great difference to outcome. Patient with a C6 lesion can drive, and those with a C7 level can be independent.

Decision to ventilate

Patients with a depressed level of consciousness, unsatisfactory airway or signs of respiratory failure (Pao_2 <70 mmHg or $Paco_2$ >52 mmHg) should be intubated and ventilated (LaSala & Frost 1990). Other causes of hypoxaemia, such as haemothorax or pneumothorax, must be excluded.

Nasal intubation should be avoided because of the associated risk of sinusitis (Bach *et al.* 1992). Suxamethonium should not be used if the injury is more than 24 h old, because of the risk of hyperkalaemic arrest.

Treatment of hypotension

Hypotension may be due to overt or concealed blood loss, cardiac contusion or tamponade and 'neurogenic' shock. Treatment of hypotension is urgent, to prevent the extension of cord ischaemia. The assessment of circulating volume can be difficult, insertion of central venous or pulmonary artery catheters is desirable but the internal jugular is often unavailable and the subclavian route carries the risk of pneumothorax. This should be considered when facilities for ventilation are not to hand. The adequacy of cardiac output can often be satisfactorily and simply assessed by catheterization of the bladder and measurement of urine output (Hirschfeld 1990).

There is no doubt that patients with ASCI often develop pulmonary oedema. In some cases this appears to be neurogenic (Poe *et al.* 1978), but in many cases it is due to overtransfusion. Soderstrom and Brumback (1986) found that hypotension was due to neural damage in 82% of their cases of ASCI. It is often more appropriate to treat hypotension with a sympathomimetic agent such as dobutamine. The use of glucose-containing fluids is controversial, since there is evidence that neuronal recovery may be impaired (Sieber *et al.* 1987).

Nutrition

A nasogastric tube should be inserted at the time of intubation, and feeding commenced as soon as intestinal function allows. Percutaneous gastrostomy is more comfortable if swallowing is impaired for lengthy periods. Intravenous feeding has to be considered if intestinal function has not returned within a few days.

Airway obstruction caused by air evacuation

With increasing transfer of spinally injured patients this phenomenon, reported by Armitage *et al.* (1990), is important to recognize. The air in pressurized aircraft is dry and there may be difficulty in achieving adequate humidification of any artificial airway. Despite regular suctioning to keep the airway clear, a plug of dried secretions may form just beyond the tip of the airway, so that *changing the airway does not relieve the obstruction*. This unpleasant complication can be avoided by frequent instillation of saline. The obstructing plugs can be broken up with a fibreoptic bronchoscope.

'Medical' treatment of ASCI

The search for an agent that will improve the outcome in ASCI continues. Most attention has been devoted to steroids, such as methyl prednisolone. Animal studies of ASCI had indicated some benefit, but no benefit was found in humans after doses of 1 g (Bracken & Collins 1985). Trials of larger doses are continuing. Other agents such as calcium channel blockers, naloxone, NMDA (*N*-methyl-D-aspartate) blockers, and neuronal gangliosides, have been or are being investigated (Hirschfeld & Young 1990). Practical problems of timely administration of agents are difficult to overcome.

CHRONIC PARAPLEGIA

Flaccid paralysis or 'spinal shock' is seen for 1–3 weeks after cord damage; following spinal shock there is a state of hyperreflexia. After transection of the cord neural connections become chaotic, and as muscle tone and reflexes return, they are discoordinated, resulting in spasticity and hyperreflexia. Visceral stimulation can trigger a mass autonomic response characterized by severe hypertension, which in turn may lead to myocardial ischaemia, cerebral or subarachnoid haemorrhage. This is sometimes associated with vasoconstriction below and vasodilatation with facial flushing above the lesion, and is accompanied by a bradycardia as a reflex response. In addition, pulmonary oedema with bizarre arrhythmias and acute left ventricular failure can occur. Where sympathetic innervation has been lost there may be abnormal tracheal reflexes which will cause profound bradycardia, myocardial ischaemia and even cardiac arrest during tracheal suction and intubation (Frazer & Edmonds-Seal 1982, Alderson 1983).

Temperature control is lost because of the inability to sweat or retain heat by vasoconstriction. The patient becomes poikilothermic, cooling being the major problem but hyperthermia is also possible (Quimby *et al.* 1973). Pulmonary embolism is another common complication; prophylaxis with subcutaneous heparin should be considered.

Postural hypotension may continue to be a problem but adaptation does develop. This may take months with a slow rise in mean plasma renin levels and an increase in the response time of plasma renin to a change in blood pressure. Good nursing and general care is essential, or the condition of the patient may deteriorate with anaemia and electrolyte disturbance due to vomiting, enemas, ileal conduits or diuretic therapy; malnourishment due to a profound negative nitrogen balance, and renal impairment as a result of chronic infection or renal amyloidosis (Walters & Nott 1977).

Anaesthesia
Monitoring may include intra-arterial measurement of blood pressure, to assess the rapid changes which can occur in association with the spinal hyperreflexia. The induction of anaesthesia can be followed by severe hypertension. A rise in pressure of 50 mmHg occurred in 42% of patients with a lesion above T4 in a series of patients reported by Alderson & Thomas (1975). It has been reported that the use of halothane or enflurane in conjunction with hypocapnia prevents the development of dysrrhythmias, and that if a hypertensive episode occurs during anaesthesia it can be controlled by adding a volatile agent (Schonwald *et al.* 1981). Alternatively, hypertensive episodes have also been effectively controlled by sodium nitroprusside and other alpha-adrenergic blocking drugs with variable success (Nieder *et al.* 1970). Following the induction of general anaesthesia hypotension occurred in 11% of patients in a series of Schonwald *et al.* (1981), which responded to an infusion of fluid, atropine or ephedrine. The incidence may be reduced by good preoperative hydration and judicious use of induction agents.

In addition to the use of general anaesthesia, or as an alternative, local techniques such as spinal anaesthesia can be used. Spinal block has also been shown to abolish the mass autonomic reflex (Barker *et al.* 1985). It has been recommended as the method of choice unless there are specific contraindications. Stimulation of the bladder is the main triggering mechanism for the mass autonomic reflex; it therefore requires drainage to avoid overdistension.

Infection

Abscesses of the cervical spine are rare in the UK, most occur as a complication of surgery. Atlanto-axial abscess can cause subluxation of the joint. The atlanto-axial complex shares the lymphatic drainage of the nasopharynx and retrograde infection is believed to occur. The condition presents with neck pain, trismus, torticollis and eventually myelopathy. It is more common in children (Van Gilder *et al.* 1987a).

Thoracic and lumbar spine

Pathology

As with the cervical spine, the majority of the pathology presenting for surgery results from degenerative disease; trauma, tumours, and congenital malformations, such as spina bifida occur. In addition there is the problem of scoliosis, which affects young adults.

Tumours are classified according to their relationship to the dura and the spinal cord and are listed in Table 11.1.

Laminectomy

This operation is performed for decompression of the spinal cord (Fig. 11.10). The extent of surgery depends on the pathology, which ranges from intradural and extradural tumours to congenital stenosis of the canal, and varies between being curative and palliative. Blood loss can

Table 11.1 Classification of spinal tumours according to their site

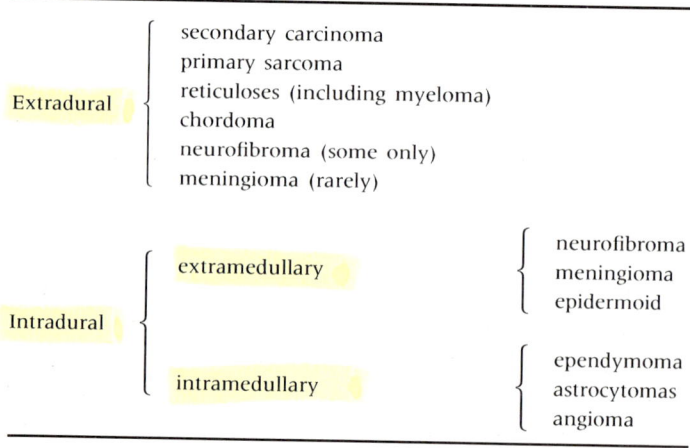

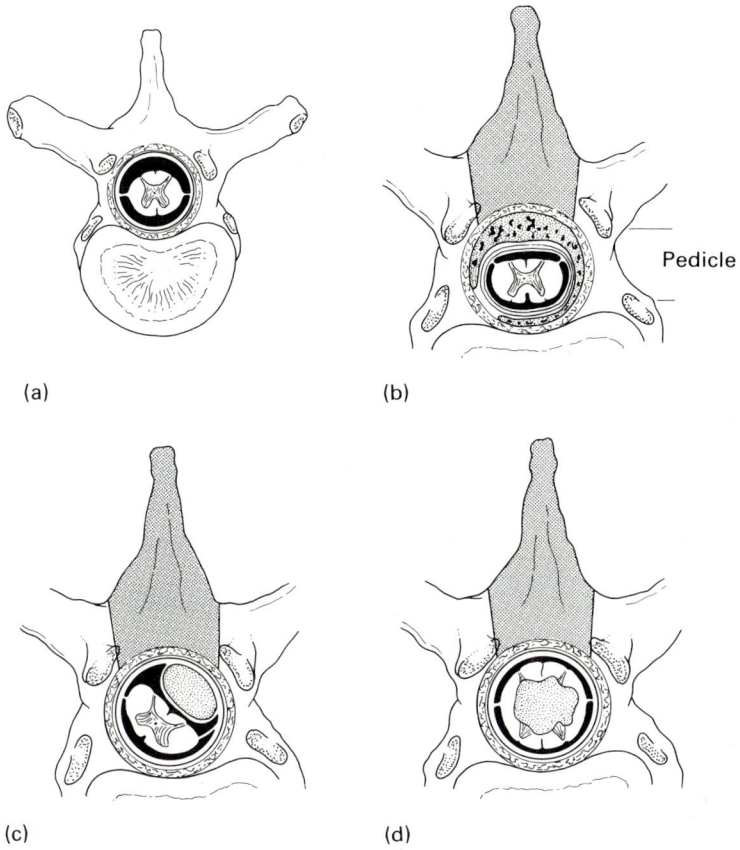

(a) (b) Pedicle

(c) (d)

Fig. 11.10 Anatomical types of spinal tumour. (a) Normal cord suspended by dentate ligaments within the subarachnoid space. (b) Extradural tumour (stippled), surrounding dural sac-like cuff. Bone removed during laminectomy (hatched). (c) Intradural (extramedullary) tumour displacing the cord. (d) Intramedullary tumour expanding the cord.

be considerable during laminectomy for bony metastases or other vascular tumours, but is rarely significant during surgery for degenerative disease.

Disc protrusion

The frequency of disc protrusions increases from top to bottom of the spine. The consequences of disc protrusion tend to be most severe in the thoracic region, since the spinal cord occupies a greater proportion of the cross-sectional area of the canal than in the cervical region. Surgical excision is particularly difficult in the thoracic spine; either a formal thoracotomy can be used or an anterolateral approach is made with excision of the head of a rib and transverse process (costotransversectomy). Under the operating microscope part of the vertebral body is removed to reach the disc.

In the lumbar region the disc can be approached posteriorly, since the spinal cord ends about L1. Damage to the aorta, inferior vena cava or iliac vessels can occur during lumbar disc surgery. Surgeons can penetrate the annulus of the disc, the anterior longitudinal ligament and the aorta, without being aware of it. In more than half the reported cases there was no bleeding from the wound (Ewah & Calder 1991).

ANAESTHESIA

Attempts have been made to perform lumbar disc surgery under local anaesthesia; however, patients find nerve root retraction unacceptably painful (Wiberg 1942). Lumbar disc excision under subarachnoid block has been reported (Rosenburg & Berner 1965). Some practitioners have attempted to dissolve disc protrusions by percutaneous injection of chymopapain, but severe anaphylactic reactions have been reported (Manchikanti *et al.* 1984).

The management of general anaesthesia is influenced by neuro-physiological monitoring. Evoked potential neural monitoring during thoracic and lumbar disc surgery can be performed with scalp electrodes and stimulation of the posterior tibial nerve. The amplitude of the positive deflection at about 40 ms after stimulation, the P40, is the usual response assessed. This deflection is less robust than that recorded after stimulation of the median nerve (the N (negative), 20 ms), which is used during cervical surgery. It may be necessary to avoid volatile agents to facilitate recordings. A propofol infusion is satisfactory; alternatively, recordings can be obtained from percutaneously or surgically placed epidural electrodes (Macon *et al.* 1982). See also Chapter 5.

More recently techniques have been developed to monitor motor function by electrical or magnetic stimulation of the motor cortex. Electrical motor monitoring appears to be very sensitive to most anaesthetic agents, including nitrous oxide but not propofol (Jellinek *et al.* 1992).

Positioning for spinal surgery

There is evidence to suggest that inappropriate positioning can cause neurological damage in patients without cervical disease. A kidnap victim became quadriparetic after being tied up, in marked neck flexion, for

12 h (Levy 1982). Hyperflexion of the neck was also blamed for quadriparesis in a child (Grundy *et al*. 1987). The risks must be greater in patients with cervical disease so that there is obvious attraction in the tactic of getting the patient to position himself or herself, before inducing anaesthesia (Lee *et al*. 1977). However, in the cases quoted above it would appear that the damage was the result of prolonged malposition. It is conceivable that a patient might be content with a position for a short time but be damaged by a lengthy period. This might be the explanation of the quadriparesis that occurred in a patient described by Deem *et al*. (1991). The patient was scheduled for surgery on his thoracic spine, but was known to have cervical spondylosis. He was intubated awake and positioned himself on the operating table. No hypotension was allowed. Nevertheless, the patient was quadriparetic on recovery from anaesthesia. Positioning the patient awake may be roughly akin to the 'wake-up' test in scoliosis surgery; providing a snapshot of cord function, but no guarantee of continuing health, and having risks of its own. Most practitioners use some form of sedation during 'awake' intubation which, it could be argued, might produce a disinhibited patient at a crucial moment, such as turning into the prone position. Continuous monitoring of sensory evoked potentials, before and after positioning, probably provides the best available guide to an acceptable position. Cord injury during positioning might be reflected in falls in blood pressure, but there is a tendency for the pressure to fall around this time because of lack of stimulation. Judicious use of a sympathomimetic drug such as ephedrine is often required.

SPECIFIC POSITIONS

Sitting position
The advantages and disadvantages of the sitting position are well known. There is some evidence that air embolism is less likely during cervical surgery in the sitting position than in cranial surgery (Losasso *et al*. 1992). The passage of sublaminar wires is not uncommonly associated with drops in blood pressure, especially at C1. The author regards the sitting position as unwise if this procedure is required.

Lateral (park-bench) position
This position can be used when transoral odontoidectomy and posterior fixation are to be performed consecutively (Crockard *et al*. 1990). It is also employed when a thoracotomy is required for an approach to a thoracic disc, and by some for lumbar discectomy.

Supine position
This position is used for the majority of anterior cervical work.

Prone position
It is a pity that the commonest position required is a difficult one
to achieve safely and efficaciously. The physical difficulties involved in
turning an unconscious patient should not be underestimated and have
been described in detail by Anderton (1991). A minimum of four staff
are required. Lee *et al.* (1977) advised 'awake pronation' for very large
patients. Specific problems with the prone position include:
1 *Risk of eye damage.* The head must be supported so that there is no
risk of pressure on the eye. An eye may be blinded by a pressure of
$20\,cmH_2O$ applied for 20 min. Horseshoe headrings are the most dangerous. The disposition of the system used for head support must be checked
after every adjustment of the table. The eye should also be taped shut
with waterproof tape to prevent cleansing solutions from reaching the
conjunctiva.
2 *Hyperextension of the neck.* It is surprisingly difficult to avoid this.
The presence of a skin crease at the back of the neck is a guide to
hyperextension.
3 *Controlling venous pressure.* The venous pressure in the lumbar venous
plexus should not be raised or troublesome bleeding will occur. However, a
reduced venous pressure raises the spectre of air embolism. The abdominal
contents should hang free, and the position that best achieves this is
probably the Tarlov seated position with the table tilted so that the back
is horizontal (Wayne 1984). Air embolism can be detected with sophisticated monitoring in any position, but clinically obvious embolism appears
very rare during spinal surgery.
4 *Compression of coronary vein grafts.* Weinlander *et al.* (1985) reported a
case of acute myocardial ischaemia due to compression of vein grafts in
the prone position.

Postoperative analgesia in spinal surgery

OPIATES AND LOCAL ANAESTHESIA

Major spinal surgery, which sometimes includes a thoracotomy, causes
significant pain in the postoperative period. The practice of continuous
narcotic infusions and patient-controlled analgesia (PCA) is well documented and has been used successfully. The increased incidence of

vomiting, which is associated with opiate PCA treatment, can be a drawback following cervical surgery. Continuous epidural and spinal techniques using narcotics with or without local anaesthetic solutions can provide excellent analgesia.

There have been several reports on the successful use of epidural narcotics and local anaesthetics following spinal surgery (Ray & Bagley 1983, Ozuna 1987, Wahab *et al*. 1986). There are difficulties when using this method in these cases. First any weakness will be difficult to assess, particularly following surgery at the thoracic level, as it may be unclear whether this is due to the local anaesthetic or a surgical complication. Secondly, as the epidural space has been disrupted, some have found the pain relief very variable (Johnson *et al*. 1989) and that PCA was equally effective.

NON-STEROIDAL ANTI-INFLAMMATORY AGENTS

Drugs such as ketoralac and diclofenac are extremely useful. Some concerns remain due to their antiplatelet activity (Power *et al*. 1990), although there is probably not a clinically important problem. Nevertheless, the author does not prescribe non-steroidal agents for 12 h after anterior cervical surgery. It must be said that many patients are already on these drugs, and it is not our practice to delay surgery.

A technique for awake fibreoptic intubation

The nasal route is often easiest in patients with stiff necks and/or poor mouth opening, since the angle of attack is better. The operator may stand in whatever position seems best and the patient can remain in the position most comfortable for him or her. In most cases we adopt the usual intubating position, and the guide below should be interpreted accordingly. Mallinkrodt metal reinforced tubes are the best in our experience (Calder 1992b). It is interesting to note that flexometallic tubes, and the benefits of rotation on insertion (see below) were advised in the first report of a series of fibreoptic intubations (Stiles *et al*. 1972).

'LANDMARKS' IN FIBREOPTIC INTUBATION

The secret of success is to start off knowing where you are, and what

you should therefore be seeing, and to carry on from landmark to
landmark (Fig. 11.12). The landmarks are:

1 The turbinates.
2 The nasopharyngeal floor.
3 The junction of the nasopharyngeal floor and the soft palate.
4 The epiglottis.
5 The glottis.
6 The anterior wall of the trachea.
7 The carina.

If you get lost, withdraw till you recognize something.

TECHNIQUE

  1 Premedicate the patient with morphine and a drying agent. The use

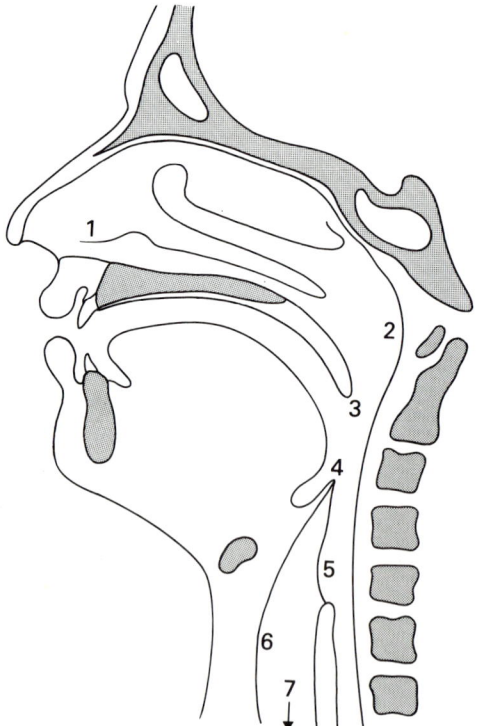

Fig. 11.11 Landmarks in fibreoptic nasotracheal intubation. 1, Turbinate;
2, nasopharyngeal floor; 3, junction of soft palate and nasopharyngeal floor;
4, epiglottis; 5, glottis, 6, anterior wall of trachea.

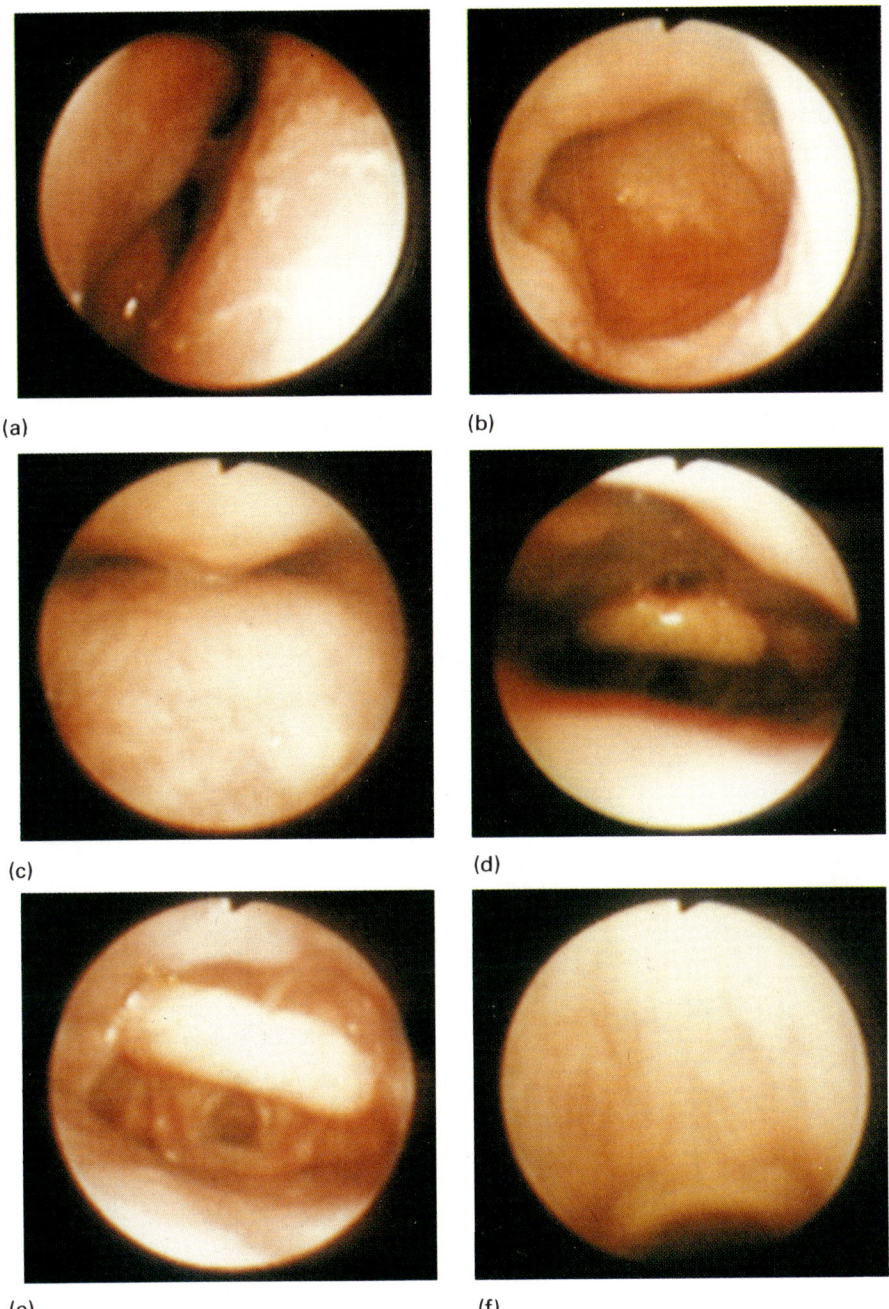

(a)

(b)

(c)

(d)

(e)

(f)

Plate 11.1 Endoscopic appearances (a–f). (a) Turbinates. (b) Floor of nasal cavity with junction of soft palate and nasal floor at top. (c) Junction of soft palate and nasal floor. (d) Epiglottis. (e) Glottis. (f) Anterior wall of trachea with tracheal lumen at bottom of field.

[facing page 308]

of a drying agent enhances the action of topical lignocaine (Watanabe *et al.* 1993).

2 Dribble 0.5 ml of xylometazoline (Otrivine™) into each nostril. Follow with 1 ml of *warm* 1% lignocaine. Wait 1 min.

3 Spray three metered doses of 10% lignocaine into the clearer nostril, and four doses into the oropharynx. The patient will inhale this lignocaine, and begin the process of anaesthetizing the glottis. If this is omitted the patient will cough when you spray the glottis with lignocaine later (see below). Place 'nasal specs' and administer oxygen. The specs are more conveniently worn as 'oral specs'.

4 Place the tip of the laryngoscope, after treating it with anti-fog solution (warm water will do; *do not put* KY *jelly on the 'scope or tube*), just into the nares and identify the first landmark — *the turbinates* (Plate 11.1a, facing p. 308).

5 Advance slowly, follow the airway (black). Try the other nostril if difficulty is encountered. Remember that bleeding is the great enemy. Continue till the airway opens out (about 4 cm) and identify the *nasopharyngeal floor*. At the top of the field you will be able to see a horizontal black line, where the soft palate approaches the nasopharyngeal floor. This is the most difficult part of the procedure; once you can recognize this landmark, you will find the rest is easy (Plate 11.1b).

6 Advance slowly, pushing the tip control *down*, so that the tip bends towards the feet. Identify the junction between the soft palate and the nasopharyngeal floor. There may be a wide gap or just a horizontal black line with a few bubbles (Plate 11.1c).

7 Advance through the gap (vision may be lost temporarily). Identify the epiglottis, which usually looks very large. Get an assistant to spray 2 ml of *warm* 4% lignocaine through the injection port. Make sure you see the lignocaine striking the epiglottis. There is often a little coughing. Wait patiently, engage the patient in conversation. If vision does not clear, ask the patient to take a deep breath (Plate 11.1d).

8 Advance towards the *glottis*, under the epiglottis. If the epiglottis is closely applied to the pharyngeal wall it can usually be raised by asking the patient to put out the tongue. Spray the glottis with further doses of 4% lignocaine until the movements of the cords are reduced. About 4–6 ml is usually enough. The patient's voice is a guide to the adequacy of anaesthesia; consonant pronunciation should be impaired e.g. '–aterham', not 'Caterham' (Plate 11.1e).

9 Advance through the cords and identify the *anterior wall of the trachea*. Pull the tip control gently up, so that the tip of the scope bends down. The tracheal lumen will be seen. Spray a further dose of 2 ml of lignocaine into the trachea. Advance and identify the carina (Plate 11.1f).

10 Give 5−10 mg of midazolam intravenously. Give the scope to an assistant to hold. Put a blob of KY jelly on the nares, *not* on the tube. Pass the tube by rotating it through many 360° turns. You should *rotate more than push.* Check the position of the tube by identifying the carina and by auscultation of the lungs.

Awake oral fibreoptic intubation

This is easier than the nasal route, provided that one can get under the epiglottis. It is probably true to say that the oral route is easier in 'easy' patients and more difficult than the nasal route in 'difficult' patients. Gagging is a problem with the oral route. A block of the lingual branch of the glossopharyngeal nerve is said to prevent this (Benumof 1991), but the author has not attempted it. The block might be technically difficult in Mallampati class 3 patients. The author has not found 'intubating airways' helpful in the awake patient.

Fibreoptic intubation under general anaesthesia

Not all patients are awake or able to cooperate with an awake procedure. The fibreoptic 'scope can be employed in much the same manner as a direct laryngoscope once the skill has been acquired, although there is no doubt that the collapse of the airway consequent upon the induction of general anaesthesia (Nandi *et al.* 1991) makes endoscopy more difficult. Oral fibreoptic intubation is easily performed with the aid of a laryngeal mask airway (Silk *et al.* 1991). This method allows paralysis and positive pressure ventilation during endoscopy, which is recommended, since endoscopy during spontaneous respiration using halothane is associated with desaturation and hypotension (Smith *et al.* 1992).

Nasotracheal intubation under general anaesthesia can be performed whilst the patient is ventilated through an oral airway.

References

Agarwal A.K., Peppelman W.C., Kraus D.R. & Eisenbeis C.H. (1993) The cervical spine in rheumatoid arthritis. *British Medical Journal* **306**, 79−80.

Aiello G. & Metcalf I. (1992) Anaesthetic implications of temporomandibular joint disease. *Canadian Journal of Anaesthesia* **39**, 610−617.

Alderson J.D. (1983) Spinal cord injuries. *Anaesthesia* **38**, 605−608.

Alderson J.C. & Thomas D.G. (1975) The use of halothane anaesthesia to control autonomic hyperreflexia during trans-urethral surgery in spinal cord injured patients. *Paraplegia* **13**, 183−188.

American College of Surgeons Committee on Trauma (1990) *Advanced Trauma Life Support Course for Physicians*. American College of Surgeons, Chicago.

Anderton J.M. (1991) The prone position for the surgical patient: a historical review of the principles and hazards. *British Journal of Anaesthesia* **67**, 452−463.

Aprahamian C., Thompson B.M., Finger W.A. & Darin J.C. (1984) Experimental cervical spine injury model: evaluation of airway management and splinting techniques. *Annals of Emergency Medicine* **13**, 584−587.

Armitage J.M., Pyne A., Williams S.J. & Frankel H. (1990) Respiratory problems of air travel in patients with spinal cord injuries. *British Medical Journal* **300**, 1498.

Bach A., Boehrer H., Schmidt H. & Geiss H.K. (1992) Nosocomial sinusitis in ventilated patients. Nasotracheal versus orotracheal intubation. *Anaesthesia* **47**, 335−339.

Barker I., Alderson J., Lydon M. & Franks C.I. (1985) Cardiovascular effects of spinal subarachnoid anaesthesia. A study in patients with chronic spinal cord injuries. *Anaesthesia* **40**, 533−536.

Benumof J.L. (1991) Management of the difficult adult airway. *Anesthesiology* **75**, 1087−1110.

Benumof J.L. & Scheller M.S. (1989) The importance of transtracheal jet ventilation in the management of the difficult airway. *Anesthesiology* **71**, 769−778.

Bivins H.G., Ford S., Bezmalinovic Z., Price H.M. & Williams J.L. (1988) The effect of axial traction during orotracheal intubation of the trauma victim with an unstable cervical spine. *Annals of Emergency Medicine* **17**, 25−29.

Bohlman H.H. (1979) Acute fractures and dislocations of the cervical spine. *Journal of Bone and Joint Surgery* **61A**, 1119−1142.

Bracken M.B. & Collins W.F. (1985) Randomised clinical trials of spinal cord injury treatment. In: Becker D.P. & Povlishock J.T. (Eds), *Central Nervous System Trauma Status Report*, pp. 303−312. National Institutes of Health, Bethesda.

Brechner V.L. (1968) Unusual problems in the management of airways: 1. Flexion−extension mobility of the cervical spine. *Anesthesia and Analgesia* **47**, 362−373.

Calder I. (1987) Anaesthesia for transoral and craniocervical surgery. In: Jewkes D.A. (Ed.), *Anaesthesia for Neurosurgery, Baillière's Clinical Anaesthesiology*, pp. 441−457. Baillière Tindall, London.

Calder I. (1988) Atlantoaxial instability in Down's syndrome. *British Medical Journal* **294**, 1549.

Calder I. (1990) Primary survey in major trauma. *British Medical Journal* **300**, 1652.

Calder I. (1992a) Predicting difficult intubation. *Anaesthesia* **47**, 528–529.

Calder I. (1992b) When the tube will not pass off the fibreoptic bronchoscope. *Anesthesiology* **77**, 398.

Calder I., Calder J. & Crockard H.A. (1991) Radiological prediction of difficult intubation: the posterior C0–1 and C1–2 'gaps'. *Anesthesiology* **75**, A190.

Calder I., Ordman A.J., Jackowski A. & Crockard H.A. (1990) The Brain laryngeal mask airway. An alternative to emergency tracheal intubation. *Anaesthesia* **45**, 137–139.

Cheshire D.J. (1969) The stability of the cervical spine following the conservative treatment of fractures and fracture–dislocations. *Paraplegia* **7**, 193–203.

Cline J.R., Scheeidel E. & Bigsby E.F. (1985) A comparison of methods of cervical immobilisation used in extrication and transport. *Journal of Trauma* **25**, 649–653.

Cloward R.B. (1958) The anterior approach for the removal of ruptured cervical discs. *Journal of Neurosurgery* **15**, 602–617.

Collins D.N., Barnes C.L. & FitsRandolph R.L. (1991) Cervical spine instability in rheumatoid patients having total hip or knee arthroplasty. *Clinical Orthopaedics and Related Research* **272**, 127–135.

Crockard H.A. (1992) Training spinal surgeons. *Journal of Bone and Joint Surgery* **74B**, 174–175.

Crockard H.A., Calder I. & Ransford A.O. (1990) One stage transoral decompression and posterior fixation in rheumatoid atlanto-axial subluxation. *Journal of Bone and Joint Surgery* **72B**, 682–685.

Deem S., Shapiro H.M., Lawrence F. & Marshall L.F. (1991) Quadriplegia in a patient with cervical spondylosis after thoracolumbar surgery in the prone position. *Anesthesiology* **75**, 527–528.

Doolan L.A. & O'Brien J.F. (1985) Safe intubation in cervical spine injury. *Anaesthesia and Intensive Care* **13**, 319–324.

Dronen S.C., Merigian K.S., Hedges J.R., Hoekstra J.W. & Borron S.W. (1987) A comparison of blind nasotracheal and succinylcholine assisted intubation in the poisoned patient. *Annals of Emergency Medicine* **16**, 650–652.

Ehni G. (1984) Cervical arthrosis. *Diseases of Cervical Motion Segments*. pp. 227–231. Year Book Medical Publishers, Chicago.

Ewah B. & Calder I. (1991) Intraoperative death during lumbar discectomy. *British Journal of Anaesthesia* **66**, 721–723.

Frazer A. & Edmonds-Seal J. (1982) Spinal cord injuries. A review of the problems facing the anaesthetist. *Anaesthesia* **37**, 1084–1098.

Funk D. & Raymon F. (1975) Rheumatoid arthritis of the cricoarytenoid joints. *Anesthesia and Analgesia* **54**, 742–745.

Grande C.M., Barton C.R. & Stene J.K. (1988) Appropriate techniques for airway management of emergency patients with suspected spinal cord injury.

Anesthesia and Analgesia **67**, 714−715.

Green B.A., Callahan R.A., Klose K.J. & de la Torre J. (1981) Acute spinal cord injuries: current concepts. *Clinical Orthopedics and Related Research* **154**, 125−135.

Grundy B., Gravenstein N. & Reid S.A. (1987) The central nervous system: Complications of positioning. In: Martin J.T. (Ed.), *Positioning in Anesthesia and Surgery*, pp. 297−315. W.B. Saunders, Philadelphia.

Gwinnutt C.L., Walsh G.R. & Kumar R. (1992) Airway obstruction after anterior cervical spine surgery. *Journal of Neurosurgical Anesthesiology* **4**, 199−202.

Hayashi H., Okada K., Hamada M., Toda K. & Ueno R. (1987) Etiologic factors of myelopathy: a radiographic evaluation of the ageing changes in the cervical spine. *Clinical Orthopedics and Related Research* **214**, 200−209.

Heeneman H. (1973) Vocal cord paralysis following approaches to the anterior cervical spine. *Laryngoscope* **83**, 17−21.

Hirschfeld A. (1990) Emergency room care of the patient with spinal cord injury. In: Alderson J.D. & Frost E.A.M. (Eds), *Spinal Cord Injuries, Anaesthetic and Associated Care*, pp. 32−46. Butterworths, London.

Hirschfeld A. & Young W. (1990) Trends in spinal cord injury research. In: Alderson J.D. & Frost E.A.M. (Eds), *Spinal Cord Injuries, Anaesthetic and Associated Care*, pp. 199−232. Butterworths, London.

Horton W.A., Fahy L. & Charters P. (1989) Disposition of cervical vertebrae, atlanto-axial joint, hyoid and mandible during X-ray laryngoscopy. *British Journal of Anaesthesia* **63**, 435−438.

Hreidarsson S., Magram G. & Singer H. (1982) Symptomatic atlantoaxial dislocation in Down's syndrome. *Pediatrics* **69**, 568−571.

James R. & Nasmyth-Jones R. (1992) The occurrence of cervical fractures in victims of judicial hanging. *Forensic Science International* **54**, 81−89.

Jellinek D., Platt M., Jewkes D. & Symon L. (1992) Effects of nitrous oxide on motor evoked potentials recorded from skeletal muscle in patients under total anaesthesia with intravenously administered propofol. *Neurosurgery* **29**, 558−562.

John R.E. & Peacock J.E. (1993) Limitations of pulse oximetry. *Lancet* **341**, 1092−1093.

Johnson R.G., Miller M. & Murphy M. (1989) Intraspinal narcotic analgesia. A comparison of two methods of postoperative pain relief. *Spine* **14**, 363−366.

Kainuma M. & Yamada S. (1985) Postextubation airway obstruction after anesthesia for posterior fusion of occipital bone and cervical spine. *Masui* **34**, 1525−1529.

Kaufman H.H., Harris J.H., Spencer J.A. & Kopansky D.R. (1982) Danger of traction during radiography for cervical trauma. *Journal of the American Medical Association* **247**, 2369.

Konttinen Y.T., Santavirta S., Kauppi M. & Moskovich R. (1991) The rheumatoid cervical spine. *Currrent Opinion in Rheumatology* **3**, 429−440.

LaSala P.A. & Frost E.A.M. (1990) Intensive care management of spinal cord injury. In: Alderson J.D. & Frost E.A.M. (Eds), *Spinal Cord Injuries, Anaesthetic and Associated Care*, pp. 72–86. Butterworths, London.

Lee C., Barnes A. & Nagel E.L. (1977) Neuroleptanalgesia for awake pronation of surgical patients. *Anesthesia and Analgesia* **56**, 276–278.

Levy L.M. (1982) An unusual case of flexion injury of the cervical spine. *Surgical Neurology* **17**, 255–259.

Lofgren R.H. & Montgomery W.W. (1962) Incidence of laryngeal involvement in rheumatoid arthritis. *New England Journal of Medicine* **267**, 193–195.

Logan A. St C. (1991) Use of the laryngeal mask in a patient with an unstable fracture of the cervical spine. *Anaesthesia* **46**, 987.

Losasso T.J., Muzzi D.A., Dietz N.M. & Cucchiara R.F. (1992) Fifty percent nitrous oxide does not increase the risk of venous air embolism in neuro-surgical patients operated upon in the sitting position. *Anesthesiology* **77**, 21–30.

McCrae R. (1981) Practical Fracture Treatment. *The Spine*, pp. 170–196. Churchill Livingstone, London.

Macon J.B., Poletti C.E., Sweet W.H., Ojemann R.G. & Zervas N.T. (1982) Conducted somatosensory potentials during spinal surgery. Part 1: Clinical applications. *Journal of Neurosurgery* **57**, 354–359.

Mallampati S.R., Gatt S.P., Gugino L.D. *et al.* (1985) A clinical sign to predict difficult tracheal intubation: a prospective study. *Canadian Anaesthetic Society Journal* **32**, 429–434.

Manchikanti L., Meriwether R.P. & Grow J.B. (1984) Anesthetic management of patients for chemonucleolysis. *Anesthesiology Review* **11**, 35–37.

Marks R.J., Forrester P.C., Calder I. & Crockard H.A. (1986) Anaesthesia for transoral cranio-cervical surgery. *Anaesthesia* **41**, 1049–1052.

Marshall L.F., Knowlton S. & Garfin S.R. (1987) Deterioration following spinal cord injury. A multicentre study. *Journal of Neurosurgery* **66**, 400–404.

Meakem T.D., Meakem T.J. & Rappaport W. (1990) Airway compromise from prevertebral soft tissue swelling during placement of halo traction for cervical spine injury. *Anesthesiology* **73**, 775–776.

Menezes A.H. (1984) 'Cranial settling' in rheumatoid arthritis. *Contemporary Neurosurgery* **6**, 1–8.

Meschino A., Devitt J.H., Koch J.P., Szalai J.P. & Schwartz M.L. (1992) The safety of awake tracheal intubation in cervical spine injury. *Canadian Journal of Anaesthesia* **39**, 114–117.

Mixter J.M. & Barr J.S. (1934) Rupture of the intervertebral disc with involvement of the spinal canal. *New England Journal of Medicine* **211**, 210–214.

Moore R.A., McNicholas K.W. & Warren S.P. (1987) Atlantoaxial subluxation with symptomatic spinal cord compression in a child with Down's syndrome. *Anesthesia and Analgesia* **66**, 89–90.

Murphy P. (1967) A fibre-optic endoscope used for nasal intubation. *Anaesthesia* **22**, 489–491.

Nandi P.R., Charlesworth C.H., Taylor S.J., Nunn J.F. & Dore C.J. (1991) Effect of general anaesthesia on the pharynx. *British Journal of Anaesthesia* **66**, 157−162.

Nieder R.M., O'Higgins J.W. & Aldrete J.A. (1970) Autonomic hyperreflexia in urological surgery. *Journal of the American Medical Association* **213**, 867−869.

Nolan J.P. & Wilson M.E. (1992) An evaluation of the gum-elastic bougie. *Anaesthesia* **47**, 878−881.

Oates J.D.L., Macleod A.D., Oates P.D., Pearsall F.J., Howie J.C. & Murray G.D. (1991) Comparison of two methods of predicting difficult intubation. *British Journal of Anaesthesia* **66**, 305−309.

Ovassapian A., Yelich S.J., Dykes M.H.M. & Brunner E.E. (1983) Blood pressure and heart rate changes during awake fiberoptic nasotracheal intubation. *Anesthesia and Analgesia* **62**, 951−954.

Ozuna J. (1987) An experience with epidural morphine in lumbar surgery patients. *Journal of Neuroscience Nursing* **19**, 235−239.

Patil V.U., Stehling L.C. & Zauder H.L. (1983) Predicting difficulty in intubation utilizing an intubation gauge. *Anaesthesiology Review* **X**, 32−33.

Pennant J.H., Pace N.A. & Gajraj N.M. (1992) Use of the laryngeal mask airway in the immobilized cervical spine. *Anesthesiology* **77**, A1063.

Podolsky S., Baraff L.J., Simon R.R., Hoffman J.R., Larmon B. & Ablon W. (1983) Efficacy of cervical spine immobilisation methods. *Journal of Trauma* **23**, 461−465.

Poe R.H., Reisman J.L. & Rodenhouse T.G. (1978) Pulmonary edema in cervical spinal cord injury. *Journal of Trauma* **18**, 71−73.

Power I., Chambers W.A., Greer I.A., Ramage D. & Simon E. (1990) Platelet function after intramuscular Diclofenac. *Anaesthesia* **45**, 916−919.

Quimby C.W., Williams R.N. & Greifenstein F.E. (1973) Anesthetic problems of the acute quadriplegic patient. *Anesthesia and Analgesia* **52**, 333−339.

Ray C.D. & Bagley R. (1983) Indwelling epidural morphine for control of post-lumbar spinal surgery pain. *Neurosurgery* **13**, 388−393.

Robinson R.A. & Smith G.W. (1955) Anterolateral cervical disc removal and interbody fusion for cervical disc syndrome. *Bulletin of the Johns Hopkins Hospital* **96**, 223−224.

Rocke D.A., Murray W.B., Rout C.C. & Gouws E. (1992) Relative risk analysis of factors associated with difficult intubation in obstetric anesthesia. *Anesthesiology* **77**, 67−73.

Rosen P. & Wolfe R.E. (1989) Therapeutic legends of emergency medicine. *Journal of Emergency Medicine* **7**, 387−389.

Rosenberg M.K. & Berner G. (1965) Spinal anesthesia in lumbar disc surgery. Review of 200 cases. *Anesthesia and Analgesia* **44**, 419−423.

Rowed D.W. (1992) Management of cervical spinal cord injury in ankylosing spondylitis: the intervertebral disc as a cause of cord compression. *Journal of Neurosurgery* **77**, 241−246.

Schneider M., Probst R. & Wey W. (1989) Magnetic resonance imaging—a useful tool for airway assessment. *Acta Anesthesiologica Scandinavica* **33**, 429–431.

Schonwald G., Fish K.J. & Perkash I. (1981) Cardiovascular complications during anesthesia in chronic spinal cord injured patients. *Anesthesiology* **55**, 550–558.

Schurno A. (1967) Halswirbelluxation als narkosefolge. *HNO* **15**, 361–363.

Semine A.A., Ertel A.N., Goldberg M.J. & Bull M.J. (1978) Cervical spine instability in children with Down's syndrome (trisomy 21). *Journal of Bone and Joint Surgery* **60A**, 648–652.

Sherk H. & Nicholson J. (1969) Rotatory atlanto-axial dislocation associated with ossiculum terminale and mongolism. *Journal of Bone and Joint Surgery* **51A**, 957–964.

Sieber F.E., Smith D.S., Traystman R.J. & Wollman H. (1987) Glucose: a re-evaluation of its intraoperative use. *Anesthesiology* **67**, 72–81.

Silk J.M., Hill H.M. & Calder I. (1991) Difficult intubation and the laryngeal mask. *European Journal of Anesthesiology* **4** (Suppl.), 47–51.

Smith J.E. (1988) Heart rate and arterial pressure changes during fibreoptic tracheal intubation under general anaesthesia. *Anaesthesia* **43**, 629–632.

Smith M., Calder I., Crockard H.A., Isert P. & Nicol M.E. (1992) Oxygen saturation and cardiovascular changes during fibreoptic intubation under general anaesthesia. *Anaesthesia* **47**, 158–161.

Soderstrom C.A. & Brumback R.J. (1986) Early care of the patient with cervical spine injury *Orthopedic Clinics of North America* **17**, 3–13.

Stannard C.F. & Goat V.A. (1990) The use of transtracheal cannulation after difficult intubation. *Anaesthesia* **45**, 790–791.

Stellin G.P., Barker S., Murdock M. & Waxman K. (1989) Oral tracheal intubation in trauma patients with cervical fractures. *Critical Care Medicine* **17**, S37.

Stiles C.M., Stiles Q.R. & Denson J.S. (1972) A flexible fibreoptic laryngoscope. *Journal of the American Medical Association* **221**, 1246–1247.

Suderman V.S., Crosby E.T. & Lui A. (1991) Elective oral tracheal intubation in cervical spine injured adults. *Canadian Journal of Anaesthesia* **38**, 785–789.

Swain A., Grundy D. & Russel J. (1985) ABC of spinal cord injury. *British Medical Journal* **291**, 1558–1560.

Tew J.M. & Mayfield F.H. (1976) Complications of surgery of the anterior cervical spine. *Clinical Neurosurgery* **23**, 24–34.

Van Gilder J.C., Menezes A.H. & Dolan K.D. (Eds) (1987a) Developmental and acquired abnormalities of the craniovertebral junction. In: *The Craniovertebral Junction and its Abnormalities*, pp. 109–158. Futura, New York.

Van Gilder J.C., Menezes A.H. & Dolan K.D. (Eds) (1987b) Inflammatory conditions of the craniovertebral junction. In: *The Craniovertebral Junction and its Abnormalities*. pp. 159–193. Futura, New York.

Wahab A.M.I., Farag H. & Naguib M. (1986) Epidural morphine for pain relief after lumbar laminectomy. *Spine* **11**, 1024–1026.

Walters F.J.M. & Nott M.R. (1977) The hazards of anaesthesia in the injured patient. *British Journal of Anaesthesia* **49**, 707−720.

Watanabe H., Lindgren P., Rosenberg P. & Randell T. (1993) Glycopyrronium prolongs topical anaesthesia of oral mucosa and enhances absorption of lignocaine. *British Journal of Anaesthesia* **70**, 94−95.

Wayne S.J. (1984) A modification of the tuck position for lumbar spine surgery. A 15 year follow up study. *Clinical Orthopedics and Related Research* **184**, 212−216.

Weinlander C.M., Coombs D.W. & Plume S.K. (1985) Myocardial ischemia due to obstruction of an aortocoronary bypass graft by intraoperative positioning. *Anesthesia and Analgesia* **64**, 933−936.

Weissman B.N., Aliabadi P., Weinfeld M.S., Thomas W.H. & Sosman J.L. (1982) Prognostic features of atlantoaxial subluxation in rheumatoid arthritis patients. *Radiology* **144**, 745−751.

Wells D.G. & Tredrea C.R. (1987) Intubation of the patient with cervical spine injury. *Anaesthesia and Intensive Care* **15**, 353−354.

White A.A. & Panjabi M.M. (Eds) (1978) Kinematics of the spine. In: *Clinical Biomechanics of the Spine*, pp. 61−90. J.B. Lippincott, Philadelphia.

Wiberg G. (1942) Anaesthesia in operation for prolapse of an intervertebral disc. *Acta Chirurgica Scandinavica* **87**, 380−384.

Wood P.R. & Lawler P.G.P. (1992) Managing the airway in cervical spine injury. A review of the Advanced Trauma Life Support Protocol. *Anaesthesia* **47**, 798−801.

Zigler J., Rockowitz N., Capen D., Nelson R. & Waters R. (1987) Posterior cervical fusion with local anaesthesia. The awake patient as the ultimate spinal cord monitor. *Spine* **12**, 206−208.

12
Anaesthesia for epilepsy and stereotactic surgery

MARTIN SMITH

Anaesthesia for epilepsy surgery

Introduction

Epilepsy is the manifestation of an underlying disorder of neuronal activity. Progress in the medical treatment of the epilepsies has been considerable in recent years, but some patients remain refractory or intolerant to therapy. Surgery may be considered in this group of patients if there is a discrete seizure focus which may be resected without producing major neurological deficit. Surgical treatment of intractable epilepsy involves careful patient selection, extensive presurgical evaluation, intra-operative electrophysiological and, in some cases, neuropsychological assessment, as well as intensive postoperative care. The anaesthetist plays a key role in the management of this particularly challenging group of patients.

Pathophysiology and medical therapy of epilepsy

PATHOPHYSIOLOGY

Sudden and excessive disordered neuronal activity is responsible for the clinical manifestations of the epilepsies (Wyler *et al.* 1982) which may present in a wide variety of seizure types. Electrical activity within the brain is normally well controlled, but in epileptogenic disorders the normal brain regulatory functions are altered.

Although the basic pathophysiology is not well understood it is clear that there is loss of postsynaptic inhibition, the introduction of significant excitatory synaptic connections and the appearance of pacemaker neurones (Prince 1985). These are a subpopulation of neurones present in the pacemaker zone of the epileptic focus which have the capacity to spontaneously produce burst discharges. This area is responsible for the characteristic interictal EEG spikes which are pathognomonic of some classes of epilepsy, as well as serving as a marker of the underlying cortical hyperactivity.

Generalized increase in cellular activity and loss of inhibitory tone around the pacemaker results in the development of frank seizure activity as the uncontrolled neuronal firing spreads to surrounding areas. Three distinct zones — the pacemaker, symptomatogenic and irritative zones — have characteristic ictal EEG appearances. The reasons for the spread of discharge outwards from the pacemaker zone is unclear, but may include alteration in ion flux secondary to membrane changes, impaired gamma-aminobutyric acid (GABA)-mediated synaptic inhibition and local alteration in neurotransmitter levels (Delgado-Escueta *et al.* 1986).

CLASSIFICATION

The epilepsies are classified into generalized or partial epilepsies (Table 12.1). Generalized epilepsies occur in 20% of patients with epilepsy and have clinical signs and EEG changes reflecting involvement of both hemispheres. They are associated with an initial impairment of consciousness, and motor activity is usually bilateral.

Partial epilepsies have clinical signs and EEG findings reflecting initial discharge limited to a discrete part of one hemisphere. The typical EEG finding in this group is the interictal spike. Simple partial seizures imply no impairment of consciousness as the seizure remains a focal discharge. Complex partial seizures, which include psychomotor or temporal lobe epilepsy, are the most common seizure disorder and occur when there is secondary loss of consciousness.

Correct classification of the seizure type is important because the natural history varies and the proper choice of anticonvulsant therapy depends upon it.

Table 12.1 Classification of the epilepsies

Generalized epilepsies
Generalized absence (petit-mal)
Generalized tonic—clonic (grand-mal)
Myoclonic
Atonic/tonic (drop attacks)

Partial epilepsies
Simple partial
Complex partial (includes psychomotor/temporal lobe)

MEDICAL THERAPY

The aim of medical treatment of epilepsy is a seizure-free patient with minimal side-effects. A variety of anticonvulsant medications exist and their correct use involves a consideration of the classification of the seizure disorder, the past seizure history, the age of the patient and the likelihood of side-effects.

Therapy is usually initiated with a single agent which is given in a dose sufficient to produce adequate plasma levels. The effect on seizure frequency or severity is then compared to plasma level and dose adjusted as required. If seizures continue, or if unacceptable side-effects develop, a second agent is substituted for the first. Should single therapy remain insufficient, combination therapy is instituted, but attention must be given to possible drug interactions.

Initial choice of anticonvulsant therapy is dependent upon seizure classification. First-line therapy for complex seizure disorders includes carbamazepine, phenytoin, phenobarbitone and primidone. Grand-mal, tonic−clonic, seizures respond well to phenytoin and sodium valproate, whereas petit-mal epilepsy is often controlled by ethosuximide. Both established and newer anticonvulsant drugs have toxicities which are of interest to the anaesthetist, and these and their therapeutic levels are shown in Table 12.2.

The exact mechanisms of action of anticonvulsant drugs are unknown but involve an action to prevent repetitive neuronal firing as well as inhibition of the spread of excitation from the focus (Macdonald & McLean 1986). It is likely that some drugs such as phenobarbitone, valproate and the benzodiazepines enhance the postsynaptic inhibitory effects of GABA, although other anticonvulsants, such as carbamazepine and phenytoin, have minimal GABA effects.

Presurgical evaluation

Despite appropriate treatment some epileptic patients remain refractory to medical therapy and have continued seizures. Others may have reasonable seizure control but suffer unacceptable side-effects from the anticonvulsant drugs to which they do respond. Patients falling into these categories may be suitable for consideration for surgical treatment (Cahan & Engel 1986).

Presurgical evaluation is a complex and time-consuming process which identifies appropriate candidates for surgery, which is generally

Table 12.2 Toxicities and therapeutic levels of anticonvulsant drugs

Drug	Therapeutic level (μmol l^{-1})	Side-effects
Phenytoin	25–80	Rash, hypersensitivity, gingival hyperplasia, ataxia, megaloblastic anaemia, neuropathy, encephalopathy, Stevens–Johnson syndrome
Sodium valproate	350–700	Tremor, weight gain, alopecia, thrombocytopenia, raised hepatic transaminase, hepatic failure
Carbamazepine	34–50	Rash, diplopia, sedation, thrombocytopenia, leukopenia, cholestatic jaundice, hyponatraemia
Phenobarbitone	65–170	Rash, hypersensitivity, sedation, megaloblastic anaemia, folate deficiency, osteomalacia
Ethosuximide	280–700	Nausea, vomiting, sedation, confusion, ataxia, photophobia, thrombocytopenia
Primidone	23–60	Ataxia, nystagmus, sedation thrombocytopenia, leukopenia
Vigabatrin	39–271	Sedation, irritability, aggression, psychosis, weight gain, mild anaemia
Lamotrigine	4–16	Rash, diplopia, dizziness, sedation, headache, ataxia, irritability, gastrointestinal disturbance, Stevens–Johnson syndrome

only considered in those with seizures of focal origin. The main aim of surgery is to improve or abolish seizures, but in some patients subsequent cessation of anticonvulsant therapy may be possible. As well as having seizures of focal onset, patients considered for surgery should have no other progressive medical or psychiatric illness. Many now consider that the intelligence of patients is unimportant as long as they are able to comprehend and cooperate with the detailed evaluation process.

The aim of presurgical evaluation is to accurately localize the area of brain responsible for the patient's seizures and to identify cortical areas which must be preserved to maintain essential neurological functions. Presurgical evaluation consists of extracranial EEG recordings, neuroradiological imaging, extensive psychometric testing and, in a small number of cases, recordings from invasively placed intracranial electrodes.

NEUROPHYSIOLOGY

The cornerstone of the evaluation process is a high-quality scalp EEG recording to localize interictal epileptiform activity. Ictal recordings are also obtained to map the spread of the epileptic discharge and associated video monitoring allows the seizure type to be examined. In some patients the scalp EEG may not be sufficient to accurately localize the epileptic focus and nasopharyngeal or percutaneously placed sphenoidal electrodes may be necessary (Spencer 1986). Even more precise localization may be achieved by the placement of intracranial electrodes with subsequent chronic recording (Engel & Crandall 1986) but this requires an additional general anaesthetic for electrode insertion. Examples include stereotactically placed depth electrodes and subdural and epidural electrodes.

NEURORADIOLOGY

Imaging studies to define structural abnormalities, such as gliomas, arteriovenous malformations, cavernous angiomas and temporal lobe or hippocampal sclerosis, are an essential part of the work up. CT has been the mainstay of neuroradiology until recently, but MRI is now the investigation of choice in this group of patients. Many patients who are CT-negative have lesions discernible on MRI, which demonstrates a structural abnormality in over 85% of cases. In patients with a temporal lobe lesion the MRI identification rate rises to over 95%. Positron emission tomography (PET) scanning, which measures glucose metabolism, may also be used to identify epileptogenic areas, although it is better at lateralization than anatomical definition. Single photon emission computerized tomography (SPECT) scanning, measuring cerebral blood flow, has also been described in epilepsy but localizes the focus best during seizures. It is difficult to imagine how radioisotopes can safely be injected into an actively fitting patient; therefore this technique is unlikely to find a place in the routine work-up.

NEUROPSYCHOLOGY

Neuropsychological assessment consists of a battery of tests to examine both verbal and non-verbal memory as well as intellectual and language function. Some tests are specific and allow lateralization and localization to one or other temporal lobe. Careful preoperative psychological assessment allows the prognosis of postoperative deficits to be made. Additional neuropsychological testing involves the selective catheterization of the carotid arteries under local anaesthesia and the injection of sodium amytal. This mimics the effects of surgery by producing selective hemispheric anaesthesia. The language-dominant hemisphere can be identified and the memory capabilities of the unaffected hemisphere determined (Wada & Ramussen 1960).

SURGICAL PROCEDURE

Ojemann (1987) outlined the criteria for selection of patients for surgical resection. The major indication is the failure to adequately control seizures with anticonvulsant medication despite trials of all appropriate anticonvulsants. A discrete seizure focus which may be resected without producing a major neurological deficit is also a prerequisite. Temporal lobe epilepsy is especially amenable to surgery.

The variety of surgical procedures undertaken for the control of epilepsy are listed in Table 12.3. The surgical resection must be extensive enough to adequately excise the epileptogenic area, but must be planned to avoid damage to surrounding language and sensorimotor areas. The extent of the resection will obviously depend upon whether or not the affected area is situated in the dominant hemisphere. In temporal lobe surgery a resection extending too far posteriorly in the lateral temporal lobe may compromise language areas, whereas extensive medial lobe resection may result in verbal memory defects.

Temporal lobectomy may be performed under general or local anaesthesia and the anaesthetic techniques are discussed below. The earliest operations, described by Horsley in 1886, were performed under local anaesthesia. Resections performed in awake patients allow topographic

Table 12.3 Surgical procedures undertaken for control of epilepsy

Temporal lobe resections
    en-bloc resection
    resection tailored with cortical EEG recordings (ECoG)
    resection tailored with stimulation
    selective procedures (amygdala—hippocampectomy under CT control)
Extratemporal resections
Lesionectomy
Hemispherectomy (in children)

localization of the epileptic focus without interference from anaesthetic
agents (Gildenberg & Katz 1990). Stimulation mapping may also be
carried out to determine the speech and sensorimotor areas which may
lie close to the resection margins. Resections carried out under general
anaesthesia offer considerable advantages to the patient in terms of
comfort, and provide superior operating conditions for the surgeon.
Although stimulation mapping is prevented during general anaesthesia,
cortical EEG recordings (ECoG) may be carried out with appropriate
anaesthetic techniques. Recordings from strip electrodes placed on the
cortex at the time of surgery supplement preoperative EEG information
(Fig. 12.1). This allows accurate mapping of the anatomical location of
the epileptogenic area (Devinsky *et al.* 1992).

Complications of temporal lobe resection include visual field defects
and third nerve palsies. Hemiplegia may rarely occur due to vascular
infarction secondary to manipulation of major vessels. A transient hemiparesis may be due to middle cerebral artery spasm and usually resolves
within 1−2 days. Postoperative seizures progressing to status epilepticus
may also occur.

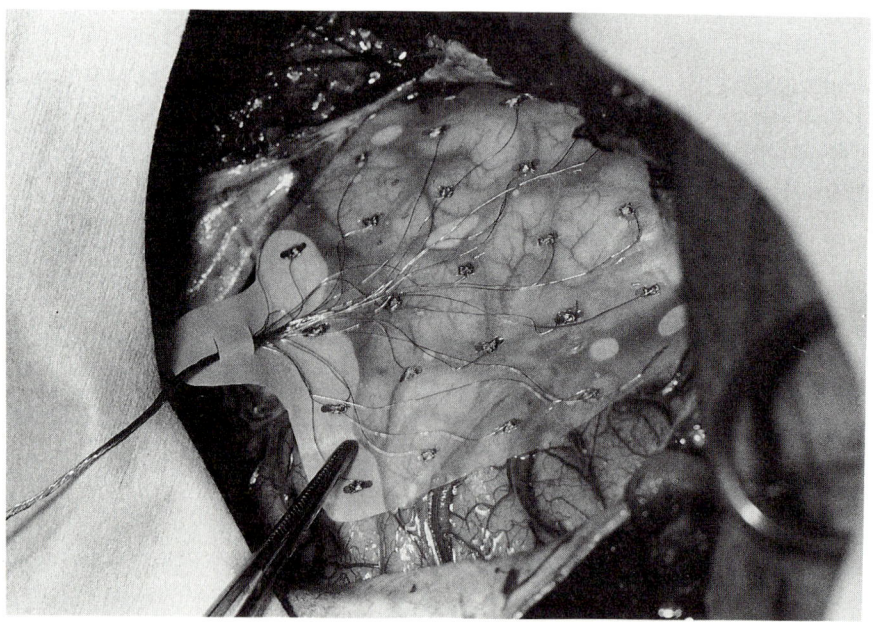

Fig. 12.1 Electrode plate in position over temporal lobe for peroperative surface
EEG recording (corticography).

Over 60% of patients may expect improvement in their seizures following temporal lobe resection. Olivier (1983) suggests that, with better selection and preoperative evaluation of patients, the improvement may be of the order of 85–90%. The risk of significant neurological morbidity is less than 4%.

Anaesthetic techniques for epilepsy surgery

The surgical treatment of epilepsy requires a coordinated approach from surgeon, neurophysiologist and anaesthetist. The role of the anaesthetist is pivotal as the anaesthetic technique must provide optimal operating conditions for the surgeon and maintenance of a safe and comfortable environment for the patient, while having minimal interference on the EEG to allow the neurophysiologist to obtain high-quality peroperative recordings. This is a challenging role as the factors affecting operating conditions may adversely affect the ability to obtain useful intraoperative ECoG information.

PREOPERATIVE ASSESSMENT

The preoperative visit of patients scheduled for epilepsy surgery has two main aims. First, the patient's history should be evaluated in relation to the epilepsy and any other medical problems. Seizure frequency, type and pattern should be established, as well as current anticonvulsant therapy. Complications of this therapy should be sought by physical examination and laboratory tests. Airway control may be difficult due to gingival hypertrophy and poor dentition secondary to chronic phenytoin therapy. Haematological and hepatic abnormalities must also be excluded. Anticonvulsant medication must be continued up to and including the day of surgery. Second, the patient must be prepared psychologically for the proposed operation. When awake craniotomy is planned the actual procedure should be discussed in detail, with particular emphasis on the parts which may be uncomfortable or distressing, the effects of intra-operative stimulation testing, potential nausea from traction on the temporal lobe and the possibility of intraoperative seizures. If craniotomy under general anaesthesia is planned, the requirement for lightening of anaesthesia with continued muscle relaxation during neurophysiological testing must be discussed. The possibility of awareness should be raised, although reassurance must be given that this would be entirely painless. This group of patients is highly motivated, has undergone several invasive procedures during presurgical evaluation and is rarely distressed by such suggestions. The risk of awareness is theoretical rather than actual, and there have been no episodes of awareness with the techniques employed at the National Hospital.

ANAESTHETIC AGENTS AND THE EEG

General anaesthetic agents may affect the EEG; some have minimal effects on the EEG, others have an anticonvulsant action whilst others may activate the EEG and cause seizures. In general, light levels of anaesthesia preserve the ability to obtain intraoperative recordings.

The intravenous agents have a variety of effects on the EEG. Short-acting barbiturates are anticonvulsants and thiopentone is often used for the treatment of postoperative seizures (Jewkes 1987). Partinen *et al.* (1981) described the use of thiopentone infusions for the treatment of status epilepticus. Methohexitone activates the EEG, especially in those with temporal lobe epilepsy (Rockoff & Goudsouzian 1981, Ford *et al.* 1982), and has been used in the evaluation of such patients (Musella *et al.* 1971). There have been varying reports of the effects of propofol on the EEG. Activation in temporal lobe epilepsy has been described (Hodkinson *et al.* 1987) as well as seizures and opisthotonos in patients with no history of seizures (DeFriez & Wong 1992, Kerz & Juntzen 1992). However, anticonvulsant effects have also been noted (al-Hader *et al.* 1992), and Mackenzie and colleagues (1990) successfully used propofol in the treatment of intractable status. Further elucidation of the effects of propofol on the normal and pathological EEG is required, as this agent is frequently used for sedation during awake craniotomy for epilepsy surgery. The benzodiazepines, especially diazepam (Browne & Penry 1973, Dejong & Heavner 1971, Macdonald & McLean 1986) and midazolam (Wroblewski & Joseph 1992, Lahat *et al.* 1992), all have anticonvulsant EEG effects.

The effects of inhalational anaesthetics on the EEG are well described. High inspired levels of isoflurane have profound effects on the EEG; at levels over two MAC the EEG becomes isoelectric (Eger *et al.* 1971, Newberg *et al.* 1983). EEG activity is maintained at levels below 1 MAC, although it has been suggested that background epileptiform activity may be reduced or suppressed and low-dose isoflurane has been used for the treatment of resistant status epilepticus (Hughes *et al.* 1992, Kofke *et al.* 1985, Sakaki *et al.* 1992). The effects of halothane are similar to isoflurane as clinically useful concentrations may suppress background epileptic activity (Avramov *et al.* 1991, Clarke & Rosner 1974, Gordon & Widen 1962). Enflurane in high concentration has a convulsant activity, especially in association with hypocarbia (Michenfelder & Cucchiara 1974). This has been used to stimulate epileptiform activity during ECoG (Flemming *et al.* 1980). Dose-dependent EEG changes secondary to nitrous oxide were first described over 40 years ago (Faulconer *et al.* 1949). More recently Stevens *et al.* (1983) demonstrated the anticonvulsant effect of nitrous oxide.

Opiates in usual clinical dosage have minimal effects on the EEG and fentanyl has been used with success during seizure surgery. However, Tempelhoff and colleagues (1992) have recently demonstrated that at moderate doses (25 μg kg^{-1}) fentanyl may cause activation of the EEG, and they suggest limiting the dose where electrocorticography is used during surgery for the purpose of determining the extent of the resection. High-dose opiate techniques, however, cause slowing of the EEG (Ochiai *et al.* 1992, Sebel *et al.* 1981).

Local anaesthetics are used during awake craniotomy and lignocaine has a biphasic effect on the EEG. At low plasma levels lignocaine may have anticonvulsant-like actions (Pascual *et al.* 1992) but at high levels it has excitatory effects on the central nervous system, including the induction of seizures (Wagman *et al.* 1968).

GENERAL ANAESTHESIA FOR EPILEPSY SURGERY

Patients in the UK prefer to undergo surgical procedures under general anaesthesia. Epileptic foci in the vicinity of sensitive areas of the dominant hemisphere may require resection with the patient awake, but the majority of epilepsy resections may safely be performed under general anaesthesia. Some patients, especially the paediatric population, will not tolerate awake procedures under any circumstances. At the National Hospital epilepsy surgery is undertaken under general anaesthesia unless there is a specific indication for an awake procedure.

Benefits of general anaesthesia include the provision of optimum operating conditions by the ability to control $PaCO_2$ and blood pressure, and the assurance of immobility. Disadvantages include the sacrifice of intraoperative memory and language assessment. The recording of intra-operative ECoG is not affected if appropriate anaesthetic techniques are employed.

Premedication is generally omitted to minimize the effects on the EEG. In particular benzodiazepines should be avoided prior to intraoperative EEG recording. General anaesthesia is induced with a short-acting barbiturate such as thiopentone and intravenous opiate (fentanyl $2 \mu g \, kg^{-1}$). Propofol is an alternative agent to thiopentone. Any EEG effects of these short-acting induction agents will have dissipated before corticography is performed. After spraying of the larynx with 4% lignocaine, tracheal intubation is achieved with the use of a short-acting non-depolarizing neuromuscular blocking agent such as vecuronium. It is essential that intubating conditions are good so that coughing and straining, with consequent adverse effects on intracranial pressure, are avoided.

During the initial craniotomy and dural opening blood pressure is controlled with additional doses of fentanyl (up to a total of $5 \mu g \, kg^{-1}$) and low-dose isoflurane. Labetolol is also used as required. Prior to recording the ECoG the inspired isoflurane concentration should be reduced to levels less than 1 MAC to minimize the effects on the EEG. This may produce light levels of anaesthesia, and unconsciousness cannot be guaranteed during corticography. The patient should have been warned of this preoperatively. It is essential during this period that muscle relaxation is maintained to prevent movement or coughing. Monitoring of neuromuscular function is mandatory because anticonvulsant medications may alter the response to neuromuscular blocking agents (Messick *et al.* 1982, Ornstein *et al.* 1986). It is possible that despite reduction or discontinuation of the inhalational anaesthetic agent adequate EEG recordings may not be obtained. In this case agents which activate the EEG may be administered; methohexitone (Musella *et al.* 1971), ketamine (Ferrer-Allado *et al.* 1973, Bennett *et al.* 1973) and enflurane (Flemming *et al.* 1980) have all been used for this purpose.

Following corticography anaesthesia may be deepened by increasing the inspired concentration of isoflurane. Following temporal lobectomy, further EEG recordings may be required from electrodes placed over the amygdyla and hippocampus. At this time isoflurane concentrations are again reduced.

Monitoring requirements are similar to those required for general anaesthesia for craniotomy discussed elsewhere in this volume. Monitoring should include direct arterial blood pressure, end-tidal carbon dioxide, end-tidal isoflurane and neuromuscular function. A urinary catheter should be inserted after induction of anaesthesia as the surgery may be protracted. A nasogastric tube is inserted in patients taking carbamezepine, as this drug has no parenteral preparation and nasogastric administration may be required.

Postoperatively the patient should be nursed in a neurosurgical intensive care unit (ICU) and invasive monitoring continued. The risk of seizures is higher in the immediate postoperative period and may progress to status epilepticus. Seizures should be aggressively treated to avoid cerebral damage (Sakaki *et al.* 1992). The use of benzodiazepines in the postoperative period may limit post-ictal neurological assessment because of a prolonged duration of action. Thiopentone is readily available in the neurosurgical ICU and small doses rapidly terminate seizures (Jewkes 1987).

LOCAL ANAESTHESIA AND SEDATION FOR EPILEPSY SURGERY

The main disadvantage of general anaesthesia for epilepsy surgery is the inability to perform intraoperative cortical stimulation. In patients with a dominant hemisphere epileptic focus whose resection margins may impinge upon nearby sensitive areas an awake procedure is essential to allow intraoperative sensorimotor mapping and neuropsychological assessment (Gildenberg & Katz 1990). Motor, sensory or language impairment and the development of verbal and non-verbal memory deficits during cortical stimulation will necessitate limitation of the resection margins to avoid damage to these vital areas.

During awake craniotomy all members of the operating team must be briefed of their duties in advance, and patient management should be carefully planned so that the procedure is smooth and uneventful. The operating theatre is a crowded place, particularly during neurophysiological monitoring (Fig. 12.2), and staff movement must be kept to a minimum. Delays and minor problems should be avoided in the presence of an awake patient. Careful positioning of the patient on a well-padded table is essential, as the procedure may last for several hours (Girvin 1986). Surgical drapes should be positioned to allow the anaesthetist access to the airway at all times, and patient contact by the neuropsychologist during intraoperative testing. The patient's eyes must be clear to allow free vision away from the operative site and the eyes should be protected during skin preparation with antiseptic solutions. The patient should be catheterized to avoid a full bladder during surgery.

Intravenous access and an arterial monitoring line should be inserted under local anaesthesia and continuous ECG and pulse oximetry initiated. The nostrils should be topically anaesthetized with cocaine and a soft nasopharyngeal airway inserted. This improves airway control during the sedation phase of the procedure and allows administration of

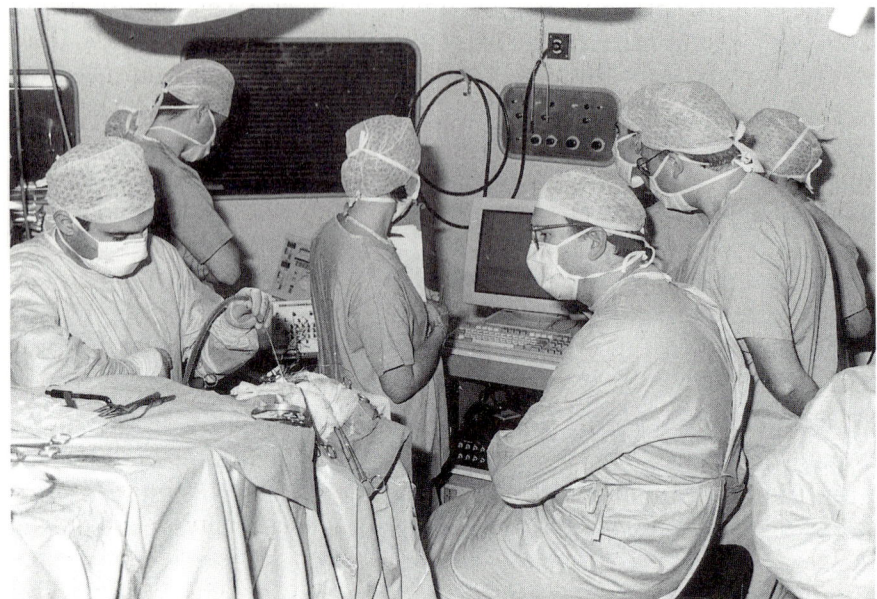

Fig. 12.2 Operating room crowded with personnel and equipment during per-operative corticography.

supplemental oxygen. Monitoring of expired carbon dioxide can also be achieved by attaching a side-stream carbon dioxide device to a small endotracheal tube connector inserted into the end of the nasopharyngeal airway.

Field block of the scalp, using lignocaine and bupivacaine, is performed by the surgeon after preparation of the operative site (Geevarghese *et al.* 1989). The skin, scalp, pericranium and periosteum of the outer table of the skull are all innervated by cutaneous nerves arising from branches of the cervical plexus and from branches of the three divisions of the trigeminal nerve. Subcutaneous infiltration with local anaesthetic in the manner of a field block, or over specific sensory nerve branches, blocks afferent input from all layers of the scalp. The skull itself has no sensation and can be drilled and opened with no discomfort to the patient (Manninen & Contreras 1986). The dura, however, is innervated by branches from all three divisions of the trigeminal nerve, the recurrent meningeal branch of the vagus and branches from the upper cervical roots. The dura may be adequately anaesthetized by application of local anaesthetic around the nerve trunk running with the middle meningeal artery and by a field block around the edges of the craniotomy.

The early part of the craniotomy until dural opening may be distressing to the patient because of incomplete local anaesthesia or noise from power tools. It is therefore appropriate to sedate patients during these early stages. Incremental fentanyl may be titrated against sedation level and respiratory rate, to a maximum of $5 \mu g \, kg^{-1}$. Repeat boluses of opiate are frequently necessary in the early stages. Some have suggested the addition of droperidol (up to $0.1 \, mg \, kg^{-1}$) to provide conscious sedation (Trop 1986, Manninen & Contreras 1986). More recently an infusion of propofol, in conjunction with fentanyl, has been used successfully at the National Hospital. As the dura is being opened the propofol infusion is discontinued and the patient returns to full consciousness and is able to cooperate with stimulation testing and neuropsychological assessment. The use of the nasopharyngeal airway allows monitoring of respiration during sedation with propofol and opiate. Airway management is generally uneventful with this technique, although the use of sedation inevitably runs a risk of apnoea and airway obstruction. Equipment should therefore be available for emergency airway control. Depending upon airway access a technique of endotracheal intubation under direct vision, blind nasal intubation or insertion of a laryngeal mask airway should all be considered.

Following stimulation testing and corticography the patient may be resedated for the surgical resection. Propofol by infusion is again the agent of choice, although benzodiazepines may be used if further EEG recording is not planned. In addition 50% nitrous oxide may be added to the inspired gas via the nasopharyngeal airway.

During awake craniotomy and stimulation testing there is an increased risk of seizures (Manninen & Contreras 1986). The development of intraoperative seizures is a major problem which should be treated aggressively. The choice of anticonvulsant depends upon the stage of the surgery. Prior to corticography long-acting anticonvulsants and benzodiazepines should be avoided, and a small dose of short-acting barbiturate such as thiopentone should be used (Manninen & Contreras 1986). Any suitable agent may be chosen postresection, and it may be appropriate to also administer a 'top-up' dose of the patient's long-acting convulsant(s).

Summary

Despite the complexities of presurgical evaluation and the surgical management of patients undergoing resection for epilepsy such techniques offer a potential benefit to those refractory or intolerant to medical therapy. The chance of a reduction in seizure frequency or severity is seized upon by this group of patients whose life is often made intolerable by this devastating condition. Furthermore, poorly controlled seizures put patients at higher risk of sudden death (Hauser *et al.* 1986); therefore until medical therapy becomes effective for all patients there will continue to be a place for surgery. The anaesthetist plays a key role in the management of this challenging group of patients.

Anaesthesia for stereotactic surgery

Introduction

There is a growing need in neurosurgical practice to make discrete lesions in, or obtain biopsies from, tissues which cannot be seen by direct vision. Such tissues may be too deep in the brain, or too intricately associated with sensitive areas, to make the risks of an open approach acceptable. A solution is the use of stereotactic surgery, which has now found an established place in the diagnosis and treatment of neurological disease. During stereotactic procedures instruments are accurately directed to a specific area of the brain using the relationship between the three-dimensional space occupied by an intracranial structure or lesion and an extracranial reference system. Biopsies may be taken, or lesions made for pain relief or the control of movement disorders, with an accuracy of approximately 1 mm. The anaesthetic management of patients undergoing stereotactic surgery involves careful coordination with the surgeon, and utilize local or general anaesthetic techniques.

Principles of stereotactic surgery

The application of geometry to the brain was described in 1908 by Horsley and Clarke, who produced focal lesions in the monkey cerebellum. It was almost four decades later that stereotactic surgery was first used in humans when Spiegel *et al.* (1947) established a system based on intracerebral landmarks. Shortly after this, other workers, notably Leksell, produced their own variations of the stereotactic apparatus (Leksell 1949). The coordinate system was initially related to intra-cerebral landmarks, in particular the third ventricle, which became the geometric localization of thalamic and basal ganglion structures. In these early days the intracranial structures were demonstrated by a pneumoencephalogram.

With the advent of CT, and more recently MRI, there has been a resurgence of stereotactic methodology. Such imaging methods provide detailed three-dimensional information about intracranial structures and mass lesions. This has allowed neurosurgeons to precisely localize and treat a variety of conditions both by conventional and stereotactic surgery. Following the advent of CT, many of the stereotactic systems already in use were modified to allow utilization of the new imaging techniques. In addition, several other systems were developed to allow incorporation of the full potential of the data available from CT.

Each element in a CT image may be defined by a set of three coordinates (Fig. 12.3), two at right angles to each other in the horizontal plane (X for left–right and Y for anterior–posterior) and one at right angles to the other two in the vertical plane (Z). Although each CT slice provides only information in the horizontal plane (X and Y), a knowledge of the spatial relationship between slices allows the position in the vertical plane (Z) to be described. The localization of structures or lesions in the X and Y coordinates is straightforward but the Z coordinate is more difficult to establish. The simplest way is to use a localizing device attached to the stereotactic headframe which remains outside the image but is included in every slice (Heilbrun 1984). Another technique utilizes stereotactic apparatus which is an integral part of the scanner (Koslow *et al.* 1981) and allows imaging and surgery to be carried out concurrently.

Indications for stereotactic surgery

STEREOTACTIC BIOPSY

The commonest indication for a stereotactic neurosurgical procedure in the UK is the need to obtain a diagnostic tissue sample from a tiny deep-seated lesion which is inaccessible by open surgery. A definitive tissue diagnosis allows the rational application of radiotherapy, chemotherapy or antimicrobial therapy. It is especially important to differentiate neo-plastic from non-neoplastic lesions as such differentiation is still not possible with 100% accuracy from radiological appearances. Furthermore, associated cystic areas may be drained to allow decompression.

The complication rate of CT-guided stereotactic biopsy is less than for open procedures. A recent study (Thomas & Nouby 1989) reported a mortality rate of less than 0.5% with the risk of significant neurological morbidity at just over 2%.

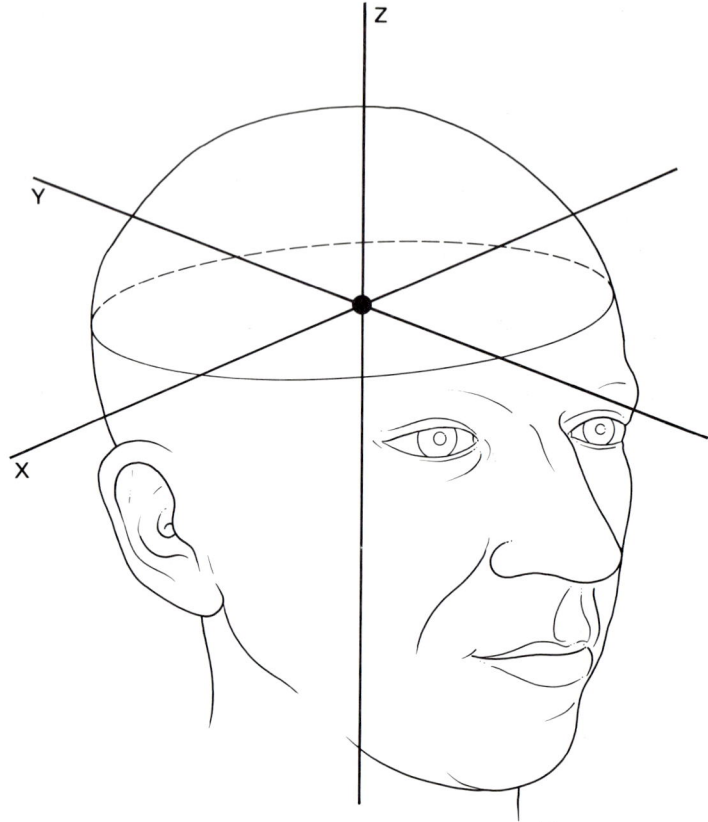

Fig. 12.3 Diagrammatic representation of the three coordinates used to define each element in a CT image.

STEREOTACTIC RESECTION

Tumours seated deep in the brain or intimately involved with important areas may not be suitable for free-hand excision. Stereotactic methodology can be applied to maintain surgical orientation during resection. Stereotactically implanted radioactive seeds are another treatment option.

FUNCTIONAL SURGERY

Stereotactic techniques may also be used to allow access to areas of the brain for ablation of nervous pathways to alter the function of specific parts of the nervous system. Such techniques are termed functional procedures.

The most frequent indication for functional ablation was lesion generation in the thalamus, basal ganglia or extrapyramidal pathways for the treatment of Parkinson's disease. However, this has become less common since the introduction of specific medical therapy. It does still have a place in the treatment of patients with intractable tremor. More recently, stereotactic procedures have been used for the implantation of dopamine-secreting neurones.

Some chronic pain conditions are amenable to stereotactic ablation of neuronal pathways. Lesions have been made in the spinothalamic tract in the midbrain and various nuclei of the thalamus for pain control. Central stimulation techniques are also possible via stereotactically placed electrodes. Stimulation of the periaqueductal grey matter reduces the sensation of chronic pain and has been used for the treatment of intractable lower back pain and some cancer pains. Thalamic stimulation may provide pain relief in specific areas because of the somatotrophic organization of the sensory thalamus.

Other applications of functional stereotactic surgery include the implantation of EEG depth electrodes for presurgical evaluation of patients with intractable epilepsy.

Application of the headframe

Application of the stereotactic headframe is carried out just before the imaging studies, and may take up to 20 min. Some frames do not obstruct the mouth, and airway access is possible at any stage. These frames may be applied using local anaesthesia and allow the imaging to be carried out with the patient awake. If the definitive procedure is to be carried out under general anaesthesia this may be induced just prior to surgery. Mask ventilation and intubation are possible with the Leksell stereotactic frame (Fig. 12.4a,b). The advantage of performing headframe application and imaging with the patient awake is that the period of general anaesthesia is short, and carried out in the environment of the operating theatre.

Other designs of stereotactic frame prevent access to the airway (Fig. 12.5) and general endotracheal anaesthesia prior to application of the frame is the preferred technique in the UK. In many other countries, however, local anaesthesia is used for the majority of stereotactic procedures.

Although there have been no reports of complications following stereotactic headframe application the procedure is similar to neuro-

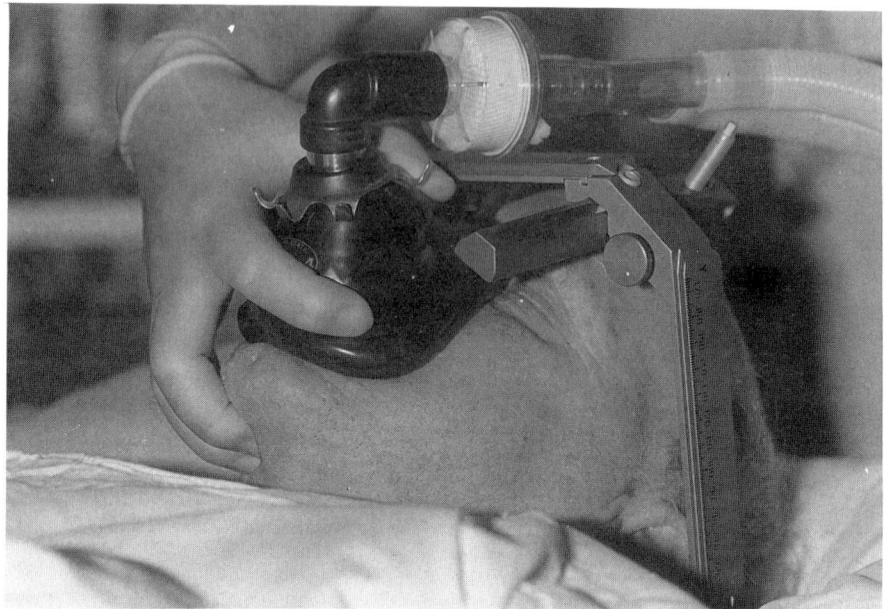

(a)

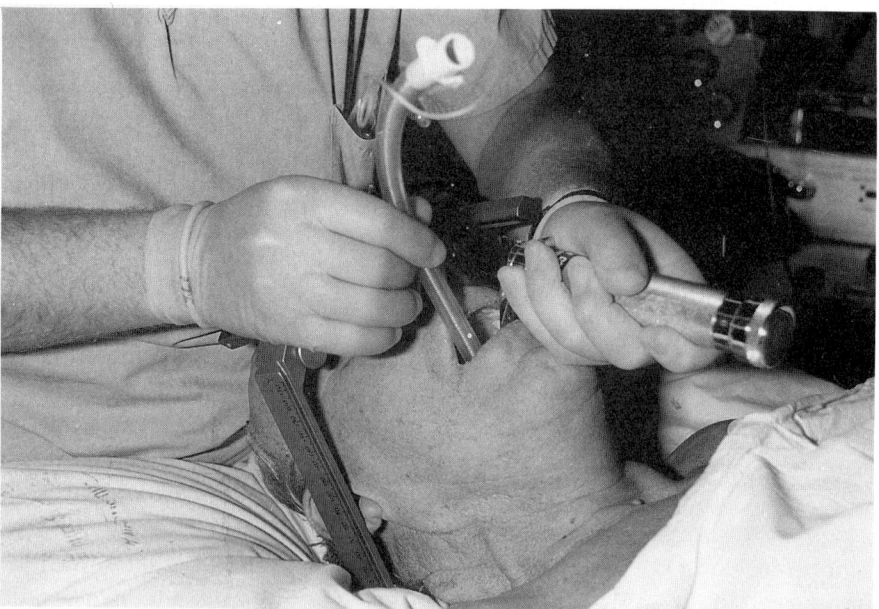

(b)

Fig. 12.4 Stereotactic frame allowing mask ventilation (a) and intubation (b) when fixed in position.

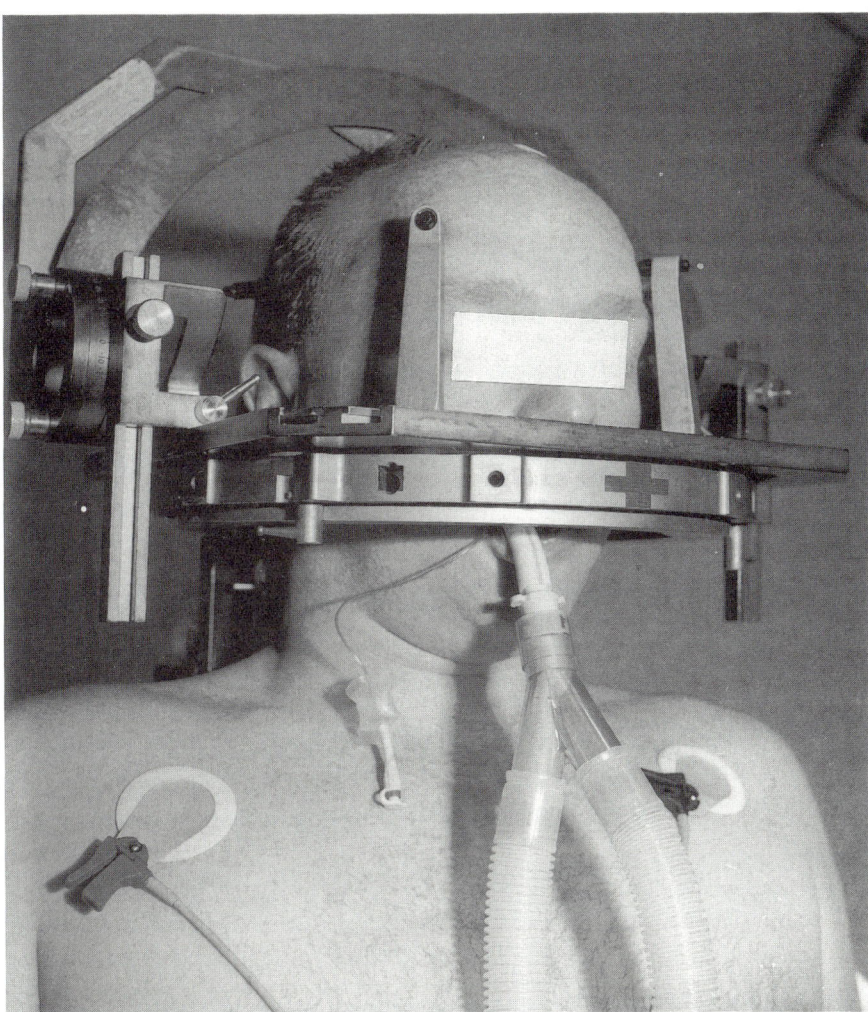

Fig. 12.5 Stereotactic frame which prevents access to the airway when fixed in position.

surgical skull clamp application which is a recognized source of complications. These include scalp haematoma, venous air embolism (Pang 1982) and perforation of the skull with subdural or extradural haematoma formation.

The imaging studies

Following application of the headframe the patient is transferred to the radiology department for the imaging studies. These may be CT or MRI, depending upon the lesion being investigated. All patients should be continuously monitored and accompanied by an anaesthetist to the radiology department. Incremental sedation may be administered as required to awake patients. The problems of conducting general anaesthesia during CT or MRI scanning have been dealt with elsewhere.

Following the collection of satisfactory images the patient is returned to the operating theatre for the surgical procedure.

Anaesthetic considerations

LOCAL ANAESTHESIA

In many countries the majority of stereotactic procedures are carried out under local anaesthesia and sedation (Perkins *et al.* 1990), whereas in the UK general anaesthesia is favoured by both neurosurgeons and patients. Some stereotactic procedures, however, must be carried out under local anaesthesia. Stereotactic thalamotomy for Parkinson's disease requires an awake, cooperative patient so that somatotrophic localization within the thalamus may be achieved. Drugs which inhibit tremor and rigidity should be avoided prior to surgery, so that the effects of the surgical lesion may be assessed peroperatively. Small doses of benzodiazepines appear to be safe.

Some designs of headframe allow general anaesthesia to be induced immediately prior to the surgical procedure, after the imaging studies have been performed (see above). In such cases the headframe must be applied under local anaesthesia. This method allows the anaesthetic time to be kept to a minimum and is well tolerated by most patients.

On arrival in the anaesthetic room an intravenous infusion should be commenced. Monitoring should be initiated and must include ECG, continuous measurement of oxygen saturation and blood pressure. Many consider that blood pressure measured non-invasively is sufficient for a straightforward stereotactic biopsy (Trop 1986). For more complicated procedures, or when some degree of hypotension is required, direct continuous blood pressure measurement via an arterial line should be employed as for craniotomy (Samuels & Larson 1987).

An anaesthetist should always be present during headframe application, to monitor vital signs and administer sedation if required (Lanier *et al.* 1987). Small doses of fentanyl and midazolam are usually sufficient. The frame is applied to the head by means of small pins which are screwed into the outer table of the skull. Local anaesthetic applied to the area of the scalp and periosteum underlying the site of the pins obtunds the cardiovascular response to frame application and renders the procedure painless.

The small scalp incision and burr-hole required for the passage of the stereotactic instrumentation can easily be carried out with local anaesthesia applied in a similar manner to that described for awake craniotomy for epilepsy surgery.

It is essential to remember to anaesthetize the dura separately, prior to making the dural incision. Lignocaine alone, or in combination with bupivacaine, is used. Adrenaline may be added to prolong the duration of action of the local anaesthetic. Bupivacaine with adrenaline reportedly provides scalp anaesthesia for between 8 and 12 h (Girvin 1986).

Monitoring is continued into the operating theatre and an anaesthetist is present throughout awake procedures. Sedation is given as required and fentanyl, midazolam and droperidol have all been used with success (Lanier *et al.* 1987). Infusion of subanaesthetic doses of propofol is now a useful alternative. Sedation should be avoided if an awake procedure is performed for a space-occupying lesion, because of the adverse effects on intracranial pressure and airway control.

When the mouth is obstructed by the stereotactic frame it is almost impossible to ventilate and intubate the patient without removing the whole frame. Equipment for emergency airway control should always be near at hand and should include a laryngeal mask airway. If the patient cannot tolerate the procedure and general anaesthesia is required an awake fibreoptic intubation may be performed.

GENERAL ANAESTHESIA

The techniques of general anaesthesia are similar to those for open craniotomy and have been discussed in detail elsewhere. The advantages of general anaesthesia for stereotactic procedures include the provision of optimal operating conditions by control of $Paco_2$ and arterial blood pressure, and comfortable conditions for the patient. General anaesthetic techniques should allow rapid wake-up and prevent brain swelling while ensuring that the brain remains 'full' if intracranial hypertension is not present. Stereotactic biopsy or excision of cerebral tumour requires the usual anaesthetic precautions for patients with space-occupying lesions.

Monitoring of patients undergoing stereotactic procedures under general anaesthesia is similar to the procedure used for local anaesthesia. However, many neuroanaesthetists consider beat-to-beat measurement of blood pressure, by direct arterial pressure monitoring, essential in the anaesthetized patient (Samuels & Larson 1987). This is mandatory if hypotension is required. Breath-by-breath end-tidal carbon dioxide measurements confirm adequate ventilation and allow controlled hyperventilation.

Careful patient positioning is essential to allow some head-up tilt and prevention of neck vein obstruction. This ensures unimpeded intracranial venous outflow and optimal intracranial pressures. However, the stereotactic headframe, or other stereotactic instrumentation, may prevent ideal positioning and other means of intracranial pressure control may be required. These have been dealt with previously, but include moderate hyperventilation and the use of modest doses of mannitol.

The risk of haemorrhage following stereotactic surgery is less than for open neurosurgical procedures. Some surgeons, however, request moderate hypotension during stereotactic procedures, but the blood pressure should not be lowered excessively. Small incremental doses of labetolol are usually sufficient. In the postoperative period sudden rises in blood pressure should be prevented and treated in the usual manner.

Summary

Anaesthesia for stereotactic procedures requires a familiarity with the techniques and instrumentation to anticipate the requirements of the surgeon and the needs of the patient. The anaesthetic demands are similar to those for other neurosurgical procedures. General anaesthesia is the preferred technique for stereotactic surgery in the UK, although in other countries local anaesthesia is favoured. The application of the stereotactic frame and the imaging may always be performed with the patient awake. Some functional procedures require an awake cooperative patient throughout.

The use of stereotactic techniques is increasing both in the numbers of centres undertaking the procedures and the applications of the technique. Stereotactic procedures for the local introduction of radioactive and chemotherapeutic substances and gamma knife technology are areas of growth. Techniques for transplantation of neuroactive tissue into discrete areas of the brain are in their infancy, but have exciting promise.

References

Anaesthesia for epilepsy surgery

Avramov M.N., Murayama T., Shingu K. & Mori K. (1991) Electroencephalographic changes during vital capacity breath induction with halothane. *British Journal of Anaesthesia* **66**, 212–215.

Bennett D.R., Madsen J.A., Jordan W.S. & Wiser W.C. (1973) Ketamine anesthesia in brain damaged epileptics. *Neurology* **23**, 449–460.

Browne T.R. & Penry J.K. (1973) Benzodiazepines in the treatment of epilepsy. *Epilepsia* **14**, 277–310.

Cahan L.D. & Engel J. (1986) Surgery for epilepsy: a review. *Acta Neurologica Scandinavica* **73**, 551–560.

Clarke D.L. & Rosner B.S. (1974) Neurophysiologic effects of general anesthetics. *Anesthesiology* **38**, 564–582.

DeFriez C.B. & Wong H.C. (1992) Seizures and opisthotonos after propofol anesthesia. *Anesthesia and Analgesia* **75**, 630–632.

Dejong R.H. & Heavner J.E. (1971) Diazepam prevents local anesthetic seizures. *Anesthesiology* **34**, 523–531.

Delgado-Escueta A.V., Ward A.A., Woodbury D.M. & Porter R.J. (1986) New wave of research in the epilepsies. *Advances in Neurology* **44**, 3–55.

Devinsky O., Canevini M.P., Sato S., Broomfield E.B., Kufta C.V. & Theodore W.H. (1992) Quantitative electrocorticography in patients undergoing temporal lobectomy. *Journal of Epilepsy* **5**, 178–185.

Eger E.L., Stevens W.C. & Cromwell T.H. (1971) The electroencephalogram in man anesthetized with Forane. *Anesthesiology* **35**, 504–508.

Engel J. & Crandall P.H. (1986) Intensive neurodiagnostic monitoring with intracranial electrodes. *Advances in Neurology* **46**, 85–106.

Faulconer A., Pender J.W. & Bickford R.G. (1949) The influence of partial pressure of nitrous oxide on the depth of anaesthesia and the electroencephalogram in man. *Anesthesiology* **10**, 601–609.

Ferrer-Allado T., Brechner V.L., Dymand A., Cazen H. & Crandall P. (1973) Ketamine-induced electroconvulsive phenomena in the human limbic and thalamic regions. *Anesthesiology* **38**, 333–334.

Flemming D.C., Fitzpatrick J., Fariello R.G., Duff T., Hellman D. & Hoff B.H. (1980) Diagnostic activation of epileptogenic foci by enflurane. *Anesthesiology* **52**, 431–433.

Ford E.W., Morell F. & Whisler W.W. (1982) Methohexital anaesthesia for surgical treatment of uncontrolled epilepsy. *Anesthesia and Analgesia* **61**, 997–1001.

Geevarghese K.P., Reiss S.J. & Garretson H.D. (1989) Alert anesthesia for intracranial surgery. *Anesthesia and Analgesia* **68** (Suppl.), S97.

Gildenberg P.L. & Katz J. (1990) Surgery for seizures. In: Frost E.A.M. (Ed.),

Clinical Anaesthesia in Neurosurgery, pp. 335–345. Butterworth-Heinemann, London.

Girvin J. (1986) Neurosurgical considerations and general methods for craniotomy under local anaesthesia. *International Anesthesiology Clinics* **24**, 89–114.

Gordon E. & Widen L. (1962) General anaesthesia with halothane for surgical interventions and electrocorticography in cases of focal epilepsy. *Acta Anesthesiologica Scandinavica* **6**, 13–28.

al-Hader A., Hasan M. & Hasan Z. (1992) The comparative effects of propofol, thiopental, and diazepam, administered intravenously, on pentylenetetrazol seizure threshold in the rabbit. *Life Sciences* **51**, 779–786.

Hauser W.A., Annegers J.F. & Elveback L.R. (1986) Mortality in patients with epilepsy. *Epilepsia* **21**, 399–412.

Hodkinson, B.P., Frith R.W. & Mee E.W. (1987) Propofol and the electro-encephalogram (correspondence). *Lancet* **ii**, 1518.

Horsley V. (1886) Brain-surgery. *British Medical Journal* **2**, 670–675.

Hughes D.R., Sharpe M.D. & McLachlan R.S. (1992) Control of epilepsia partialis continua and secondarily generalised status epilepticus with isoflurane (letter). *Journal of Neurology, Neurosurgery and Psychiatry* **55**, 739–740.

Jewkes D.A. (1987) The postoperative period—some important complications. *Clinical Anesthesiology* **1**, 517–531.

Kerz T. & Juntzen J.P. (1992) A myoclonic seizure during propofol-alfentanil anesthesia? *Anaesthetist* **41**, 426–430.

Kofke W.A., Snider M.T., Young R.S.K. & Ramer J.C. (1985) Prolonged low flow isoflurane anaesthesia for status epilepticus. *Anesthesiology* **55**, 203–211.

Lahat E., Aladjem M., Eshel G., Bistritzer T. & Katz Y. (1992) Midazolam in treatment of epileptic seizures. *Pediatric Neurology* **8**, 215–216.

Macdonald R.L. & McLean M.J. (1986) Anticonvulsant drugs: mechanisms of action. *Advances in Neurology* **44**, 713–736.

Mackenzie S.J., Kapadia F. & Grant I.S. (1990) Propofol infusion for control of status epilepticus. *Anaesthesia* **45**, 1043–1045.

Manninen P. & Contreras J. (1986) Anesthetic considerations for craniotomy in awake patients. *International Anesthesiology Clinics* **24**, 157–174.

Messick J.M., Maass L., Faust R.J. & Cucchiara R.F. (1982) Duration of pancuronium neuromuscular blockade in patients taking anticonvulsant medication. *Anesthesia and Analgesia* **61**, 203–204.

Michenfelder J.D. & Cucchiara R.F. (1974) Canine cerebral oxygen consumption during enflurane anaesthesia and its modification during induced seizures. *Anesthesiology* **40**, 575–580.

Musella L., Wilder B.J. & Schmidt R.P. (1971) Electroencephalographic activation with intravenous methohexital in psychomotor epilepsy. *Neurology* **21**, 594–602.

Newberg L.A., Milde J.H. & Michenfelder J.D. (1983) Systemic and cerebral effects of isoflurane at and above concentrations that suppress cortical activity. *Anesthesiology* **59**, 23−28.

Ochiai R., Sato K., Koitabashi T., Takeda J., Sekiguchi H. & Fukushima K. (1992) Electroencephalographic changes during induction of high-dose fentanyl anesthesia−evaluation by Lifescan EEG monitor. *Masui* **41**, 799−804.

Ojemann G.A. (1987) Surgical therapy for medically intractable epilepsy. *Journal of Neurosurgery* **66**, 489−499.

Olivier A. (1983) Surgical management of complex partial seizures. In: Nistico G., Di Perri R. & Meindardi H. (Eds), *Epilepsy−an Update on Research and Therapy*, pp. 309−324. Alan R. Liss, New York.

Ornstein E., Matteo R.S., Silverberg P.A., Schwartz A.E., Young W.L. & Diaz J. (1986) Chronic phenytoin therapy and non-depolarizing muscular blockade. *Anesthesiology* **63**, A331.

Partinen M., Kovanen J. & Nilsson E. (1981) Status epilepticus treated by barbiturate anaesthesia with continuous monitoring of cerebral function. *British Medical Journal* **282**, 520−521.

Pascual J., Ciudad J. & Berciano J. (1992) Role of lidocaine (lignocaine) in managing status epilepticus. *Journal of Neurology, Neurosurgery and Psychiatry* **55**, 49−51.

Prince D.A. (1985) Physiological mechanisms of focal epileptogenesis. *Epilepsia* **26** (Suppl.), S3−S14.

Rockoff M.A. & Goudsouzian N.C. (1981) Seizures induced by methohexital. *Anesthesiology* **54**, 333−334.

Sakaki T., Abe K., Hoshida T. *et al.* (1992) Isoflurane in the management of status epilepticus after surgery for lesion around the motor area. *Acta Neurochirurgica (Wien)* **116**, 38−43.

Sebel P.S., Bovill J.G., Wauquier A. & Rog P. (1981) Effects of high dose fentanyl anaesthesia on the electroencephalogram. *Anesthesiology* **55**, 203−211.

Spencer S.S. (1986) Surgical options for uncontrolled epilepsy. *Neurology Clinics* **4**, 669−695.

Stevens J.E., Oshima E. & Mori K. (1983) Effects of nitrous oxide of the epileptogenic properties of enflurane in cats. *British Journal of Anaesthesia* **55**, 145−154.

Tempelhoff R., Modica P.A., Bernardo K.L. & Edwards I. (1992) Fentanyl-induced electrocorticographic seizures in patients with complex partial seizures. *Journal of Neurosurgery* **77**, 201−208.

Trop D. (1986) Conscious−sedation analgesia during the neurosurgical treatment of epilepsies−practice at the Montreal Neurological Institute. *International Anesthesiology Clinics* **24**, 175−184.

Wada J. & Ramussen T. (1960) Intracarotid injection of sodium amytal for the lateralisation of cerebral speech dominance. *Journal of Neurosurgery* **17**, 266−282.

Wagman I.H., DeJong R.H. & Prince D.A. (1968) Effects of lidocaine on spontaneous cortical and subcortical electrical activity. *Archives of Neurology* **18**, 277−290.

Wroblewski B.A. & Joseph A.B. (1992) Intramuscular midazolam for treatment of acute seizures or behavioural episodes in patients with brain injuries. *Journal of Neurology, Neurosurgery and Psychiatry* **55**, 328−329.

Wyler A.R., Ojemann G.A. & Ward A.A. (1982) Neurons in human epileptic cortex: correlation between unit and EEG activity. *Annals of Neurology* **11**, 301−308.

Anaesthesia for stereotactic surgery

Girvin J.P. (1986) Neurosurgical considerations and general methods for craniotomy under local anaesthesia. *International Anesthesiology Clinics* **24**, 89−114.

Heilbrun M.P. (1984) Computed tomography-guided stereotactic systems. *Clinical Neurosurgery* **31**, 564−581.

Horsley V. & Clarke R.H. (1908) The structure and functions of the cerebellum examined by a new method. *Brain* **31**, 45−124.

Koslow M., Abele M.G., Griffith R.C., Mair G.A. & Chase N. (1981) Stereotactic surgical system controlled by computed tomography. *Neurosurgery* **8**, 72−82.

Lanier W.L., Hool G.J., Faust R.J. *et al.* (1987) Sedation for stereotactic headframe application; a randomized comparison of two techniques. *Applied Neurophysiology* **50**, 227−232.

Leksell L. (1949) A stereotactic apparatus for intracerebral surgery. *Acta Chirurgica Scandinavica* **99**, 229−233.

Pang D. (1982) Air embolism associated with wounds from a pin-type head holder. *Journal of Neurosurgery* **57**, 710−713.

Perkins W.J., Kelly P.J. & Faust R.J. (1990) Stereotactic surgery. In: Cucchiara R.F. & Michenfelder J.D. (Eds), *Clinical Neuroanaesthesia*, pp. 379−419. Churchill Livingstone, New York.

Samuels S.I. & Larson C.P. (1987) Principles of anaesthesia for craniotomy. *Clinical Anaesthesiology* **1**, 279−294.

Spiegel E.A., Wycis H.T., Marks M. *et al.* (1947) Stereotactic apparatus for operations on the human brain. *Science* **106**, 349−350.

Thomas D.G.T. & Nouby R.M. (1989) Experience in 300 cases of CT directed stereotactic surgery for lesion biopsy and aspiration of haematoma. *British Journal of Neurosurgery* **3**, 321−326.

Trop D. (1986) Conscious-sedation analgesia during neurosurgical treatment of epilepsies−practice at the Montreal Neurologic Institute. *International Anesthesiology Clinics* **24**, 175−184.

13
Anaesthesia for paediatric surgery

ANGELA M. MACKERSIE

Introduction

Paediatric neuroanaesthesia requires an intimate knowledge not only of the scientific basis of modern neuroanaesthesia but also of the physiology and pathology of small children and how they differ from adults. Major surgery in small children, which includes nearly all neurosurgical procedures, requires an anaesthetist familiar with the management of small children and an acute awareness of the potential problems which can arise at any time in infants with limited physiological reserves and small blood volumes. The techniques utilized must therefore sometimes be a compromise between the theoretical ideal for controlled neuroanaesthesia and the practical problems of the management of sick infants and children.

General considerations

Children with intracranial pathology differ from adults in certain ways which may be advantageous. The fontanelles and non-fused sutures, which can separate even in early adolescence, provide protection from gradual changes in intracranial volume resulting in an increased head size prior to a rise in pressure. Acute changes are not absorbed in this way because of the rigidity of the fibrous tissue bridging the sutures and fontanelles. Children of all ages are fortunate in having healthy blood vessels devoid of atheroma, and therefore are less likely to suffer focal ischaemia during treatment for intracranial pathology.

Unlike other systems of the body which only increase in size after birth, the central nervous system not only grows but becomes massively more complex. At birth the number of neurones is almost complete, but glial growth with dendritic arborization and synoptic formation, and also myelination, continues postnatally. At birth about one-quarter of the cells are present with two-thirds present by 6 months, and growth completed by 2 years. Differential rates of growth occur, with the

345

cerebellum less developed at birth but achieving full development within the first year of life, before the cortex and brainstem. Nutrition both prenatally and postnatally is important for full cerebral development. Malnutrition results in reduced numbers of cells and dendritic connections, and also reduced cerebral lipid and protein contents.

Intracranial physiology

The upper limit of normal intracranial pressure in children of different ages is not yet accurately defined, but the improvement in intracranial pressure monitoring devices such as the Camino system, and the relatively non-invasive nature of the procedure, means that some information is available from children with cranial abnormalities, but for ethical reasons this cannot be obtained from normal children. Again absolute values for cerebral blood flow (CBF) are not known for normal small children, but in older children the values are almost double those for adults, and the oxygen consumption is increased by approximately one-third (Kennedy & Sokoloff 1957). CBF in children with severe head injury or encephalopathy from Reye's syndrome has been measured in children using a nitrous oxide dilution technique with simultaneous arterial and jugular venous bulb blood sampling, but again such an invasive technique would be unethical in normal children (Swedlow & Lewis 1980).

The same effects of hypocarbia and hypercarbia on CBF have been assumed from clinical experience. Wyatt *et al.* 1986 have demonstrated the linear relationship between $PaCO_2$ and changes in CBF using near-infrared spectrophotometry in sick newborns.

Transcranial Doppler is increasing in popularity because of its non-invasive nature and ease of use. However, the results expressed as CBF velocity have not yet been clearly related to CBF or intracranial pressure.

The lower limit of autoregulation again is unknown in small children, but is assumed to be related to normal systemic blood pressure (Table 13.1). Sick newborn infants with respiratory distress syndrome or birth asphyxia are well known to have impaired autoregulation with CBF following systemic pressure, which may explain the susceptibility of these infants to intraventricular haemorrhage (Lou *et al.* 1979).

CONTROL OF INTRACRANIAL PRESSURE (ICP)

Good operative conditions for neurosurgery are produced by controlling

Table 13.1 Normal blood pressure and heart rate

Age	Blood pressure (mmHg)	Heart rate (beats min^{-1})
Birth	80/50	135 ± 20
6 months	90/60	140 ± 20
1 year	95/65	120 ± 20
2 years	100/65	110 ± 20
5 years	95/55	90 ± 20
10 years	110/60	80 ± 20

the ICP. Raised pressure caused by obstructive hydrocephalus and tumours associated with large cysts is little affected by the anaesthetist's skills, and therapeutic manoeuvres and conditions are changed only by removal of the encysted fluid. Reduction in the normal brain volume should be reserved for critical rises in ICP.

Steroids can provide dramatic improvement in the clinical condition by reducing peritumour oedema. Dexamethasone 0.25 mg kg^{-1} as a loading dose with 0.1 mg kg^{-1} 6-hourly is still used perioperatively for tumour surgery in most units, despite lack of definite studies into its benefits. Recent work on the effects of hyperglycaemia and outcome in head injury and surgery may lead to controlled studies finally being performed.

Cerebral dehydration with reduction in both intracellular and extra-cellular fluid volume is achieved with diuretics. Twenty per cent mannitol, apart from its use in the treatment of acute rises in ICP, is usually reserved for operations where surgical access to small solid lesions is particularly difficult. Children have excellent renal function with small blood volumes so that a maximum dose of mannitol 1 g kg^{-1} is recommended with careful monitoring of urine output, using an indwelling urinary catheter. If urine output exceeds the infused volume plus 10% of the estimated blood volume increased intravenous replacement will be urgently required. A vigorous and rapid response to the mannitol, leading to a marked reduction in intracerebral volume prior to opening the dura, may lead to tearing of the dural veins and haematoma formation. Cerebral dehydration can also be produced with frusemide 0.5 mg kg^{-1} which, despite its advantages of not providing an osmotic load to the circulation, has not replaced mannitol as the agent of choice in most units.

POSITIONING AND VENTILATION

Low cerebral venous pressure during surgery results from good positioning of the patient. This is much harder to achieve in small children due to their relatively short necks and large heads, which can lead to kinking of the neck veins. A moderate head-up position should be used routinely, but this is associated with an increased risk of air embolism, especially in the presence of hypovolaemia. The children also need to be supported in their chosen position using sandbags or strapping to prevent movement during surgery, as a result of surgical manipulation. Positive end-expiratory pressure (PEEP) is avoided during ventilation of all neurosurgical patients except in those with poor respiratory function. Manual ventilation of neonates and small infants, still a recognized technique in general surgery, should be avoided because of the difficulty in not applying PEEP, and reserved only for high-risk infants with decreased compliance where further changes may be critical, for example in ex prems with bronchopulmonary dysplasia, during tunnelling of the VP shunt system.

Moderate hyperventilation should be employed to control intracranial pressure, but may be difficult with ventilators of the T-piece occluder pattern popular in paediatric anaesthesia, as increasing the rate results in rebreathing unless very high fresh gas flows are employed (Nightingale *et al.* 1965). With larger tidal volumes the expiratory time needs to be increased to avoid rebreathing and the application of PEEP. Children over 20 kg, and those with abnormal lungs, are better ventilated with a non-rebreathing system. Adequate oxygenation is also essential at all times, and there is some evidence from neurointensive care suggesting that hyperoxia PaO_2 greater than 20 kPa may have a beneficial effect, increasing tissue oxygenation in areas of poor flow due to gross cerebral oedema (Swedlow 1983). During anaesthesia in patients with normal lungs and a fractional inspiratory oxygen (FIO_2) of 0.35, these levels are usually attained. However, care should be taken to avoid hyperoxia in newborns and ex prems where high levels result in retrolental fibroplasia.

INDUCED HYPOTENSION

Induced arterial hypotension must be associated with deep anaesthesia, adequate muscle relaxation, good oxygenation and normovolaemia. Hypotensive agents should not be administered to small children without direct arterial pressure monitoring, especially in a situation where sudden or heavy blood loss is expected. Good operative conditions are best achieved with a relatively slow heart rate for a particular size of patient, in a neonate 110 beats per minute would be considered slow but in an 8-year-old tachycardiac (Table 13.1). If the heart rate is fast initial measures of deepening anaesthesia, increasing the infusion rate and checking blood gases should be done prior to embarking on active measures. Control of heart rate with beta-blockers either alone (propranolol incrementally up to $0.5\,mg\,kg^{-1}$), or in combination with an alpha-blocker (labetalol incrementally up to $1\,mg\,kg^{-1}$) is sufficient to provide moderate hypotension and improved surgical conditions. Where the patient already has a relatively slow heart rate, or more profound falls in pressure are required, vasodilator agents such as sodium nitroprusside $0.5\,\mu g\,kg^{-1}\,min^{-1}$ can be used, with a maximum dose of $1\,mg\,kg^{-1}$ every 24 h. Induced hypotension should be used only where surgical conditions are inadequate, and where all other measures have failed to achieve the desired effect. It should never be used to achieve a blood pressure thought optimal. In general children are more resistant to hypotensive agents than adults.

In practice the main differences in paediatric neuroanaesthesia are due to the small size of the patient with an increased metabolic rate, greater oxygen demands and resultant rapid development of hypoxia during acute events. Secondly normal children have relatively large heads compared to adults (Table 13.2) and, as already described, children with intracranial pathology have increased head sizes due to separation of the sutures, so that in some neurosurgical patients the head may be almost half the total surface area, which contributes to the increased blood losses and difficulty with temperature control.

Anaesthetic management

PREOPERATIVE ASSESSMENT

All neurosurgical patients require an accurate assessment of their neurological status including evidence of raised intracranial pressure, alteration in conscious level and any focal findings, in particular cranial nerve palsies. Bulbar palsies associated with brainstem lesions may result in reduced reflexes and impaired swallowing, leading to silent aspiration with pulmonary consolidation and hypoxaemia.

Raised intracranial pressure commonly presents with vomiting which is

Table 13.2 Surface area of the head of normal children

Age (years)	Percentage
0−1	19
1−4	17
5−9	13
10−14	11
Adult	7

frequently attributed to an infectious origin in a child but may become sufficiently severe to cause dehydration and electrolyte disturbance; this can result in hypotension following the induction of anaesthesia if not treated.

Pathology in other systems is rare in children with CNS neoplasia; however, certain neurosurgical patients are likely to have multisystem disease such as ex prems with bronchopulmonary dysplasia and hydro-cephalus, cerebral abscess in patients with cyanotic heart disease, renal disease in children with major spinal defects, and those with congenital syndromes having cranio-facial surgery.

Preoperative investigations should include a full blood count for all patients, and electrolyte estimation in those with a history of vomiting or with a ventricular drain. Children with chronic shunt infections frequently become severely anaemic due to poor intake and toxic bone marrow depression, and may require preoperative transfusion. Lesser degrees of anaemia can be corrected perioperatively. The physiological anaemia of infancy as fetal haemoglobin (HbF) is replaced by adult haemoglobin (HbA) may result in a normal haemoglobin of $9-10\,g\,dl^{-1}$ in the first year of life, gradually increasing to adult levels through childhood. In the presence of dehydration from vomiting the initial haemoglobin estimation may be falsely high, by $1-2\,g\,dl^{-1}$. All children having neurosurgical operations should be cross-matched.

The preoperative visit is when discussion should take place with the children able to understand. The nature of their induction technique and postoperative course and monitoring equipment should be explained in simple terms, without frightening them about details of which they will not be aware. In younger children without verbal communication skills, alleviation of parental anxiety, as far as possible, will help in prevention of its transmission to the child.

PREMEDICATION

Sedative premedication should be avoided in all children having intracranial surgery. Children with raised ICP, especially those with blocked ventricular shunts, may appear remarkably well, apart from complaining of headache and occasional vomiting. However, many of these children have markedly raised ICP, and minor triggers such as sedative premedication may cause a sudden spiralling effect with a massive increase in pressure and the potential for coning.

Atropine is administered according to weight (Table 13.3) intramuscularly at least 30 min prior to surgery in all infants and those older children having surgery in the sitting or prone position where salivation may result in dislodgement of the endotracheal tube, despite great care being taken with its fixation.

While the intramuscular route is not encouraged in children, the advantages of improved antisialogogue properties with less tachycardia, while still providing the cardiostability, outweigh the disadvantages. Use of antisialogogues is still recommended in paediatric practice because of the small airways and greatly increased resistance to flow with any reduction in size by secretions.

Children not having intracranial or cervical spinal surgery can receive a standard sedative premedication, e.g. trimeprazine $2\,mg\,kg^{-1}$; papaveretum $0.4\,mg\,kg^{-1}$; or pethidine 25 mg, promazine 6.25 mg, chlorpromazine 6.25 mg in 1 ml, at $0.07\,ml\,kg^{-1}$ to a maximum dose of 1.5 ml, again all combined with an antisialogogue. EMLA topical local anaesthetic mixture of lignocaine (50%) and prilocaine (50%) cream is used routinely, applied over suitable veins, but is most effective in those children able to understand its properties and tolerate removal of the adhesive covering.

Parental presence in the anaesthetic room, especially with an unsedated child, can provide great support and comfort to the young patients.

Table 13.3 Atropine dosage for premedication

Weight (kg)	Intramuscular (mg)	Oral (mg)
Under 2.5	0.15	—
2.5–8	0.2	0.4
8–15	0.3	0.6
15–25	0.4	0.8
Over 25	0.5	1.0

However, with infants too small to be aware of their parent's presence, or in situations where the parents are too distressed to support their child, it may be preferable to induce the child alone. The anaesthetist in charge must be the final arbiter to the presence of a parent during induction and also to when the parent should leave.

INDUCTION

The effects of different anaesthetic agents on intracranial pressure are well known. Despite the use of EMLA cream and sensitive handling of the young patient an inhalational induction may have less deleterious effect on the ICP than an intravenous injection associated with crying and breath-holding in an already cerebrally irritable child.

Isoflurane has better properties as an inhalational agent in neuro-anaesthesia, but the longer induction time and potential for breath-holding and coughing, if not frank laryngeal spasm, in the author's opinion precludes it from routine use as an induction agent. Halothane at present is still the agent of choice for an inhalational induction. Once induced, venous access can be rapidly secured and the concentration of inhalational agent reduced. If necessary a small dose of thiopentone $1-2\,\mathrm{mg\,kg^{-1}}$ and/or fentanyl $1-2\,\mathrm{\mu g\,kg^{-1}}$ can be administered to obtain deep anaesthesia prior to muscle relaxation and intubation. The latter is achieved with either suxamethonium $1-2\,\mathrm{mg\,kg^{-1}}$, or atracurium $0.4-0.5\,\mathrm{mg\,kg^{-1}}$. Suxamethonium rarely causes fasciculation in small children, and enables the patient to be intubated rapidly. The longer period of mask ventilation prior to the development of intubating conditions with non-depolarizing agents may lead to gastric distension and diaphragmatic splinting and reduced compliance in small children, and certainly moderate hyperventilation is much harder to achieve.

The airway is secured with an uncuffed endotracheal tube of the correct size (age divided by 4, plus 4) which has a small leak at cricoid level; too large a leak may cause hypoventilation. The author's preference for neurosurgery is to use a reinforced silastic tube; although slightly more difficult to insert they provide excellent security once in place. The tubes are thicker-walled and therefore a smaller size may be required. After intubation it is essential to check for bilateral ventilation with the head both in a neutral position and its position for surgery, as in a small child 1 cm may be the difference between a good position and endo-bronchial intubation. Preformed south-facing tubes such as Mallinkrodt RAE and Portex polar tubes are extremely popular in paediatric use.

However, it must be remembered that just because a preformed tube is the correct size for the larynx it is not necessarily the correct length; endobronchial intubation is not uncommon with these tubes, while others may be dangerously short especially for neurosurgery (Black & Mackersie 1991).

MAINTENANCE

Maintenance of anaesthesia is with a balanced technique of muscle relaxation, analgesia and anaesthesia with moderate hyperventilation. The choice of muscle relaxant is a matter of personal preference based on experience. d-Tubocurarine $0.4-0.5\,\mathrm{mg\,kg^{-1}}$ still has a place in paediatric anaesthesia for major surgery, as significant falls in blood pressure are not seen in this population, and it results in excellent cardiovascular stability, prolonged relaxation with no sudden reversal, and conditions which are always able to be reversed with neostigmine. For short procedures, especially in high risk patients, e.g. ex prems having VP shunts inserted, atracurium $0.4-0.5\,\mathrm{mg\,kg^{-1}}$ is the agent of choice because of its very predictable metabolism; however, because of its abrupt spontaneous reversal, neuromuscular function must always be monitored. Vecuronium $0.08-0.1\,\mathrm{mg\,kg^{-1}}$ provides excellent cardiovascular stability and has little histamine release, but in small children may have an unpredictable dose response and therefore a relaxograph is recommended especially if it is being administered by infusion.

Analgesia is provided with fentanyl up to $5\,\mathrm{\mu g\,kg^{-1}}$ initially with increments of $1\,\mathrm{\mu g\,kg^{-1}\,h^{-1}}$ after approximately $2\,\mathrm{h}$. A maximum dose of $6-7\,\mathrm{\mu g\,kg^{-1}}$ is usually sufficient unless surgery is prolonged, more than $4\,\mathrm{h}$. Higher doses are used when postoperative ventilation is planned.

Anaesthesia is supplemented with low-dose isoflurane, usually $0.5-1.0\%$, with higher doses intermittently as required. Bisonette & Leon (1992) have demonstrated cerebrovascular stability in children during isoflurane anaesthesia which did not change with time when isoflurane was administered up to 1.5 MAC. In a parallel study (Leon & Bisonette 1991) on the effect of nitrous oxide, increased CBF was demonstrated, which was reversed when air/oxygen mixtures were administered.

A total intravenous technique also has its proponents, but it is questionable whether propofol will continue to be used in this way in children, following the recommendation to ban its use for intensive care sedation as a result of deaths or near-deaths occurring from a 'Reye syndrome-like' illness in children admitted with croup (CSM 1992).

At the end of surgery residual muscle relaxation should always be reversed with neostigmine 0.05 mg kg^{-1} and atropine 0.025 mg kg^{-1} unless postoperative ventilation is planned. Extubation is performed only when the child is breathing well and awake.

CONCLUSION

In practice what is required for paediatric neuroanaesthesia is a balanced technique which provides good analgesia and anaesthesia with stable cardiovascular conditions, but which will allow rapid compensation during periods of reduced cardiac output due to excess bleeding, so common in major neurosurgical procedures in small children. The author's choice of agents which best fit these criteria is a combination of nitrous oxide, oxygen and fentanyl supplemented by low-dose isoflurane.

Monitoring

Routine monitoring is standard with a stethoscope, either precordial or oesophageal, ECG, non-invasive blood pressure, pulse oximetry, capnography, temperature probe and peripheral nerve stimulator. The blood pressure cuff should be the largest that easily fits the upper arm of the child, making allowance for the relatively greater forearm and axillary subcutaneous fat, to provide an accurate reading. All major cases should have direct arterial pressure measurement.

Capnography has a dual role in neurosurgery, to monitor both for adequate moderate hyperventilation and also for air embolism. The latter can occur in all neurosurgical cases, especially if there is heavy blood loss and the patient becomes slightly hypovolaemic. There are basically two types of capnographs, in-line and side-stream. The in-line machine with an infant cuvette (Hewlett-Packard) has been available for more than a decade. Children with normal lungs and pulmonary blood flow have demonstrated a good correlation between arterial and end-tidal carbon dioxide (Lindahl *et al.* 1987), but the added dead space may make reductions in end-tidal carbon dioxide more difficult to achieve in some patients.

Side-stream machines sample at volumes greater than 120 ml min^{-1}, and several studies, especially those from Toronto Children's Hospital, have shown excellent correlation with distal endotracheal tube sampling. Proximal sampling is more valuable, and depends on the nature of the circuit and the ventilator with partial rebreathing systems being less accurate. Correlation in many patients, compared to arterial levels, is within 2 mmHg. However, while capnography is an excellent breath-to-breath monitor of adequate ventilation, and a good trend monitor, if there is any doubt about absolute values arterial blood gas analysis must be performed.

Central venous pressure (CVP) lines are recommended for all major general surgery in children, but the most reliable route for insertion in infants and children is via the internal jugular vein, which might result in obstruction to cerebral venous drainage in a small child, especially when positioned with the neck flexed or extremely extended. Percutaneous long lines inserted via the antecubital fossa are rarely successful in children under 5 years of age. The most appropriate route may be via the femoral vein. In experienced hands intraoperative fluid balance can be accurately assessed without CVP monitoring by other cardiovascular parameters (Uppington & Goat 1987). However, good venous access with at least two good peripheral cannulas is essential.

Urinary catheters are not used routinely, but are reserved for patients in whom a large urine output may produce fluid balance problems, either after diuretics or in patients at risk for developing diabetes insipidus.

Temperature control

The large head surface area of most child neurosurgical patients contributes to heat losses. Children have much larger surface area to weight ratios than adults, and also have less subcutaneous fat. Heat losses by conduction, convection and radiation, and from the latent heat of vaporization, must be minimized and active measures available for rewarming as required. The hot air mattress (Howarth Air Engineering Company) gives the anaesthetist the ability to rewarm the patient if necessary. Passive measures to prevent heat loss include wrapping the child in aluminum foil and covering in gamgee. If rapid transfusions are required, greater than 20% of the blood volume per hour, an in-line blood warmer should be used. Close monitoring of body temperature is essential, both central and peripheral. Hypothermia with peripheral circulatory shutdown and metabolic acidosis may be very difficult to reverse even with increased transfusion rates. Ideally a temperature between 36°C and 36.5°C should be maintained. However, when there are surgical difficulties a lower temperature may have a cerebral protective effect by lowering cerebral metabolism, enabling surgery to be completed while the cerebral perfusion is somewhat compromised. Temperatures over

34.5°C may provide protection without putting the child at jeopardy from cardiac arrhythmias and metabolic changes (Berntman *et al.* 1981). This degree of hypothermia is usually achieved by cessation of warming and does not require active cooling.

POSTOPERATIVE HYPERPYREXIA

Hyperpyrexia is more likely after craniopharyngioma resection and hypothalamic, pontine and midbrain manipulations, and if not treated vigorously has a poor prognosis, especially if the temperature exceeds 40.5°C. Initial active cooling methods include increased transfusion of room temperature fluids and fanning, and administration of paracetamol 15 mg kg^{-1} rectally. If these measures are not successful peripheral vasodilatation can be achieved using small doses of chlorpromazine 0.1−0.2 mg kg^{-1} intravenously or other vasodilator drugs of choice, while closely monitoring and correcting any fall in blood pressure. If the temperature is still resistant to lowering, and remains over 40°C, other steps which can be taken are to use ice packs placed over large vessels and the liver, and also rectal, bladder or gastric washouts with ice-cold saline. Frequent blood gas analysis is required to ensure adequate venti-lation during a period of increased metabolism. Electrolyte imbalance is also likely due to both cellular dysfunction and rapid transfusion, and will require correction.

Fluid balance

The recurring theme of paediatric neurosurgery is the relatively large size of the patient's head, and this results in proportionately larger blood losses. In children under 20 kg undergoing craniotomy blood transfusion is almost invariable, even in the present climate of avoiding blood transfusion. The exception is surgery performed in the sitting position where, even in children under 10 kg, less than half the patients at Great Ormond Street require blood transfusion.

Table 13.4 Estimate blood volume (ml kg^{-1})

Newborn	80−85
6 weeks−2 years	75−80
2 years−15 years	70−75

Blood loss in neurosurgery is notoriously difficult to measure due to contamination of the drapes and mixing of the blood with saline used during the bone work and cerebrospinal fluid (CSF). The use of the ultrasonic suction device, with its continuous spray of saline, also adds to this difficulty.

Replacement, in experienced hands, is performed accurately using all cardiovascular parameters, in particular heart rate and arterial pressure trace. Exchange transfusions are not unusual in small children, and are extremely well tolerated provided clotting factors, blood gases and in particular K^+ levels are checked regularly and normal values maintained. Fresh-frozen plasma at approximately 10% of the blood volume should be administered for each exchange transfusion, to ensure adequate clotting factors. Calcium supplements are usually required only with rapid transfusions greater than 40% of the blood volume per hour (Abbott 1983).

Rapid transfusion of blood stored for more than 12 days and low cardiac output, a situation not that uncommon in small neurosurgical patients having craniofacial or large tumour surgery, has a high risk of hyperkalaemia, which should be actively treated otherwise cardiac arrest may ensure (Brown *et al.* 1990). It should be remembered that the definition of a massive transfusion is an exchanged blood volume transfused within 24 h. It is not uncommon for high-risk patients to receive two or three exchange volumes intraoperatively, and a single exchange within 1 h. Of course, active intervention to maintain normal blood parameters is much more likely to be needed in such situations.

Hyperglycaemia is recognized in head injuries to be associated with an adverse outcome. Adult neuroanaesthetists usually avoid glucose-containing infusions for the first 24 h. However, small children are more likely to develop perioperative hypoglycaemia, especially if there has been a prolonged period of vomiting and reduced food and fluid intake prior to surgery which may have depleted reserves. Blood sugar should be monitored regularly during long operations and postoperatively, and glucose-containing infusions administered accordingly. Postoperative fluids are usually administered as 4% glucose 0.18% saline to avoid hypoglycaemia at a rate of $2.5-3.0\,\mathrm{ml\,kg^{-1}\,h^{-1}}$ reducing to $2.0\,\mathrm{ml}$ $\mathrm{kg^{-1}\,h^{-1}}$ by about 20 kg and $1.0-1.5\,\mathrm{ml\,kg^{-1}}$ as adult size is approached. If nasogastric losses are significant normal saline with potassium added will be required as replacement. Continuing blood losses should be expected and replaced.

0 – 10 kg	4 ml/kg/hr
10 – 20 kg	40 ml + ((weight – 10) + 2 ml/kg)/hr
20 – 30 kg	60 ml + ((weight – 20) ml/kg)/hr
>30	70 ml + ((weight – 30)/2 ml/kg)/hr

POSTOPERATIVE CARE

Ventilation is usually reserved for patients with particular indications. Airway problems, either from a craniofacial anomaly or central causes such as bulbar lesions or obtunded central control of reflexes, are indications for intubation and usually postoperative ventilation for the first 24 h. Otherwise only if the operation has been particularly prolonged, or there has been cardiovascular instability or a particular neurosurgical indication, are children ventilated at Great Ormond Street.

All patients are closely monitored postoperatively; following craniotomy direct arterial pressure monitoring is continued until the next day and regular evaluation of the neurological status and cardiorespiratory function is carried out, together with an accurate assessment of fluid balance.

Traditionally postoperative analgesia has been administered as codeine phosphate $1 \, mg \, kg^{-1}$ intramuscularly 4-hourly, as in many adult neurosurgical units. This provides good pain relief without altering consciousness and pupil size. It should not be administered intravenously due to the potent cardiac depressant effect (Shanahan *et al.* 1983). Recently diclofenac $1.0-1.5 \, mg \, kg^{-1}$ rectally 8−12-hourly, inserted at the end of surgery, has provided excellent analgesia in craniotomy patients who subsequently only require simple analgesics. However, it should not be used where there is a high risk of bleeding or impaired renal function. Paracetamol $10-15 \, mg \, kg^{-1}$ with a maximum dose of $60 \, mg \, kg^{-1} day^{-1}$ administered orally or rectally is usually substituted after the first 24 h.

Children ventilated postoperatively will require analgesics and sedation, which is usually provided by low-dose morphine infusion maximum rate $10 \, \mu g \, kg^{-1} h^{-1}$, which still allows neurological assessment. Additional sedation can be provided either with midazolam infusions $2-5 \, \mu g \, kg^{-1} min^{-1}$ or diazepam $0.1 \, mg \, kg^{-1}$ by bolus injection, if required. Children having spinal surgery receive morphine infusions either as patient-controlled analgesia or nurse-controlled analgesia, which has a higher background infusion level with a longer shut-out period. This latter is particularly effective in toddlers who are reluctant to lie flat after surgery unless well sedated.

Antiemetics are not routinely prescribed in children under 5 years of age unless vomiting is troublesome; prochlorperazine $0.15-0.2 \, mg \, kg^{-1}$ or metoclopramide $0.15 \, mg \, kg^{-1}$ may be prescribed.

Anaesthesia for specific surgical procedures

Neonatal surgery

Neurosurgery in the neonatal period, which is now defined as less than 44 weeks gestation, is usually performed for neural tube defects, especially spina bifida and encephalocoels, hydrocephalus, or elevation of depressed fractures caused during a traumatic delivery.

NEURAL TUBE DEFECTS

Neural tube defects occur around the 26th day of gestation at the time of anterior neural tube closure. Lesions involving meningeal structures only may occur at a later developmental stage. While much is known about the incidence of all these defects, including anencephaly, there are still many unanswered questions (Sellar 1987). There is considerable geographical variation in incidence both within and between countries. Many areas of the world have reported a spontaneous decrease in incidence which cannot be explained by early antenatal diagnosis and therapeutic abortion. Approximately 10% of neural tube defects may result from a genetic mutation or chromosomal abnormality, while the remainder have a multifactorial origin. It is this latter group which gives rise to the geographical and racial variation, while genetic cases have a similar incidence worldwide. Recent work published by the MRC Vitamin Research Group (1991) showed a 72% reduction in the incidence of neural tube defects in subsequent pregnancies conceived after treatment with daily supplements of folic acid, but no such benefit from multi-vitamins. The aetiology of these defects still requires considerable unravelling.

Antenatal diagnosis of neural tube defects can either be from maternal alpha-fetoprotein levels (αFP) or by routine ultrasonography. The former is reliable only for open defects, which is more likely with anencephaly and meningomyeloceles than encephaloceles. Ultrasound not only makes the diagnosis but also gives some indication of the contents of the lesion and the presence of other abnormalities such as hydrocephalus. Early diagnosis by 12–14 weeks enables discussion of therapeutic abortion. Detection late in pregnancy allows discussion of the optimal mode of delivery and its timing. Non-vaginal delivery may be recommended to avoid rupture of flimsy meningeal sacs, or with the probability of pelvic disproportion with large solid lesions. Early delivery is sometimes recommended where hydrocephalus is present, to minimize the detrimental effect of the large ventricles on the cortical mantle and subsequent cerebral function. However, the risks of prematurity and considerably greater need for intensive care, with the concomitant potential for complications, must outweigh any advantage of an early planned delivery. Fetal surgery has potential for transamniotic aspiration of CSF, but the risk of infection has precluded its routine use. Emergency surgery for neural tube lesions is now thought to be unnecessary except for uncovered defects, allowing formal investigation of the lesion at least with ultrasound, but preferably with CT and/or MRI scans, and the ability to confirm the presence and the magnitude of other CNS abnormalities. Early surgery is recommended for large lesions and those with very flimsy coverings where there is a risk of rupture and subsequent development of meningitis, but other lesions can have surgery deferred if necessary.

Preoperative assessment should include an assessment of the ease of intubation, especially for larger spinal lesions or occipital encephaloceles. The traditional suggestion is that the left lateral position be used, but the author uses the more common supine position with the lesion surrounded by a stack of 'doughnut' head rings so that there is no pressure on the coverings and the remainder of the head and body are supported on foam pads or folded gamgee so that the head, neck and thorax are in a neutral position and well supported. This position not only provides optimal conditions for intubation, but also ensures an unobstructed airway during preoxygenation and induction of anaesthesia.

Vitamin K should be administered preoperatively to reduce the risk of bleeding from haemorrhagic disease of the newborn. There is recent evidence (Golding *et al.* 1990, 1992), that intramuscular vitamin K is associated with an increased risk of childhood cancer whereas the oral route is not, but it is too early to abandon the use of the intramuscular route before full knowledge of the efficacy of oral administration is known (Hull 1992).

ANAESTHESIA

Intravenous cannulation should be instituted prior to anaesthesia; many of these babies will require intravenous fluids prior to surgery to maintain blood glucose because of slow feeding from their neurological state. *Awake intubation* should be performed if there is any doubt about the ease of intubation or the abilities of an inexperienced paediatric anaesthetist in these circumstances, otherwise a standard neonatal technique of gaseous induction with oxygen and low-dose halothane or intravenously with thiopentone $2-3\,\mathrm{mg\,kg^{-1}}$ can be performed. Usually a gaseous induction is used with a muscle relaxant given as soon as light anaesthesia is induced, for even with low-dose thiopentone there is some residual depressant effect postoperatively.

Anaesthesia should be maintained with nitrous oxide in oxygen with supplemental isoflurane as necessary, usually only during skin incision to avoid the stress response to surgery (Anand *et al.* 1987). In this first of many papers, Anand *et al.* have demonstrated an improved outcome when the stress response to surgery is blocked either by anaesthesia or analgesia. Opiates should be avoided in this very high-risk group of patients unless postoperative ventilation is planned. It is well recognized that infants under 46 weeks gestation are at risk of postoperative apnoea (Steward 1982) and this will, of course, be much higher in a neurosurgical population who already have reduced cerebral activity.

The operations are usually performed in the prone position; great care is needed to avoid inferior vena caval compression leading to engorgement of the paraspinal veins. Many of the neural tube defects have associated haemangiomas in the surrounding tissues and skin which may increase the bleeding. Meningomyeloceles are unlikely to require blood transfusion unless the base of the lesion is more than 5 cm. Large lesions may need rotational flaps, or rarely tissue expanders are used to produce adequate skin cover. The bases of encephaloceles are frequently associated with a leash of vessels which may cause massive haemorrhage from the dural veins, which can be very difficult to control due to the small size of the cranial defect.

HYDROCEPHALUS

Treatment of hydrocephalus is the commonest procedure in paediatric neurosurgery. It is either primary or secondary to intraventricular haemorrhage (IVH), meningitis or the Arnold—Chiari malformation usually associated with spina bifida. There is evidence that primary or antenatal hydrocephalus is caused by intrauterine infection or haemorrhage. The diagnosis of progressive hydrocephalus is made by increasing head circumference. The clinical picture of the massively enlarged head, bulging fontanelles, engorged veins and sunsetting eyes is rarely seen nowadays.

After a trial period of early surgery for premature infants with hydrocephalus from IVH, these patients are now treated with repeated ventricular taps, either direct or after insertion of a Rickham cap and ventricular drain because of the high surgical complication rate from raised protein levels in the CSF and low flow. Many of these infants will still be less than 44 weeks gestation despite having survived 3 months stormy intensive care treatment, and may well have other complications of prematurity such as bronchopulmonary dysplasia or incompletely resolved necrotizing enterocolitis which may affect both surgical and anaesthetic decisions.

Ventriculoperitoneal shunts are the usual choice but coexisting inguinal hernias, very common in premature babies, have to be repaired to prevent CSF accumulating in the sacs. The peritoneal route is avoided if there is intra-abdominal pathology for which future surgical treatment is likely. Atrial shunts are no longer used routinely because of the rare but disastrous complication of bacterial endocarditis with pulmonary emboli and resultant pulmonary hypertension. Alternatively the pleural route is used, but is usually reserved for cyst or subdural haematoma drainage. If large volumes of fluid drain into the pleural cavity respiratory embarrassment can occur.

When inserting peritoneal shunts blood loss is usually less than 10 ml and transfusion is not required. With atrial shunts the blood loss is greater, but still transfusion is not routine. There is also a risk of air embolism as the catheter is inserted. However, cross-matched blood should be available for all children having shunts in case the enlarged dural veins are damaged during burr-hole drilling, when control can be difficult to achieve with limited access.

Central control of temperature may also be reduced compared with normal neonates; therefore every attempt to conserve heat is required. Surgical access is required to head, thorax and abdomen, and the infant should be completely wrapped in aluminium foil with monitoring attached, leaving just sufficient access for the surgeon.

Postoperatively both preterm infants and those with neural tube defects will require very close monitoring, not only for central apnoeic spells but also excessive drainage of CSF may affect central cardiac stability and result in a low cardiac output. Any preoperative respiratory support, either with oxygen therapy or pressure support, is likely to need upgrading, e.g. oxygen therapy to nasal continuous positive airway pressure (CPAP), nasal CPAP to intubation with pressure support or ventilation. At the same time the risks of hyperoxia should be remembered in preterm infants. Postoperative transcutaneous oxygen monitor or pulse oximetry should be used routinely maintaining saturations between 90% and 92%.

Infants under 5 kg should not receive codeine phosphate. Paracetamol 10 mg kg^{-1} rectally can be used. Phenobarbitone 1–1.5 mg kg^{-1} is extremely effective in treating the symptoms of cerebral irritability presumably produced by blood in the CSF, and is more effective than analgesics.

Tumours

Malignancy is the second most common cause of death in children after accidents. CNS tumours are second only to the leukaemias in the malignancy table in the paediatric population. Despite this, however, they are still rare, with less than 200 new cases diagnosed each year in the UK.

There have been no major breakthroughs in chemotherapy and radiotherapy, which is not recommended in the younger patients because of the detrimental effect on brain development, but survival has improved largely due to better general care of the child and the massive advances in imaging techniques leading to earlier diagnosis and treatment. More than 50% of children with medulloblastomas now survive more than 5 years, but younger children and those with spinal seedlings at presentation have a worse outcome.

POSTERIOR FOSSA TUMOURS

The majority of brain tumours in children occur in the posterior fossa and are midline, so that the sitting position is usually the position of choice, producing excellent conditions with less than half of 100 consecutive patients at Great Ormond Street between 1984 and 1987 requiring blood transfusions, even those weighing less than 15 kg. Only three patients required more than 30% of their blood volume. More recently, in the current atmosphere of greater reticence about blood transfusion, only 20% of patients required intra-operative transfusions and only 3% postoperative 'top-ups'.

Postural hypotension is very rare in children unless they are clinically dehydrated, when they rapidly respond to 5 ml kg^{-1} of crystalloid. Despite this they should be moved gradually to the full sitting position over a period of 3–4 min while monitoring the blood pressure. Careful positioning is very important both for maintaining the venous pressure and preventing air embolism, and to ensure a free airway as extremes of head flexion may result in bevelling of the end of the endotracheal tube against the tracheal wall. The sitting position can be used in all ages, but is harder to achieve in those infants who do not sit independently and have no secondary lumbar curve. The smaller children all sit with flexed legs, the smallest cross-legged in a very natural and stable position on the seat of the chair, larger ones have flexed knees and feet supported at the same level as the buttocks. Only those approaching small adult size are required to have their legs semidependent, and the legs are then strapped with elastic bandages. There is no antigravity device available for small children.

Venous air embolism (VAE) is the major disadvantage of the sitting position but, as already said, it can also occur in other positions although less commonly. Most units in the UK monitor for VAE using end-tidal carbon dioxide; Doppler is also in some units but tends to be oversensitive and noise interference during diathermy precludes its use during certain periods of the operation. There is some evidence that transoesophageal echocardiography may be helpful in the early detection of VAE, and especially of paradoxical emboli (Cucchiari *et al.* 1984).

Significant VAE (i.e. those causing cardiovascular symptoms) are

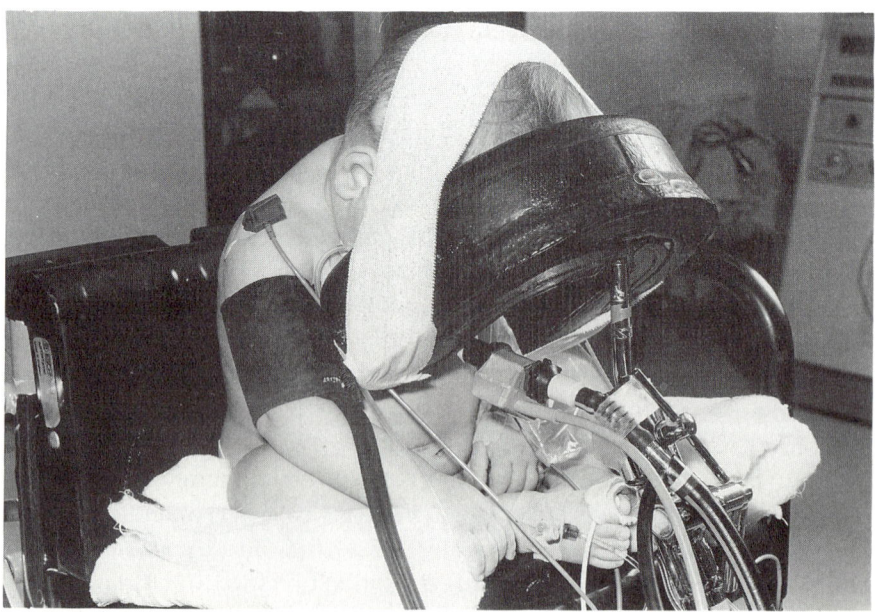

Fig. 13.1 The sitting position for posterior fossa exploration in a child.

thought to be caused by emboli greater than $0.5\,ml\,kg^{-1}\,min^{-1}$ and therefore more significant emboli should be expected in children. This is not confirmed either at the Mayo Clinic (Cucchiara and Bowen 1982) or at Great Ormond Street. We have a VAE incidence of 15% in 200 consecutive cases similar to other units performing large numbers of sitting operations. Only three patients had significant emboli with a change of blood pressure or heart rate more than 20% from the base level. All three patients had end-tidal carbon dioxide levels of 15 mmHg (2 kPa) or less, emphasizing the importance of minimizing the size of the embolus with immediate action by both anaesthetist and surgeon to prevent more air entering. In our patients VAE had no effect on outcome.

CRANIOPHARYNGIOMA

This is a rare tumour in childhood, with a similar incidence to adults, and the perioperative problems are usually related to fluid balance due to diabetes insipidus (DI). Both central venous pressure monitoring and an indwelling catheter are essential as urine volumes up to 25% of the blood volume can be produced in 1 h. Synthetic vasopressin (DDAVP) is invariably required at some stage in the postoperative course in children (Yasargil *et al.* 1990) and also in our experience. The DI has been shown to be due to large amounts of inactive neurohypophyseal peptides excreted in the early postoperative phase (Seckl *et al.* 1987). More recently evidence of a vasopressin antagonist has been shown (Seckl *et al.* 1990).

OTHER TUMOURS

In infants primitive neuroectodermal tumuors may be extremely vascular. Despite paying meticulous detail to providing optimal conditions there is still a small but significant operative mortality from these procedures, even in the best units. As already described, morbidity from massive transfusions in children is low provided good oxygenation is maintained both before and during periods of low cardiac output. Some lesions may be appropriate for preoperative embolization of large feeding vessels.

Craniofacial surgery

Rapid and continuing advancements in surgery are taking place since the pioneering work of Tessier *et al.* (1967), who showed that the cranial and facial bones could be completely mobilized and rearranged with good bone survival, and that, despite gross external abnormalities of the orbits, the optic foramina are normally positioned allowing orbital reconstruction without affecting vision.

Craniosynostosis arises from the premature fusion of one or more sutures. Combined with defective growth of the skull base and mid-face it is a craniofacial synostosis. The craniofacial syndrome, Apert's, Crouzon's, etc., are diagnosed by their characteristic facial features and associated abnormalities, usually of the hands and feet such as the complex syndactyly in Apert's syndrome. The deformities give rise to a number of secondary disorders such as raised ICP, restriction of brain growth, upper airway obstruction and extreme proptosis. Early surgery is now geared to these problems, in particular cranial vault remodelling which is usually performed in the first 6 months of life, with the best results in the youngest patients.

The development of the multidisciplinary craniofacial team and national centralization of these services has led to rapid development of the optimal treatment for these complex patients. At Great Ormond Street there is a formal assessment period including intracranial pressure monitoring and airway assessment related to rises in ICP before planning the subsequent surgical intervention.

Simple craniectomy is performed for sagittal synostosis, a relatively short operation but again with the potential for brisk haemorrhage with an average transfusion of 30% of the blood volume to a 5 kg infant, making allowance for continuing postoperative blood loss.

More formal multiple craniectomies are performed for the craniofacial syndromes and multiple suture synostosis, with surgical development continuing to optimize the cosmetic results. Despite optimal anaesthesia and changing surgical practices to decrease blood loss these procedures are invariably associated with considerable blood losses. The surgeons at Great Ormond Street have now abandoned infiltration with adrenaline in favour of complete diathermy dissection, a manoeuvre which has markedly reduced skin loss but unfortunately has little effect on bone edge loss. In a recent survey of 126 craniofacial patients in a 5-year period (in press) more than 20% received intraoperative exchange transfusions and another 56% received more than 50% of their blood volumes.

Maxillary surgery is usually performed on older patients either as a second procedure or as a combined operation on those who have not had early cranial surgery. These operations were originally performed postpubertally after final facial growth had commenced. They are now frequently performed on preschool children to optimize the cosmetic and psychological advantage. Surprisingly the children with the most major lesions, and their families, suffer less psychological trauma than those with relatively minor defects, where psychological problems may be severe.

Preoperative assessment must include an upper airway assessment. In infants failure to thrive is often an indication of a poor airway, and extreme cases of upper airway obstruction may require nasogastric feeding. Some patients have indwelling nasopharyngeal airways and the worst lesions may require treatment with long-term tracheostomy to prevent recurrent airway obstruction. Intercurrent upper respiratory tract infection is a contraindication to surgery, as wound infection and breakdown is disastrous due to loss of bone flaps. Routine antibiotic prophylaxis is administered.

Children with craniofacial abnormalities invariably suffer airway obstruction during light anaesthesia, but this can be relieved in most cases with a Guedel airway. Intubation is not usually difficult with maxillary hypoplasia, but if there is any doubt about its ease intubation should be performed under spontaneous ventilation and deep anaesthesia. Producing a good seal with a face mask can be difficult with major facial abnormalities, especially gross proptosis and facial clefts. A suitable neuroanaesthetic technique is then employed, with standard monitoring. Radial arterial puncture can be difficult in these patients due to their hand abnormalities, and the femoral route may need to be used. Despite premedication with atropine reflex hypotension with or without arrhythmias can occur during orbital manipulation or traction on the skin flaps with tarsorraphies in place (Flandin-Bléty 1982) an extreme variation of the oculocardiac reflex.

Postoperatively with greater confidence, almost no patients are now ventilated. Those with poor airways may require nasopharyneal airways or rarely intubation. Where major facial surgery is planned coincidentally elective tracheostomy may be performed.

Spinal surgery

Congenital spinal abnormalities are relatively common, frequently with cutaneous manifestations such as a hair tuft, capillary or pigmented naevus or dermal pits as the only clinical feature. Investigations are usually with CT or MRI scans and myelography. Surgery usually is for untethering of the cord and debulking of subcutaneous lesions, with minimal bony surgery to prevent further spinal distortion with growth.

These lesions are usually avascular with minimal transfusion requirements. Spinal tumours in childhood can either be primary or secondary, and these are very different, being extremely vascular and, despite optimal positioning, avoiding IVC compression and induced hypotension, they may require large transfusions. All surgical manipulations of the spinal cord are very potent stimuli, and may be associated with arrhythmias and hypotension if there is inadequate anaesthesia.

Neuroimaging

This rapidly developing field with both non-invasive and invasive procedures can provide a considerable challenge in paediatric practice. Great Ormond Street, as in some other paediatric specialist units, has a long tradition of major investigative procedures being performed under sedation which needs to be tailored to the specific procedure, for example to the type and likely duration, CT scan usually requires lighter sedation than MRI scans (Table 13.5).

General principles should apply to all patients being sedated for investigations. They should be starved, and require to be observed by someone trained in paediatric resuscitation with the equipment readily available. Minimal monitoring should always be pulse oximetry, as the problems with oximetry in MRI scanners have now been overcome. Sedation is contraindicated for patients with raised ICP, airway obstruction (actual or potential), respiratory failure including potential failure due to muscle weakness or central causes, and severe hepatic or renal dysfunction, in whom recovery may be prolonged.

In units where fewer procedures are performed on children, the time involved in achieving a good working practice for sedation may be excessive to requirements, and general anaesthesia is probably more appropriate. Angiography and myelography routinely are performed under general anaesthesia, though those over 12 years and of normal intelligence may tolerate myelography under local analgesia and light sedation.

Invasive radiology and embolization techniques are a fertile area of development. Intracranial vascular lesions are routinely treated by embolization in our unit, in particular vein of Galen aneurysms. The latter is a lesion associated with a large mortality and morbidity whatever the treatment. Patients with such lesions present at various stages depending on the size and blood flow. In the neonatal period patients present as cardiac failure, initially high output, and on investigation

Table 13.5 Sedation for imaging

CT scan

< 5 kg + < 3/12 corrected for prematurity	No sedation; feed and swaddle
< 5 kg + > 3/12	Inj. Peth. Co. 0.06 ml kg^{-1} IM
5–15 kg	Inj. Peth. Co. 0.08 ml kg^{-1} IM
> 15 kg	{ Trimeprazine 2 mg kg^{-1} po { Papaveretum 0.4 mg kg^{-1} IM

Older children usually require proportionally less sedation

MRI scan

<5 kg	No sedation; feed and swaddle
5–15 kg	{ Triclofos 50 mg kg^{-1} po { Inj. Peth. Co. 0.06 ml kg^{-1} IM { Trimeprazine 2 mg kg^{-1} po { Papaveretum 0.4 mg kg^{-1} IM

EMLA cream should be applied to all children

Intravenous diazepam 0.1 mg kg^{-1} to a maximum of 0.3 mg kg^{-1} may also be administered by a suitably skilled doctor who remains with the patient until recovered.

Inj. Peth. Co. contains:	Pethidine	25 mg	
	Promethazine	6.25 mg	} in 1 ml
	Chlorpromazine	6.25 mg	

have a normal heart. They invariably have a loud cranial flow murmur or bruit. Infants usually present with increasing head size from associated hydrocephalus, or from fitting due to cerebral ischaemia of the remainder of the brain. Older children usually present with neurological deficit, again from the effect of vascular steal.

In a 5-year period to 1989, 15 patients with vein of Galen aneurysm underwent 36 embolizations with the variable results shown in Table 13.6. Other vascular lesions had a better outcome. Since then we have had considerably more experience with neonatal lesions as more patients are referred for this treatment. It is now obvious that some lesions are much more amenable to treatment and cure than others. This observation is confirmed by the sporadic cases in the literature of good results from surgery. The difficulty still seems to be patient selection, as until the

Table 13.6 Results of intracranial embolization

	Vein of Galen aneurysm	Other lesions
Dead	4	1
Worse	1	0
No change	4	0
Improved	6	7

embolization is performed the presence of other feeding vessels cannot be demonstrated. The lesions best treated by this technique have several, but not too many, feeders, and do not open up other vessels after treatment. If there are only one or two feeders the effect of the procedure is extremely dramatic. Either myocardial failure occurs due to the cardiac output now going to a much larger circulation, or cerebral haemorrhage occurs from vessels previously unperfused and now subjected to a high cardiac output. If too many vessels are present, or new feeders open up each time another embolus is placed, again the overall treatment will be a failure despite individual embolizations being successful.

The procedure itself can be hazardous, with risks of intracerebral bleeding or movement of the embolus material especially passing through the venous system into the lungs. Strict fluid balance needs to be measured, especially the volume of contrast administered and blood loss estimated during sheath and catheter insertion or by syringe during the investigation. Neonates usually need blood transfusions, and blood should always be cross-matched for all small patients.

The actual embolization may be associated with cardiovascular instability due to direct stimulation, as the embolus is disconnected from the catheter or due to dramatic alterations in blood flow to the malformation. These procedures are extremely technically demanding for the radiologist, and can be very prolonged with all the concomitant problems. These patients also make considerable demands on intensive care both pre-treatment and after treatment.

References

Abbott T.R. (1983) Changes in serum calcium concentrations during massive blood transfusions and cardiopulmonary bypass. *British Journal of Anaesthesia* **55**, 753–760.

Anand K.J.S., Sippell W.G. & Aynsley-Green A. (1987) Randomized trial of fentanyl anaesthesia in preterm babies undergoing surgery: effect on the stress response. *Lancet* **i**, 243−248.

Berntman L., Welsh F.A. & Harp J.R. (1981) Cerebral protective effect of low grade hypothermia. *Anesthesiology* **55**, 495−498.

Bisonnette B. & Leon J.E. (1992) Cerebrovascular stability during isoflurane anaesthesia in children. *Canadian Journal of Anaesthesia* **39**, 128−134.

Black A.E. & Mackersie A.M. (1991) Accidental bronchial intubation with Rae tubes. *Anaesthesia* **46**, 42−43.

Brown K.A., Bisonnette B. & McIntyre B. (1990) Hyperkalaemia during rapid blood transfusion and hypovolaemic cardiac arrest in children. *Canadian Journal of Anaesthesia* **37**, 747−754.

Committee on Safety of Medicines (1992) *Current Problems*, Number 34, June.

Cucchiara R.F. & Bowen B. (1982) Air embolism in children undergoing sub-occipital craniectomy. *Anesthesiology* **57**, 338−339.

Cucchiara R.F., Nugent M., Seward J.B. & Messich J.M. (1984) Air embolism in upright neurosurgical patients: detection and localization by two-dimensional transesophageal echocardiography. *Anesthesiology* **60**, 353−355.

Flandin-Bléty C. (1982) Anesthesia and intensive care for craniofacial surgery in children. In: Marchac D. & Renier D. (Eds), *Craniofacial Surgery for Craniosynostoses*, pp. 39−45. Little Brown, Boston.

Golding J., Paterson M. & Kinlen L.J. (1990) Factors associated with childhood cancer in a national cohort study. *British Journal of Cancer* **62**, 304−308.

Golding J., Greenwood R., Birmingham K. & Mott M. (1992) Childhood cancer, intramuscular vitamin K, and pethidine given during labour. *British Medical Journal* **305**, 341−346.

Hull D. (1992) Vitamin K and childhood cancer. *British Medical Journal* **305**, 326−327.

Kennedy C. & Sokoloff L. (1957) An adaption of the nitrous oxide method to the study of cerebral circulation in children: normal values for cerebral blood flow and cerebral metabolic rate in childhood. *Journal of Clinical Investigation* **36**, 1130−1136.

Leon J.E. & Bisonnette B. (1991) Transcranial doppler sonography: nitrous oxide and cerebral blood flow velocity in children. *Canadian Journal of Anaesthesia* **38**, 974−979.

Lindahl S.G.E., Yates A.P. & Hatch D.J. (1987) Relationship between invasive and non invasive measurements of gas exchange in anesthetized infants and children. *Anesthesiology* **66**, 168−175.

Lou H.C. & Friis-Hansen B. (1979) Impaired autoregulation of cerebral blood flow in the distressed newborn infant. *Journal of Pediatrics* **94**, 118−121.

MRC Vitamin Research Group (1991) Prevention of neural tube defects: results of the Medical Research Council Vitamin Study. *Lancet* **338**, 131−135.

Nightingale D.A., Richards C.C. & Glass A. (1965) An evaluation of rebreathing in a modified T-piece during controlled ventilation of anaesthetised children. *British Journal of Anaesthesia* **37**, 762−771.

Seckl J.R., Dunger D.B. & Lightman S.L. (1987) Neurohypophyseal function during early postoperative diabetes insipidis. *Brain* **110**, 737−746.

Seckl J.R., Dunger D.B., Bevan J.S. *et al.* (1990) Vasopressin antagonist in early postoperative diabetes insipidus. *Lancet* **335**, 1353−1356.

Sellar M.J. (1987) Unanswered questions on neural tube defects. *British Medical Journal* **294**, 1−2.

Shanahan E.C., Marshall A.G. & Garrett C.P.O. (1983) Adverse reactions to intravenous codeine phosphate in children. *Anaesthesia* **38**, 40−44.

Steward D.J. (1982) Preterm infants are more prone to complications following minor surgery than are term infants. *Anesthesiology* **56**, 304−306.

Swedlow D.B. (1983) Anaesthesia for neurosurgical procedures. In: Gregory G.A. (Ed.), *Pediatric Anesthesia*, Vol. 2, pp. 679−706. Churchill Livingstone, New York.

Swedlow D.B. & Lewis L.E. (1980) Measurement of cerebral blood flow in children. *Anesthesiology* **53**, S160.

Tessier P., Guiot G., Rougerie J., Delber J.P. & Pastoriza J. (1967) Ostéotomies cranio-naso-orbito-facial. Hypertélorisme. *Annales Chirogie Plastique* **12**, 103−118.

Uppington J. & Goat V. (1987) Anaesthesia for major craniofacial surgery: a report of 23 cases in children under 4 years of age. *Annals of the Royal College of Surgeons of England* **69**, 175−178.

Wyatt J.S., Cope M., Delpy D.T., Wray S. & Reynolds E.O. (1986) Quantification of cerebral oxygenation and haemodynamics in sick newborn infants by near infrared spectrophotometry. *Lancet* **ii**, 1063−1066.

Yasargil M.G., Curcic M., Kis M., Siegenthaler G., Teddy P.J. & Roth P. (1990) Total removal of craniopharyngiomas. *Journal of Neurosurgery* **73**, 3−11.

14

Head injuries

SUSAN MIDGLEY AND MARK DEARDEN

Handwritten annotations:

Aims: N or supranormal CO
aggressive fluid regimen (does not worsen brain injury)
vasopressors/inotropes (only consider drug venodilation (USA))
CPP>70mmHg

a) IVI
b) vasopressors
c) ventriculo...
d) mannitol (late)

(Rosner et al J. Neurosurg. 1995 83, 949)

"CPP-directed therapy"   CBF   nl- hypoxia
CMRO₂ - CBF relationship   ↑CPP (r? PaO₂ !!)   nl. hyperaemia   CMRO↑

INCIDENCE

Head injuries constitute an important health problem in all industrialized nations. The incidences of mild and severe traumatic brain lesions for the UK are shown in Table 14.1. Less than 1% of hospital attendances and 5% of hospital admissions are cases of major brain trauma. Intracranial mass lesions demanding neurosurgical intervention occur in about 0.3% of all hospital attendances and in less than 2% of all head-injured patients admitted to hospital (*British Journal of Neurosurgery* 1988). The mortality from severe head injury is up to 50%. Many of the survivors are left with permanent brain damage; their average age is 30 years and many will never be employed (Jennett 1987). In youth, road traffic accidents account for the majority while in later life falls predominate (Jennett *et al.* 1977). More than 50% of severe head injuries suffer associated trauma (Miller *et al.* 1992).

Pathophysiology of head injury

Brain damage remains the most important consequence of head trauma and may arise both as a direct result of primary impact and from avoidable secondary systemic or intracranial events. Damage to the scalp and skull may give an indication of the possibility of underlying brain pathology and is a portal of infection. However, fatal brain damage can occur without a blemish on the scalp or a fracture in the skull. Head injuries include: skull fractures, focal brain injuries, diffuse brain injuries and secondary brain damage.

Skull fractures

Skull fractures are common, but do not by themselves cause neurological disability. The significance of a skull fracture is that it identifies the

Table 14.1 Frequency of head injuries

	Incidence per million population
Hospital attendances	15 000
Hospital admissions	2 500
Major injuries	136
Surgical haematomas	45

patient with a higher probability of having or developing an intracranial haematoma and, if compound, may permit outward leakage of cerebro-spinal fluid (CSF) or ingress of air and/or bacteria (Teasdale *et al.* 1990).

LINEAR, NON-DEPRESSED FRACTURES

These are often seen on X-ray as a lucent line and require no specific treatment; management is directed towards the underlying brain injury. Fractures across vascular arterial grooves or suture lines should increase suspicion of the possibility of extradural haematoma formation.

DEPRESSED SKULL FRACTURE

This occurs when a blow lacerates the scalp and drives bone fragments into the intracranial cavity, sometimes tearing the dura mater. A depressed fracture that is displaced inwards more than 1 cm, or more than the full thickness of the skull, should be elevated within the first 24 h for cosmetic reasons, as well as to reduce possible damage to the underlying brain. When the wound is believed to have been contaminated with dirt, hair, gravel, etc., elevation of the depressed fragments is necessary so that the wound can be cleaned adequately, necrotic brain removed and the dura repaired. Although the presence of a depressed skull fracture is one of the prognostic factors in the prediction of post-traumatic epilepsy, it is not the bony depression itself which is responsible for the abnormal activity but the cerebral component of the injury.

BASAL SKULL FRACTURES

These are often not apparent on skull radiographs, although the presence of intracranial air or a fluid level in the sphenoid sinus may give a clue.

Diagnosis is more often based on physical findings such as CSF leaking from the ear (CSF otorrhoea) or the nose (CSF rhinorrhoea). When CSF is mixed with blood it may be difficult to detect. An aid is the 'ring sign', detected by allowing a drop of leaking fluid to fall on to a piece of filter paper. If CSF is present, blood remains in the centre, and one or more concentric rings of clearer fluid develop.

Ecchymosis in the mastoid region (Battle's sign) also indicates a basal skull fracture, as does blood behind the tympanic membrane (haemotypanum) Cribriform plate fractures are often associated with periorbital ecchymosis (raccoon eyes). However, these signs may take several hours to develop. Evidence of basal skull fracture should alert the clinician to the dangers of airway instrumentation with the potential for intracranial penetration. The oral route should be used in preference to the nasal route for tracheal and gastric tubes (Fremstad & Martin 1978).

Focal brain injuries

Macroscopic damage occurs in a relatively local area comprising contusions and haematomas which may require emergency surgery because of their mass effects. Early post-injury detection and surgical treatment of lesions is important to minimize morbidity and mortality. Thirty per cent of head-injured patients in coma have an intracranial haematoma (Becker *et al.* 1977, Teasdale *et al.* 1990).

Contusions

These are caused by contact, particularly at the frontal and temporal poles, between the surface of the brain and interior ridges of the skull. They may occur beneath the area of impact or in areas remote from impact (contre-coup). The contusion itself may produce focal neurological deficit if it occurs near the sensory or motor areas of the brain. Large contusions or those associated with significant pericontusional oedema may, by their mass effect, cause herniation and brainstem compression, resulting in delayed neurological deterioration.

Extradural haematomas

These occur almost always from a tear in a dural artery, usually the middle meningeal artery, although a small percentage occur after perforation of a dural venous sinus. Primary brain damage can be minimal and early detection and evacuation should minimize mortality and morbidity due to secondary cerebral compression. One-third of patients in hospital with fatal head injuries have talked at some time after injury (Reilly *et al.* 1975). In 75% of these an intracranial haematoma was found at autopsy (Rose *et al.* 1977).

Textbook symptoms and signs of extradural haematoma occur in only 45% of cases. These are loss of consciousness followed by an intervening lucid interval (the lucid period may not be a return to full consciousness), a secondary depression of conscious level and development of a contralateral hemiparesis and ipsilateral pupil dilatation with loss of reaction to light (although in 10% of cases the opposite pupil dilates). Figure 14.1 shows the lens-shaped appearance of an extradural haematoma on CT scan.

Acute subdural haematomas

These are more common than extradural haematomas and occur predominantly in older patients from rupture of bridging veins between the cerebral cortex and dura. They may also be due to lacerations of the brain's surface. In addition to the problems caused by the mass of subdural blood, underlying primary brain injury is often severe. In

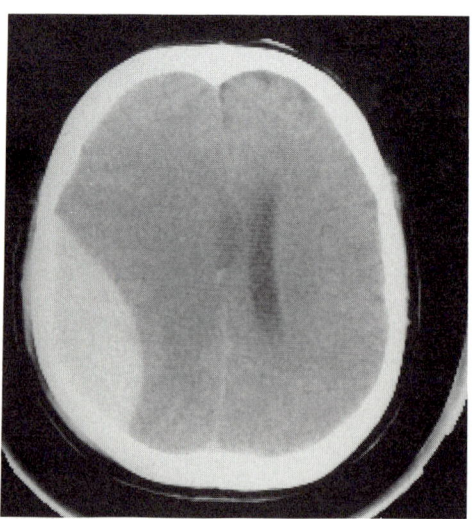

Fig. 14.1 CT scan showing the lens-shaped appearance of a right-sided temporoparietal extradural haematoma.

younger patients acute subdural haematoma is associated with coma from the outset. Outcome is improved with early evacuation (Seelig *et al.* 1981). Figure 14.2 shows the typical CT scan apperance of an acute subdural haematoma.

Intracerebral haematomas

These often occur at the poles of the brain and may be associated with severe primary brain damage. Neurological deficit depends on the size and location of the haematoma. Figure 14.3 shows the CT scan appearance of an intracerebral haematoma.

Diffuse brain injuries

Rapid head motions (acceleration or deceleration) cause widespread interruption of brain function. Distortion of the brain caused by internal shearing leads to stretching and tearing of the axonal tracts within the white matter. Mild stretch injury with reversible loss of function is called concussion. There is temporary loss of brain function with a brief loss of consciousness, confusion or amnesia. In contrast, diffuse axonal injury is characterized by prolonged coma. On CT scan minute haemorrhages may be seen deep within the brain substance, especially the posterior

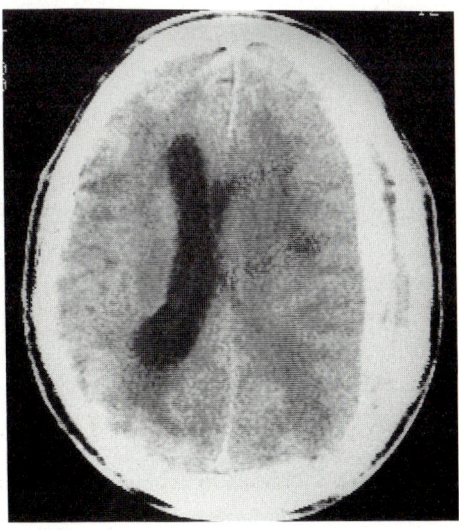

Fig. 14.2 CT scan appearance of an acute left-sided subdural haematoma.

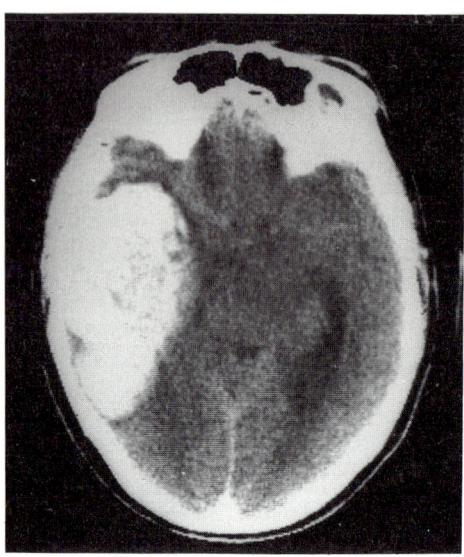

Fig. 14.3 CT scan appearance of a right-sided traumatic intracerebral haematoma.

corpus callosum. However, this is not pathognomonic and the diagnosis is usually only confirmed at postmortem when microscopic retraction balls are detected within the white matter.

Secondary brain damage

The brain requires continuous adequate perfusion by well-oxygenated blood. Permanent ischaemic nueronal damage occurs if this is reduced below a critical threshold of $10-15\,\mathrm{ml\,min^{-1}\,100\,g^{-1}}$ for more than a few minutes (Dearden 1990). Normally the brain regulates its own blood supply to maintain constant perfusion despite wide variations in systemic blood pressure; when injured, the brain may lose this capacity and be particularly vulnerable to ischaemic damage when hypotension or hypoxia occur. Secondary damage will further insult the already damaged brain and compromise outcome. Cerebral perfusion pressure (CPP), which is the difference between mean arterial blood pressure (MAP) and intracranial pressure (ICP) (CPP = MAP − ICP) may be compromised either by hypotension or by a rise in intracranial pressure leading to cerebral hypoperfusion (Table 14.2). In the management of head injury the clinician must aspire to prevention of secondary brain

Table 14.2 Causes of raised intracranial pressure after head injury

1 Cerebrovascular engorgement
2 Cerebral oedema — focal (around a contusion) or diffuse
3 Haematoma
4 Hydrocephalus

damage by ensuring adequate CPP, blood oxygenation and avoiding factors that increase cerebral metabolic rate.

Assessment of head injuries

Head injuries may be classified as severe, moderate and minor from the post-resuscitation Glasgow Coma Scale (GCS) sum score, which provides a quantitative measure of the patient's level of consciousness. The GCS is derived from adding three separate areas of assessment: eye opening, best motor response and verbal response (Teasdale & Jennet 1974). Clinically more useful information is gained by listing each component separately (Teasdale *et al.* 1983). To give a chronological picture of a patient's response after injury the GCS can be recorded sequentially at regular time intervals. A decrease in GCS of two or more points clearly means that the patient has deteriorated. More subtle signs of deterioration which should alert the physician are: an increase in size or decrease in reaction of a pupil, deviation of the eyes to one side and development of weakness on one side. Alcohol ingestion should never be assumed to be the sole cause of a deterioration in conscious level.

The Glasgow Coma Scale

EYE-OPENING (E SCORE)

Scoring of eye-opening is not valid if the eyes are closed by swelling (C). This fact should be documented by 'C'.
1 Spontaneous — already open; E = 4.
2 To speech (not necessarily a request for eye-opening); E = 3.
3 To pain; E = 2.
4 None: E = 1.

BEST MOTOR RESPONSE (M SCORE)

The best response from the upper limb is recorded. The worst motor response may also be important for determining focal deficits but is not used in determination of GCS. For patients not following verbal command, a graduated painful stimulus is applied to the nailbed. Pressure may be applied in the area of the trigeminal nerve, over the supraorbital nerve or at the angle of the jaw to assess whether the patient localizes to these stimuli.

1 Obeys — moves limb to command; M = 6.
2 Localizes — makes purposeful movement towards a stimulus; M = 5.
3 Withdraws — pulls away from painful stimulus; M = 4.
4 Abnormal flexion; M = 3.
5 Extensor response; M = 2.
6 No movement; M = 1.

VERBAL RESPONSE

Scoring of verbal response is invalid if speech is impossible due to the presence of a tracheal tube (T). This must therefore be documented by 'T'.

1 Orientated — knows name, age; V = 5.
2 Confused conversation — still answers questions; V = 4.
3 Inappropriate words; V = 3.
4 Incomprehensible sounds — grunts and groans are produced, no words are uttered. Not to be confused with partial respiratory obstruction; V = 2.
5 None; V = 1.

The maximum sum score is 15, the minimum is 3. If the patient is intubated, paralysed and ventilated this should be documented.

Patients in coma have no eye-opening (E1), have inability to follow commands (M1−5) and utter no words (V1−2). Coma is therefore defined as GCS <9 with E1. The GCS can be used to classify the severity of head injury:

severe head injury	GCS <9 with E1
moderate head injury	GCS 9−12, or <9 with at least E2
minor head injury	GCS 13−15.

Modifications of the GCS may be used in children (Table 14.3).

Table 14.3 Paediatric Glasgow Coma Scale

	>1 year	<1 year
Eye opening		
4	Spontaneously	Spontaneous
3	To speech	To shout
2	To pain	To pain
1	None	None
Best motor response		
5	Obeys commands	
4	Localizes	Localizes
3	Flexion to pain	Flexion to pain
2	Extension to pain	Extension to pain
1	None	None

	>5 years	2−5 years	0−2 years
Best verbal response			
5	Oriented and converses	Appropriate words and phrases	Smiles and cries appropriately
4	Disoriented but converses	Inappropriate words	Cries
3	Inappropriate words	Cries	Inappropriate crying
2	Incomprehensible sounds	Grunting	Grunting
1	None	None	None

Normal aggregate score

<6 months	12
6−12 months	12
1−2 years	13
2−5 years	14
>5 years	14

ASSESSMENT OF PUPILLARY FUNCTION

The pupils are examined for their size and response to light. A difference in pupil size of more than 1 mm is abnormal. It is important to rule out intracranial pathology even if the eye signs are thought to be due to eye injury. The briskness of the light response is important as a more sluggish response may indicate intracranial pathology. Sedative and analgesic drugs may mask such subtle signs, but their effects are bilateral.

LATERALIZED EXTREMITY WEAKNESS

Spontaneous movements are observed for equality. If spontaneous motion is minimal the response to painful stimulus is assessed. A delay in onset of movement, less movement or need for more stimulus on one side is significant. A clearly lateralized weakness suggests an intracranial mass lesion. In patients recovering from sedative or analgesic drugs it is frequently noticeable that the dominant side recovers first.

The above clinical signs should be documented on a neurological observation chart at frequent intervals. The observations should be repeated regularly to determine whether a patient is deteriorating or improving.

Immediate care

Anaesthetists will not normally be required for early care of patients with minor head injury but will mainly be involved in the management of patients with severe and moderate injuries. Their skills will be valuable during initial resuscitation, transfer to a regional neurosurgical centre, CT scan, theatre and intensive care of these patients. Initial management should follow the ABC sequence of resuscitation.

Airway and breathing

The airway should be protected by positioning or intubation if necessary. This may entail insertion of an oropharyngeal airway, turning the patient on to his or her side or intubation. Intubation should take the form of a rapid sequence induction using preoxygenation, cricoid pressure and tracheal intubation facilitated by suxamethonium preceded by, for example, thiopentone. Emergency intubation should be via the oral route as a basal skull fracture may be present. The tracheal tube should be secured with adhesive strapping and not by tape around the neck, thus avoiding venous compression. The possibility of neck injury should always be borne in mind. A cervical spine injury should always be assumed until it has been confidently excluded by a good-quality lateral cervical spine X-ray demonstrating the entire cervical spine, including the C7–T1 interspace. An injury of the cervical spine may be present despite a normal X-ray. The head should be held immobile in line with the body by an assistant, and the neck should not be allowed to flex or to rotate. It should then be secured with tape and sandbags and a hard cervical collar applied. A properly applied cervical collar should not impede cerebral venous drainage significantly. The indications for intubation and ventilation in the accident and emergency department are listed in Table 14.4. Severe trauma is associated with gastric dilatation and therefore an orogastric tube (preferably double-lumen) must be inserted also. Associated injuries, especially those causing hypoxia such as pneumothorax, should be dealt with promptly.

Circulation

Brain injury should never be assumed to be the cause of hypotension. Scalp bleeding may cause haemorrhagic shock, particularly in young children or the elderly, but one should always make that diagnosis by exclusion. The history of the nature of the injury is important as thoracic and abdominal injuries may occur in high-velocity accidents. A head-injured patient with unexplained hypotension should always have a peritoneal lavage. Patients with hypotension should have at least two large-bore intravenous cannulae inserted and be resuscitated with colloid solutions, normal saline or possibly hypertonic saline (large volumes of crystalloid, particularly 5% dextrose, should be avoided). Cervical spinal cord transection may be a cause of intractable hypotension associated with a slow pulse rate.

Table 14.4 Guidelines for intubation and ventilation of head-injured patients (in Accident and Emergency Department)

1 No response to pain (GCS 3)
2 Spontaneous extensor posturing (GCS 4)
3 Repeated convulsions. IPPV with full muscle paralysis must be accompanied by anticonvulsant therapy and EEG monitoring when possible
4 Spontaneous hyperventilation ($Paco_2$ less than 26.3 mmHg)
5 Cyanosis (Pao_2 less than 67.7 mmHg on air, or less than 97.7 mmHg while receiving oxygen from a disposable, conventional mask, e.g. MC mask)
6 Ventilatory inadequacy or respiratory arrythmia
7 Associated pathology indicating a need for IPPV, e.g. chest injury

ECG, pulse oximetry and direct measurement of blood pressure should be established. A urinary catheter should be inserted to monitor urine output and an accurate record of fluid balance kept. Consideration should be given to inserting a central venous line for monitoring progress of resuscitation in multiply injured patients.

After this period of immediate care a full examination (secondary survey) and neurological assessment should be carried out. Neurological examination at this stage allows quantification of the effects of resuscitation on the Glasgow Coma Scale, allowing estimation of the relative contributions of primary and secondary insults to the brain. All patients with a history of head trauma should have skull X-rays as the presence of a fracture greatly increases the likelihood of the presence of an intracerebral haematoma (Teasdale *et al.* 1990). Table 14.5 gives the indications for skull X-ray after head injury. Good-quality anteroposterior (AP) and lateral cervical spine X-rays should be obtained. Following this the decision will need to be made regarding referral to a neurosurgical centre and the need for CT scanning. The criteria for referral to a neurosurgical centre are listed in Table 14.6 (Briggs *et al.* 1984).

It is important to establish priorities in the patient's management with senior help from appropriate disciplines. Patients with intrathoracic

Table 14.5 Criteria for skull X-ray after recent head injury

1 Loss of consciousness or amnesia at any time
2 Neurological symptoms or signs
3 Cerebrospinal fluid or blood escaping from nose or ear
4 Suspected penetrating injury or scalp bruising or swelling
5 Scalp laceration, or bruising

Table 14.6 Criteria for consultation with a regional neurosurgical centre concerning patients admitted to a district general hospital

1 Coma continuing after resuscitation
2 Neurological deterioration after admission
3 Depressed skull fracture
4 Linear fracture of skull in combination with either confusion or other depression of the level of consciousness or focal neurological signs or fits
5 Suspected fracture of base of skull (CSF rhinorrhoea or otorrhoea, bilateral periorbital ecchymosis, mastoid haematoma) or evidence of a penetrating type of injury such as spike or gunshot.

or intra-abdominal trauma may need surgical intervention before full resuscitation can be achieved. If a head-injured patient requires another surgical procedure prior to CT scan or neurosurgical intervention it is important for the anaesthetist to continue resuscitation and frequent neurological observations. Anaesthesia should be established according to the guidelines below. In paralysed and ventilated patients pupillary size and responsiveness to light will usually be the only signs of intra-cranial compression available. Unilateral pupillary changes associated with intracranial compression are not obtunded by anaesthesia and should be treated with mannitol 20%, $0.5-1\,g\,kg^{-1}$, over 20 min and the response documented. The neurosurgeon should be informed immediately.

Special investigations

CT scan

Guidelines for the use of CT scan following head injury are based upon the observation that intracranial haematomas occur in 40% of comatose head-injured patients and in noncomatose patients, the presence of a skull fracture greatly increases the probability that a haematoma will be present (Teasdale *et al.* 1990, Becker *et al.* 1977). In adults the absolute risk of haematoma in patients without skull fracture who are fully conscious is 1 in 7900, 1 in 180 if consciousness is impaired and 1 in 27 if in coma. In adults with skull fracture the risk of haematoma is 1 in 45 if fully conscious, 1 in 5.1 if consciousness is impaired and 1 in 3.6 if the patient is in coma (Teasdale *et al.* 1990). In children the same increasing risk of haematoma is observed with altered conscious level and the presence of a skull fracture. Table 14.7 outlines the indications for CT scan after head trauma.

Once the need for a CT scan has been determined it is important to establish that resuscitation is complete. The patient must be fully resuscitated and attended closely throughout transport and imaging. Vital signs must be monitored (invasive blood pressure (BP), pulse oximetry and ECG) and pupil signs observed.

Patient movement results in artifact and a poor-quality scan. Movement artifact can be eliminated by sedating restless or uncooperative patients. However, extreme caution must be exercised in sedating patients whose airway may not be protected adequately, and in whom restlessness

Table 14.7 Guidelines for CT scan in head injury (after resuscitation is completed)

1 Patient in coma (GCS <9 with E1)
2 Patient with skull fracture and GCS <15 or seizures or focal neurological signs
3 Patient with depressed conscious level and multiple injuries requiring surgery under anaesthesia. Rule out intracerebral haematoma by CT before surgery but only if airway and circulation are secure (i.e. establish priorities)
4 Neurological deterioration or unexplained elevation of ICP
5 GCS <15 persisting for more than 24 h
6 Severely disabled head injury survivors—CT at 3 months to assess ventricular size and areas of established atrophy

is a sign of hypoxia. Tracheal intubation with sedation, analgesia and paralysis therefore provides the safest and best conditions, and in the Edinburgh unit patients are anaesthetized, intubated and ventilated with continuous monitoring of arterial oxygen saturation (pulse oximeter), BP and ECG from the resuscitation room through CT scan and the operating theatre to the recovery room, and if appropriate, to the intensive-care unit (ICU).

Transporting patients with head injuries

Patients presenting to District General Hospitals without neurosurgical facilities may require transfer between hospitals.

The events associated with interhospital transfer are a potent cause of avoidable mortality and morbidity after head injury (Gentleman & Jennett 1990). Problems may be caused by delay in arranging transfer, inadequate resuscitation before transfer, inadequate preparation for the journey and inadequate care during the journey. The recommendations for transfer to a neurosurgical unit are outlined in Table 14.8.

When the referral is made to the neurosurgical centre a clear description of the patient's injuries should be given and a detailed description of any procedures carried out. If an injury is suspected, its presence should be assumed and appropriate action taken for transfer, e.g. hard collar for suspected cervical spine injury. The airway is particularly vulnerable during transfer. All patients in coma should be intubated and ventilated. However, other patients may require intubation to protect the airway. These may include patients who have fitted or whose conscious level is at all depressed. Patients who are intubated should receive sedation and analgesia and be paralysed and ventilated. If the CT

Table 14.8 Recommendations for transfer of patients to a neurosurgical unit

1 Initial resuscitation for extracranial injuries and complications should be completed, e.g. blood loss, impaired ventilation, splinting of fractures
2 Establish appropriate monitoring
3 Attach identification tag to patient
4 Give a clear description of all injuries, conscious level (GCS), pupil size and response, BP and all drugs and IV fluids given
5 Send notes and X-rays
6 Reduce to a minimum the risks en route—adequately equipped ambulance and trained escort. Smooth slow journey. Patient in head-up position if possible

scan proves to be normal anaesthesia can be reversed at the neurosurgical centre. Before departing, the neurosurgical unit should be contacted to give some estimation of the time of arrival.

Anaesthetic considerations

Head-injured patients may require anaesthesia for CT scan, general and neurosurgical procedures including craniotomy or the insertion of an ICP monitor. Anaesthetic agents and techniques have marked effects on these patients due to their effect on cerebral blood flow, cerebral metabolic rate for oxygen, ICP, systemic BP, CPP and pressure autoregulation. Furthermore, anaesthesia may be administered in several differing environments including the operating theatre, CT scan and accident and emergency department. The anaesthetist should be familiar with all the areas in which anaesthesia may have to be administered. Anaesthesia should be induced only in well-equipped and adequately staffed areas.

The anaesthetic technique should provide a smooth induction and intubation. A rapid sequence induction with preoxygenation and cricoid pressure and oral intubation facilitated by suxamethonium should be employed. The hypertensive response to intubation should be obtunded by the administration of a hypnotic agent (thiopentone) and narcotic (fentanyl $1.5\,\mu g\,kg^{-1}$ or alfentanil $15\,\mu g\,kg^{-1}$). Ideally, monitoring should be established prior to induction and should comprise ECG, direct measurement of blood pressure and pulse oximetry. The operating table should be placed $15-30°$ head-up. Anaesthesia should be maintained by mild hypocapnic intermittent positive pressure ventilation (IPPV) under full muscle paralysis using nitrous oxide and at least 30% oxygen.

Ventilation should be adjusted to maintain $Paco_2$ of 26−33 mmHg with end-tidal carbon dioxide being monitored continuously. Volatile agents are best avoided in diffuse head injury and should only ever be used in low concentrations as they all cause cerebral vasodilatation and interfere with cerebral pressure autoregulation, especially when combined with nitrous oxide. Isoflurane appears to be the agent with the least adverse effects. If intracranial air is visible on X-ray or CT scan nitrous oxide should be avoided, and ideally a total intravenous technique should be used using hypnotic, narcotic, relaxant and oxygen in air for diffuse head injury or air, oxygen and isoflurane for evacuation of an intracranial haematoma (Frost 1984). Hypertension due to surgical stimulation should be avoided by the administration of adequate analgesia.

Following a decision to evacuate surgically an *intracerebral haematoma*, mannitol 20%, 1 g kg^{-1}, or frusemide 0.5−0.7 mg kg^{-1} should be given (if not previously administered) to minimize risk of intracranial compression during transfer to the operating theatre. The bladder should also be catheterized as the stimulus of a full bladder will lead to an increase in blood pressure and possible elevation in ICP. Colloid solutions (plasma protein solution, PPS) should be given to prolong ICP reduction and maintain circulating blood volume following the diuretic. The surgeon should warn the anaesthetist prior to evacuation of the haematoma as the blood pressure may decrease at this time. When ICP is reduced by surgical decompression, the stimulus to hypertension (Cushing response) is precipitously removed and hypovolaemic hypotension may be unmasked. At the end of the procedure an ICP monitor may be inserted if the patient was in coma preoperatively, had signs of increased ICP on admission CT (Teasdale *et al.* 1984) or if the brain appeared tight at craniotomy. Such patients are usually transferred ventilated to the ICU postoperatively. At the end of the procedure, prior to transfer, pupillary responses should be checked and adequate sedation, analgesia and paralysis administered to cover transport and setting up in the ICU.

Similar anaesthetic considerations apply to patients requiring *elevation of depressed skull fractures*. The bone fragment should be elevated within 24 h to prevent infection. It is imperative to optimize operating conditions to avoid loss of brain tissue through a dural tear. Mannitol 20%, 0.5 g kg^{-1}, or frusemide 0.3−0.5 mg kg^{-1} may be given at the start of the operation. Again, the anaesthetist must ensure that the patient has been catheterized.

Chronic subdural haematomas may be evacuated through a burrhole under local anaesthesia with or without sedation. Patients should be monitored adequately during this procedure (ECG, non-invasive blood pressure and pulse oximetry), and should be given supplemental oxygen. In patients with a reduced level of consciousness evacuation of a chronic subdural haematoma may be associated with a rapid improvement necessitating additional sedation.

Patients with *diffuse brain injury* may require anaesthesia for insertion of an ICP monitor. Many units now use the Camino fibreoptic system for measuring brain tissue pressure (Crutchfield *et al.* 1990). This system can be inserted at the bedside in the ICU. This and other systems are discussed in Chapter 2.

Patients with an apparently *minor head injury* may require anaesthesia for an extracranial procedure such as orthopaedic fixation or laparotomy; they present a particular hazard. These patients require the same meticulous care as a patient undergoing a neurosurgical procedure. They should be paralysed, intubated and ventilated during surgery, which should be delayed whenever possible for several days after head injury. These patients should be closely observed by experienced staff for 24 h after surgery.

Postoperative and intensive care

Indications for continuing controlled ventilation in the ICU are given in Table 14.9. In the authors' view BP, ICP and derived CPP should be monitored continuously. The basic aspects of intensive care are similar to those of other neurosurgical patients and are discussed in Chapter 15.

With the exception of patients who have had a chronic subdural evacuated, who should be nursed in a head-down position to prevent reaccumulation, patients should be nursed in a $15-30°$ head-up position.

Table 14.9 Indications for continuing controlled ventilation in the intensive-care unit

1 Any previously comatose patient requiring a significant intracranial operation should be ventilated for a minimum period of $12-24$ h prior to reassessment
2 Patients with the clinical features described in Table 14.4 as indicative of a need for controlled ventilation should be ventilated for a minimum of 3 days prior to reassessment. After assessment, persistence of these features indicates the need for a further period of IPPV
3 In patients whose prognosis is considered extremely poor, IPPV without relaxants or sedation may be considered appropriate during continued resuscitation in the ICU. However, in the event of any improvement more active therapy will be required

The head should be kept in a neutral position and the tracheal tube secured with elastic strapping, thus preventing cerebrovascular engorgement due to venous congestion.

To promote cardiovascular stability sedative drugs, usually a combination of benzodiazepine and opiate (e.g. fentanyl) should be given by continuous infusion. It is particularly important to give analgesic drugs to patients with multiple injuries. Additional slow bolus doses of analgesia and sedation may be necessary prior to stimulating procedures such as physiotherapy, although it is the practice in Edinburgh to use such techniques to control ICP only when significant rises are observed, and not as a routine because of the risk of compromising CPP. The authors paralyse all-head injured patients on IPPV, but many centres ventilate without paralysis. Some units use a propofol infusion as sedation for patients receiving IPPV because it is short-acting and neurological assessment is possible shortly after stopping the infusion, the rate of the infusion can be increased temporarily for physiotherapy and other stimulating procedures and it has some free radical scavenging action. However, profound decreases in blood pressure and hence CPP may occur readily, and this agent should be used with care. There is further reference to propofol in Chapter 15.

Ventilation should be adjusted to maintain a PaO_2 of greater than 97 mmHg and $PaCO_2$ of 26−34 mmHg. Concern is often expressed as to the effects of positive end-expiratory pressure (PEEP) on ICP. However, in some patients it may be necessary to use up to 15 mmHg of PEEP to correct hypoxaemia. Provided the patient is nursed in a head-up position of up to 30° the adverse effects of PEEP on ICP are minimal, and are outweighed by the beneficial effect of improving $PaCO_2$ (Frost 1977). The effects of posture on BP and CPP should be observed closely, although if CPP is greater than 60 mmHg, CBF is preserved with 30° head-up tilt (Feldman et al. 1992). Patients should be ventilated at a slow respiratory rate with large tidal volumes to prevent atelectasis. Head-injured patients should have regular chest physiotherapy because of their propensity to retain secretions in association with paralysis.

Elevation of ICP during intensive care is frequently attributable to avoidable causes (Table 14.10). Because of the difficulty in assessing these patients clinically, multimodality monitoring is being used increasingly to detect and correct adverse events, and to monitor the effects of ICP treatment. The monitoring which may be used in head-injured patients is listed in Table 14.11. Some of the more specialized forms of monitoring are discussed below.

Table 14.10 Checklist for remediable causes of raised ICP

1 Position and calibration of transducer
2 Patency of ICP monitor
3 Position of patient
4 Posture of head and neck
5 Level of sedation/analgesia
6 Level of neuromuscular blockade
7 Ventilation (Pao_2, $Paco_2$, inflation pressure, PEEP)
8 Pyrexia
9 Seizure activity
10 Arterial hypertension/hypotension
11 Hyponatraemia
12 Hypoproteinaemia

Table 14.11 Indications for ICP monitoring in head-injured patients

1 Coma with intracranial haematoma/contusion
2 Coma with loss of 3rd ventricle and perimesencephalic cisterns on CT
3 Coma with abnormal motor responses (GCS < 6)
4 Tight brain at operation after evacuation of a haematoma
5 Associated multiple trauma requiring IPPV

Measurement of ICP

The indications for ICP monitoring in patients with head injury are given in Table 14.11. In patients with focal pathology the ICP monitor should be placed on the opposite side, as this will give a better indication of the stress being applied to the normal brain. The measurement of ICP is discussed in Chapter 2.

Jugular venous oxygen saturation monitoring

Some neurosurgical units now measure cerebral oxygen flux (Robertson *et al.* 1987, 1989, Dearden 1991). A catheter can be placed in the jugular bulb and cerebral venous blood sampled. Recently, a fibreoptic system has been developed which permits continuous measurement of jugular venous oxygen saturation (SjO_2). This works on the principle of reflectance oximetry (Oximetrix 3, Abbott Critical Care Systems, USA). The catheter is inserted percutaneously and passed in a retrograde fashion into the jugular bulb. The normal value for SjO_2 is 54–75%. Decreasing SjO_2 reflects increasing oxygen extraction and may herald cerebral ischaemia. If the brain becomes ischaemic anaerobic metabolism takes place, and leads to the production of lactic acid. The lactate oxygen index (LOI) can be calculated (Robertson *et al.* 1989). This is $AJDL/AJDO_2$ where AJDL is the arteriojugular difference for lactate (in $\mu mol\, ml^{-1}$) and $AJDO_2$ is the arteriojugular difference for oxygen (in $\mu mol\, ml^{-1}$). A low SjO_2 in association with a LOI greater than 0.08 indicates brain ischaemia. A low SjO_2 alone indicates a state of compensated hypoperfusion where increased oxygen extraction compensates for reduced oxygen delivery and if not corrected ischaemia may follow.

In the absence of hypoxaemia and anaemia increased oxygen extraction can be observed during seizure activity, systemic hypotension or intracranial hypertension (comprising CPP) and severe hyperventilation ($PaCO_2$ <23 mmHg).

CPP management

During the past decade many centres have directed therapy towards reducing intracranial hypertension after severe head injury. Recently, however, there has been a greater interest in maintaining or elevating CPP. It appears that compromised CPP rather than raised ICP carries the greater risk to the injured brain (Rosner & Daughton 1990). Unpublished data from Edinburgh have shown that the duration of compromised CPP below 60 mmHg during intensive care was the most important predictor of mortality in a group of head-injured patients. There is increasing evidence that maintaining CPP above 70 mmHg is paramount during ICP therapy (Chan *et al.* 1992).

When considering maintenance of CPP it is important to consider both BP and ICP.

BP should be measured directly from an arterial line. Hypovolaemia should be corrected. Respiratory swing on the arterial trace suggests that the patient is underfilled. Anaemic patients benefit from transfusion as the increase in blood viscosity associated with a higher haematocrit increases diastolic BP, which has a greater effect on mean BP than a similar increase in systolic pressure. Patients with intact cerebral pressure autoregulation will get a secondary rise in ICP in the presence of compromised CPP due to arteriolar dilatation in an attempt to maintain constant cerebral blood flow.

ICP and derived CPP should be monitored continuously. ICP may increase after head injury due to four principal factors: cerebrovascular engorgement, cerebral oedema, haematoma formation and hydrocephalus (Table 14.2). However, before starting specific ICP reduction therapy it is important to detect and correct remediable factors (Table 14.10).

If the ICP increases soon after return from theatre the possibility of a recurrent or new haematoma should be considered, especially if the patient has had a period of hypotension or has developed a coagulopathy. Detection of a haematoma will require transfer of the patient to the CT scan. The clinician is therefore faced with the dilemma of balancing the value of detecting a haematoma against the risks of transferring a patient with raised ICP from the ICU. Patients with uncontrolled ICP in the ICU prior to transfer to CT have more insults on return. Attempts should therefore be made to control ICP below 20 mmHg but maintain CPP above 60 mmHg before leaving the ICU (Andrews *et al.* 1990).

In the first 48 h following severe head injury it is the authors' practice to treat ICP at a threshold of 25 mmHg (20 mmHg in children). Several days after head injury some patients appear to tolerate a higher ICP without evidence of brain dysfunction (pupil changes or reduction in SjO_2) and in these patients the ICP is allowed to rise to 30 mmHg or more provided that the CPP is maintained at over 70 mmHg and the pupils remain equal and reacting.

Hyperventilation

Head-injured patients are often ventilated to reduced $PaCO_2$ which produces a degree of cerebral vasoconstriction. After experimental head injury the rate of formation of cerebral oedema is reduced by hyperventilation, and dissipation of oedema fluid from the grey matter via the white matter extracellular spaces to the ventricles is increased. However, vigorous hyperventilation to $PaCO_2$ <23 mmHg may produce excessive cerebral vasoconstriction with the risk of producing cerebral ischaemia. In addition, hyperventilation may produce systemic hypotension, particularly if the patient is hypovolaemic thus compromising CPP.

From experimental work it appears that the vasoconstrictor effect of hyperventilation is only sustained for about 6 h. This may be due to CSF lactic acidosis reversing the pH changes of respiratory alkalosis (Muizelaar *et al.* 1988). In general hyperventilation should be used only as a temporary measure in the control of ICP, for example, in an emergency situation with hand ventilation on 100% oxygen when a patient develops a fixed dilated pupil. However, the authors have noticed that in certain groups of patients, notably children and young adults with increased ICP in association with cerebral hyperaemia, hyperventilation to a $Paco_2$ of less than 26 mmHg may have a more prolonged effect without inducing lactic acidosis.

CSF drainage

ICP monitoring through a ventricular catheter permits drainage of CSF. Although ICP can be reduced and CPP increased, drainage may accentuate brain shift, particularly in a patient with a unilateral lesion and contralateral ventricular dilatation. It is therefore important to drain CSF against a positive back pressure of 10–15 mmHg (with reference to the external auditory meatus) to prevent excessive shifts and ventricular collapse.

Osmotherapy

The agent which is used most commonly is mannitol 20%. This is the alcohol of the 6-carbon sugar, mannose. It is not metabolized to any great extent and, in the absence of damage to the blood–brain barrier, appears to remain entirely in the body's extracellular compartment.

Mannitol appears to reduce ICP by a number of mechanisms. First, it reduces brain water content by maintaining an osmotic gradient between brain extracellular fluid and plasma (Albright *et al.* 1984). Previously, it was thought that this was in areas where the blood–brain barrier was intact. However, more recent work using magnetic resonance imaging (which enables an index of brain water content to be obtained) has demonstrated that mannitol withdraws water from oedematous brain where the blood–brain barrier is deranged (Bell *et al.* 1987). Secondly mannitol reduces blood viscosity and thus increases cerebral blood flow (CBF). If pressure autoregulation is preserved this leads to compensatory vasoconstriction to preserve constant CBF. The decrease in cerebral blood volume results in a reduction in ICP (Muizelaar *et al.* 1984). A third mechanism of action is a reduction in the rate of formation of CSF (Takagi *et al.* 1983). Fourthly, mannitol may act as a scavenger of free radicals which may be implicated in the formation of cerebral oedema. The vascular mechanism may account for the rapid onset of action, while the more sustained effect may be due to the reduction in brain water or the reduced rate of production of CSF.

Mannitol 20% should be given by infusion at a dose $0.25-1\,g\,kg^{-1}$ over $15-20\,min$. Intravenous frusemide $0.3-0.6\,mg\,kg^{-1}$ given with the mannitol potentiates its effects and may prevent rebound (Pollay *et al.* 1983) After completion of the mannitol, plasma protein solution $(3\,ml\,kg^{-1})$ may be given over the next hour to preserve circulatory normovolaemia during the diuresis and prolong ICP reduction. The total daily dose of mannitol should not exceed $2\,g\,kg^{-1}$. It is important to monitor the serum osmolality in patients receiving mannitol because, if this exceeds $320\,mosmol\,l^{-1}$ mannitol will be ineffective and may cause renal failure. In areas of brain injury, the blood−brain barrier may be deranged so that mannitol diffuses into the surrounding brain, bringing water with it and thus increasing brain swelling. This may become a problem in patients receiving repeated doses or infusions of mannitol.

Hypnotic agents

These drugs reduce ICP by depressing cerebral metabolic rate, thus inducing cerebral vasoconstriction. If cerebral metabolism is already very depressed these agents will be ineffective. They are therefore contraindicated if the lower border voltage on the cerebral function monitor (CFM) is less than $5\,\mu V$. Vascular responsiveness to carbon dioxide must also be retained (Nordstrom *et al.* 1988). These drugs may cause hypotension so a fall in ICP may not necessarily be accompanied by a net improvement in CPP. This problem will be accentuated in patients with hypovolaemia. Patients in whom hypnotic therapy is being considered should have direct monitoring of BP, central venous pressure and possibly also measurement of pulmonary artery occlusion pressure. Hypnotic agents should be administered through a central venous catheter. Hypnotics should be continued only if ICP is reduced and CPP improved. Reduced BP in the absence of hypovolaemia may be treated with inotropic support.

A commonly used hypnotic agent is thiopentone. This is given by infusion at a dose of $15\,mg\,kg^{-1}$ for the first hour, $8\,mg\,kg^{-1}$ for the next $2\,h$ and thereafter at a rate of about $5\,mg\,kg^{-1}\,h^{-1}$. Brain electrical activity should be monitored continuously and the dose adjusted to maintain 'burst suppression'. The CFM at this point shows bursts of activity interspersed with periods of no activity, and this is the level where there is an optimal reduction of cerebral metabolic rate without excessive cardiovascular depression. Gamma hydroxybutyrate and etomidate have been used also, although there is concern about excessive sodium load with the former and adrenocortical suppression with the latter agent. Propofol has been used to treat raised ICP (Vandesteene *et al.* 1988), but must be used with great care as profound falls in BP may occur with rapid administration increasing the risk of cerebral ischaemia (Andrews *et al.* 1991). Patients receiving hypnotic infusions may become immunocompromised and be at increased risk of infection. Infection may go unrecognized as these patients may not mount a leucocytosis or develop a pyrexia. Prolonged hypnotic infusions can also lead to hepatic and renal impairment. In the authors' opinion hypnotic agents have a limited role after cerebral trauma in the management of increased ICP, although on occasions it may be the only method of reducing ICP and improving CPP.

? Propofol superior to barbiturates? Rx hypoten. c̄ IVI + NAdr ?

Other agents

Dihydroergotamine has been reported as being effective in the treatment of raised ICP (Grande 1989). This is thought to be the result of a marked reduction in cerebral blood volume, due predominantly to constriction of venous capacitance vessels. Intravenous infusion of indomethacin has also been reported as being an effective treatment (Jensen *et al.* 1991). Steroids have no place in the treatment of raised ICP in patients with head injury. Indeed, these patients fare worse if given steroids (Dearden *et al.* 1986).

Selecting therapy for raised ICP

An understanding of the mechanism of raised ICP should allow a rational choice of therapy.

If remediable causes have been excluded, an increasing ICP after completion of resuscitation during the first 36 h after a severe head injury is often due to *cerebrovascular dilatation* and engorgement associated with failure of autoregulation. This occurs most frequently in young patients with a diffuse head injury. Prolonged hyperventilation to less than 26 mmHg is often effective in these patients and does not induce cerebral lactic acidosis. If further treatment is required infusion of a hypnotic should be considered.

If *autoregulation is preserved* compromised CPP will result in arteriolar dilatation. If cerebral blood flow is compromised the SjO_2 will fall, indicating hypoperfusion. Patients with focal head injury often show these characteristics. Optimal therapy may be to raise the BP using

↑ICP → ↓ICBV   CSF drainage
↓CMRO₂ - drugs   hyperventilation aim to PaCO₂ 4.5 kPa
Osmotic agents   (or maint SvjO₂ if
*   PaO₂ < 4.5)*

volume loading, inotropic agents or vasoconstriction with methoxamine or phenylephrine. Mannitol may also be useful as autoregulation is preserved (Muizelaar *et al.* 1984, Rosner & Coley 1986). Hyperventilation and hypnotic agents are contraindicated in these patients as they will increase the risk of cerebral ischaemia.

Patients with predominantly *cerebral oedema* should probably be treated with osmotic agents and/or elevation of BP since oedema is most likely to be ischaemic in origin in the first week after injury. Again, in this group of patients, hyperventilation and hypnotic agents are contraindicated because of the likelihood of inducing cerebral ischaemia.

Discontinuing ICP therapy and weaning from IPPV

ICP therapy should probably be continued until ICP has been stabilized below 20 mmHg for 24 h with CPP over 70 mmHg. If ICP remains below this level, without therapy, for a further 24 h weaning from IPPV may be considered. In some patients, after 72 h of intensive care, ICP may exceed 20 mmHg, but if it no longer rises during stimulating procedures, there are no localizing signs, CPP remains well preserved and SjO_2 remains normal these patients may also be considered for weaning.

Once ICP and CPP have stabilized, the $PaCO_2$ is allowed to increase in stages. This may be accomplished by increasing the amount of dead space in the ventilator circuit or by reducing the respiratory rate (to maintain constant tidal ventilation) thus reducing the risk of atelectasis. ICP and SjO_2 commonly increase with each elevation in $PaCO_2$. Thereafter, the ICP and SjO_2 levels slowly return to the initial values in those patients ready for weaning. If there is a progressive increase in ICP or SjO_2, or if focal signs develop, the $PaCO_2$ should be reduced again rapidly. Once $PaCO_2$ is normal, and if ICP and CPP remain satisfactory, paralysis is discontinued and subsequently sedation stopped or reduced as appropriate. It is the authors' practice to transfer patients on to a continuous positive airway pressure (CPAP) system ($5-10$ cmH$_2$O) and spontaneous ventilation is assessed. Some patients remain on CPAP for several days and require to be sedated with an infusion of diazemuls to suppress hyperventilation and hypertonic spasms. Once spontaneous ventilation is established, provided ICP and CPP remain satisfactory, the ICP monitor can be removed after 6 h. Depending on the patients' state they will either be extubated or may require a tracheostomy if protection of the airway is in doubt. Percutaneous tracheostomy can now be performed readily in the ICU (Ciaglia *et al.* 1985). Weaning of head-injured patients with other injuries or chest complications often requires a period of assisted ventilation with sedation and analgesia after paralysis is discontinued.

Temperature control

The optimum temperature for the head-injured patient is 35–37°C. Pyrexia increases the cerebral metabolic rate (CMRO$_2$) and thus may be a cause of elevated ICP (Clasen *et al.* 1974). On no account should pyrexia be permitted. If infection is suspected cultures should be taken of sputum, urine and blood and appropriate antibiotics commenced. Blood cultures should be taken through all monitoring lines. All monitoring should be reviewed and unnecessary monitoring lines removed. If invasive monitoring lines are still required then these should be changed. A sample of CSF should be sent for culture if the patient has a CSF access device or ventricular catheter *in situ*. All reasonable means should be used to reduce temperature, such as tepid sponging and placing ice-packs in the groins and axillae. Small doses of chlorpromazine ($0.1-0.2\,\mathrm{mg\,kg^{-1}}$) by intramuscular injection may help, but it is important to observe the BP. Paracetamol by suppository may also be beneficial.

[handwritten annotation: Moder hypothermia (33-34°C) protective (not due to ↓ CMRO$_2$) ? effect on free radicals, EAAS, lipid peroxidation?]

Fluid balance

The patient with acute head injury exhibits a pattern of metabolic response similar to that found after other types of trauma with conservation of sodium and water. Administration of hypotonic solutions will lead to a reduction in serum sodium concentration which may lead to aggravation of cerebral oedema (hypo-osmotic oedema). Five per cent dextrose solution, which although isotonic to plasma, on administration will swiftly be made hypotonic as the dextrose is metabolized, should be avoided. Head-injured patients should not be allowed to become hypovolaemic or dehydrated. As a guide the hourly fluid input in adults should equal the previous hour's urine output plus 30 ml to replace insensible losses to a maximum of $150\,\mathrm{ml\,h^{-1}}$. It is the authors' practice to use dextrose 5% in saline 0.45% with 40 mmol potassium chloride per litre initially. Serum electrolytes should be measured daily. Patients receiving frequent mannitol treatments should also have the serum osmolality measured.

Damage to the hypothalamus and pituitary axis can produce diabetes insipidus due to failure of secretion of antidiuretic hormone (ADH). The patient passes large quantities of dilute urine, which can lead to hypernatraemia and dehydration. If urine output exceeds $4\,ml\,kg^{-1}\,h^{-1}$ for more than 2 h with specific gravity below 1005, in the absence of glycosuria or diuretics, deamino-D-arginine vasopressin (DDAVP) $1-4\,\mu g$ should be given intramuscularly 8-hourly as required. It is useful to remember that patients recently weaned from IPPV often have a diuresis for 2−3 h.

Head-injured patients should have CVP monitored and normovolaemia maintained with colloid solutions or blood as appropriate. Sedated patients nursed in a head-up position often require additional fluids to maintain normotension.

Nutrition

The metabolic rate is increased after severe head injury, and early orogastric feeding should be used if at all possible. However, patients on IPPV receiving opiate infusions often have an ileus and therefore do not absorb from the enteral route and require parenteral nutrition. Patients in coma with abnormal motor responses often have large gastric aspirates and do not readily absorb food. However, neurological improvement often heralds a return of gastrointestinal function. Before commencing enteral feeding the position of the stomach tube should be checked by X-ray. In patients who do not cooperate with orogastric feeding, and who cannot be fed orally because of abnormal swallowing reflexes, a feeding gastrostomy should be considered.

Management of seizures

Control of seizures is of paramount importance. Neuromuscular blocking drugs mask the peripheral manifestations while the neuronal disturbance continues with increasing CBF leading to anaerobic respiration and further deterioration unless the focus is suppressed. It is the opinion of the authors that paralysed head-injured patients should have some form of cerebral electrical monitoring such as the cerebral function analysing monitor (CFAM) or CFM.

In Edinburgh all patients with an intracerebral haematoma or history of multiple post-traumatic convulsions receive prophylactic anticonvulsants, e.g. phenytoin. If intravenous phenytoin is given it is important to monitor the ECG and BP.

Seizures occurring within the first week carry a low risk of late

Table 14.12 Monitoring during intensive care

Systemic	Craniocerebral
Arterial pressure	Intracranial pressure
Heart rate and ECG	Cerebral perfusion pressure
Central venous pressure	Pupils
Pulmonary artery pressure	Jugular venous oxygen saturation
Arterial oxygen saturation	Cerebral electrical activity
End-tidal carbon dioxide	Transcranial Doppler sonography
Core temperature	
Peripheral temperature	
Arterial blood gases	
Fluid balance	
Haematology	
Biochemistry	
Bacteriology	

epilepsy but may cause hypoxic brain damage. Early seizures are seen, particularly in the first 24 h, and are most common in children where a generalized convulsion can complicate even a mild injury. Seizure activity occurring later is usually related to other complications such as meningitis, CSF leakage or a subdural haematoma, and carries a greater risk of late epilepsy.

Rehabilitation

Advances in immediate resuscitation and intensive care have led to ever-increasing numbers of survivors from severe head injury (Miller *et al.* 1992). Many of these are young adults with a near-normal life expectancy. In the past emphasis was placed on the physical impairments but research over the past 20 years has highlighted the cognitive and behavioural problems which affect the long-term social functioning of these patients. After acute care these patients benefit from a period spent in a rehabilitation unit where a multidisciplinary approach can identify the physical and mental problems and can help the patients and their families adapt and come to terms with residual disabilities and maximize their functional abilities (Oddy *et al.* 1989). It is important to emphasize to the relatives of head-injured patients that recovery from head injury is slow, but that there is often improvement up to 2 years after the injury.

CONCLUSION

Severe head injury remains the commonest cause of death and disability in the Western world in people under the age of 40 years. Early detection and evacuation of intracerebral haematomas and prevention of secondary insults provide the mainstay of management. Anaesthetists, with their skills in resuscitation and interest in intensive care, can contribute a great deal as members of a team concerned with the management of these challenging patients.

References

Albright A.L., Latchaw R.E. & Robinson A.G. (1984) Intracranial and systemic effects of osmotic and oncotic therapy in experimental cerebral edema. *Journal of Neurosurgery* **60**, 481–489.

Andrews P.J.D., Dearden N.M & Miller J.D. (1991) Comparison of thiopentone and propofol at two rates of administration in patients with severe head injury. *British Journal of Anaesthesia* **67**, 212P.

Andrews P.J.D., Piper I.R., Dearden N.M. & Miller J.D. (1990) Secondary insults during intrahospital transport of head-injured patients. *Lancet* **335**, 327–330.

Becker D.P., Miller J.D., Ward J.D., Greenberg R.P., Young H.F. & Sakalas R. (1977) The outcome from severe head injury with early diagnosis and intensive management. *Journal of Neurosurgery* **47**, 491–502.

Bell B.A., Smith M.A., Kean D.M. *et al.* (1987) Brain water measured by magnetic resonance imaging: correlation with direct estimation and changes after mannitol and dexamethasone. *Lancet* **i**, 66–69.

Briggs M., Clarke P., Crockard A. *et al.* (1984) Guidelines for initial management after head injury in adults. *British Medical Journal* **288**, 983–985.

Chan K.H., Dearden N.M., Miller J.D., Andrews P.J.D. & Midgley S. (1993) Multimodality monitoring as a guide to treatment of intracranial hypertension after severe head injury. *Neurosurgery* **32**, 547–552.

Ciaglia P., Firsching R. & Syniec C. (1985) Elective percutaneous dilatational tracheostomy. A new simple bedside procedure; preliminary report. *Chest* **87**, 715–719.

Clasen R.A., Pandolfi S., Laing I. & Casey D. (1974) Experimental study of relation of fever to cerebral edema. *Journal of Neurosurgery* **41**, 576–581.

Crutchfield J.S., Narayan R.K., Robertson C.S. & Michael L.H. (1990) Evaluation of a fiberoptic intracranial pressure monitor. *Journal of Neurosurgery* **72**, 482–487.

Dearden N.M. (1990) The management of the post-ischaemic brain. *Current Anaesthesia and Critical Care* **1**, 105–114.

Dearden N.M (1991) Jugular bulb venous oxygen saturation in the management of severe head injury. *Current Opinion in Anaesthesiology* **4**, 279–286.

Dearden N.M., Gibson S., McDowall D.G., Gibson R.M. & Cameron M.M. (1986) Effect of high-dose dexamethasone on outcome from severe head injury. *Journal of Neurosurgery* **64**, 81–88.

Feldman Z., Kanter M.J., Robertson C.S. *et al.* (1992) Effect of head elevation on intracranial pressure, cerebral perfusion pressure, and cerebral blood flow in head-injured patients. *Journal of Neurosurgery* **76**, 207–211.

Fremstad J.D. & Martin S.H. (1978) Lethal complication from insertion of nasogastric tube after severe basilar skull fracture. *Journal of Trauma* **18**, 820–822.

Frequency of neurosurgical disorders in the UK. (1988) *British Journal of Neurosurgery* **2**, 281–283.

Frost E.A.M. (1977) Effects of positive end-expiratory pressure on intracranial pressure and compliance in brain-injured patients. *Journal of Neurosurgery* **47**, 195–200.

Frost E.A.M. (1984) Some inquiries in neuroanesthesia and neurological supportive care. *Journal of Neurosurgery* **60**, 673–686.

Gentleman D. & Jennett B. (1990) Audit of transfer of unconscious head-injured patients to a neurosurgical unit. *Lancet* **335**, 330–334.

Grande P-O. (1989) The effects of dihydroergotamine in patients with head injury and raised intracranial pressure. *Intensive Care Medicine* **15**, 523–527.

Jennett B. (1987) Medical aspects of head injury. In: Stearn M. and Macken J. (Eds), *Medicine International* **38**, 1595–1601.

Jennett B., Teasdale G., Galbraith S. *et al.* (1977) Severe head injuries in three countries. *Journal of Neurology, Neurosurgery and Psychiatry* **40**, 291–298.

Jensen K., Christrom J., Cold G.E. & Astrup J. (1991) The effects of indomethacin on intracranial pressure, cerebral blood flow and cerebral metabolism in patients with severe head injury and intracranial hypertension. *Acta Neurochirurgica (Wien)* **108**, 116–121.

Miller J.D., Jones P.A., Dearden N.M. & Tocher J.L. (1992) Progress in the management of head injury. *British Journal of Surgery* **79**, 60–64.

Muizelaar J.P., Lutz H.A. & Becker D.P. (1984) Effect of mannitol on ICP and CBF and correlation with pressure autoregulation in severely head-injured patients. *Journal of Neurosurgery* **61**, 700–706.

Muizelaar J.P., Henk G., van der Poel H.G., Li Z., Kontos H.A. & Levasseur J.E. (1988) Pial arteriolar vessel diameter and CO_2 reactivity during prolonged hyperventilation in the rabbit. *Journal of Neurosurgery* **69**, 923–927.

Nordstrom C.H., Messeter K., Sundbarg G., Schalen W., Werner M. & Ryding E. (1988) Cerebral blood flow, vasoreactivity and oxygen consumption during barbiturate therapy in severe traumatic brain lesions. *Journal of Neurosurgery* **68**, 424–431.

Oddy M., Bonham E., McMillan T., Stroud A. & Rickard S. (1989) A comprehensive service for the rehabilitation and long-term care of head injury survivors. *Clinical Rehabilitation* **3**, 141–147.

Pollay M., Fullenwider C., Roberts P.A. & Stevens F.A. (1983) Effect of mannitol and furosemide on blood–brain osmotic gradient and intracranial pressure. *Journal of Neurosurgery* **59**, 945–950.

Reilly P.L., Graham D.I., Adams J.H. & Jennett B. (1975) Patients with head injury who talk and die. *Lancet* **ii**, 375–377.

Robertson C.S., Grossman R.G., Goodman J.C. & Narayan R.K. (1987) The predictive value of cerebral anaerobic metabolism with cerebral infarction after head injury. *Journal of Neurosurgery* **67**, 361–368.

Robertson C.S., Narayan R.K., Gokaslan Z.L. *et al.* (1989) Cerebral arteriovenous oxygen difference as an estimate of cerebral blood flow in comatose patients *Journal of Neurosurgery* **70**, 222–230.

Rose J., Valtonen S. & Jennett B. (1977) Avoidable factors contributing to death after head injury. *British Medical Journal* **2**, 615–618.

Rosner M.J. & Coley I.B. (1986) Cerebral perfusion pressure, intracranial pressure, and head elevation. *Journal of Neurosurgery* **65**, 636–641.

Rosner M. & Daughton S. (1990) Cerebral perfusion pressure management in head injury. *Journal of Trauma* **30**, 933–941.

Seelig J.M., Becker D.P., Miller J.D., Greenberg R.P., Ward J.D. & Choi S.C. (1981) Traumatic acute subdural hematoma: major mortality reduction in comatose patients treated within four hours. *New England Journal of Medicine* **304**, 1511–1518.

Takagi H., Saito T., Kitahara T., Morii S., Ohwada J. & Yada K. (1983) The mechanism of the ICP reducing effect of mannitol. In: Ishii S., Nagai H. & Brock M. (Eds), *Intracranial Pressure*, vol. V, pp. 729–773. Springer-Verlag, Berlin.

Teasdale G. & Jennett B. (1974) Assessment of coma and impaired consciousness. A practical scale. *Lancet* **ii**, 81–84.

Teasdale E., Cardoso E., Galbraith S. & Teasdale G. (1984) CT scan in severe diffuse head injury: physiological and clinical correlations. *Journal of Neurology, Neurosurgery and Psychiatry* **47**, 600–603.

Teasdale G., Jennett B., Murray L. & Murray G. (1983) Glasgow Coma Scale: to sum or not to sum? (Letter) *Lancet* **ii**, 678.

Teasdale G.M., Murray G., Anderson E. *et al.* (1990) Risks of acute traumatic intracranial haematoma in children and adults: implications for managing head injuries. *British Medical Journal* **300**, 363–367.

Vandesteene A., Trempont V., Engelman E., Deloof T., Focroul M., Schoutens A. & De Rood M. (1988) Effect of propofol on cerebral blood flow and metabolism in man. *Anaesthesia* **43** (Suppl.), 42–43.

15
Postoperative care and aspects of intensive care

ALEX MANARA

Introduction

While neurosurgery may be regarded as a relatively small and seemingly expensive speciality, it has been shown that in Britain neurosurgical management compares favourably with the costs of other branches of medicine and, with the exception of severe diffuse head injury and malignant brain tumours, the cost per quality adjusted life year (QALY) is unexpectedly low (Pickard et al. 1990). Appropriate postoperative care is essential if a successful outcome from intracranial surgery is to be achieved. The postoperative period is critical for the neurosurgical patient who may be at risk of persistent effects of the primary lesion, as well as complications of the intracranial surgery itself. Close monitoring is essential to identify and treat problems promptly, and is best achieved with high-dependency nursing care in the recovery room, on a neuro-surgical ward or in the intensive-care unit (ICU). Criteria for admission to the ICU will vary according to the local availability of beds, trained nursing staff and finance. At Frenchay Hospital, in Bristol, 75% of neurosurgical patients admitted to the ICU have intracranial haemorrhage or severe head injuries, a further 20% are patients with combined head injuries and multiple trauma, and the final 5% include patients admitted after intracranial tumour or spinal surgery. It must be stressed that admission to an ICU should not be dependent on a patient requiring mechanical ventilation; similarly it should not be necessary to ventilate electively postoperative neurosurgical patients simply to ensure adequate high-dependency care. Ideally peroperative monitoring should be con-tinued into the immediate postoperative period. In the recovery room monitoring the pulse rate, blood pressure, respiratory rate and pattern, pulse oximetry, conscious level and fluid balance are mandatory. Some aspects of care are specific to neurosurgical or head-injured patients, although many of the principles of good postoperative and intensive care are applicable to the neurosurgical as well as any other postoperative patient. In particular many of the recent advances in the care of critically ill patients are equally beneficial to neurosurgical or head-injured patients receiving mechanical ventilation on the ICU and are discussed briefly. In the author's opinion it is wrong to treat the intensive-care management of these patients as merely an extension of intraoperative care.

Routine postoperative and intensive care

Airway and ventilation

A clear unobstructed airway is essential after any neurosurgical procedure. Hypoxia, hypercarbia and straining will contribute to secondary neurological damage and must be avoided or treated aggressively. All that is usually required in the recovery room is the insertion of an oropharyngeal or nasopharyngeal airway and the administration of oxygen until the patient recovers consciousness. If concerns about the adequacy of the airway, or of the adequacy of gas exchange, persist it is safer to reintubate in the recovery room and nurse the patient in the ICU.

Most of the patients admitted to the ICU for continued postoperative mechanical ventilation will be patients with severe head injuries, patients with a large amount of peroperative oedema, those developing cerebral oedema postoperatively and patients with hypoxaemia. Other indications for elective postoperative ventilation differ among various centres. Elective ventilation after prolonged surgery in the posterior fossa remains controversial. Valid reasons in favour of elective ventilation include the prevention of hypoxia and hypercarbia, control of the intracranial pressure (ICP), and improvement of blood flow to areas of brain with impaired autoregulation. The alternative view is that sedating these patients to allow mechanical ventilation will mask the early indicators of the development of significant oedema or haematoma within the posterior fossa, such as a deterioration in the level of consciousness and an abnormal respiratory pattern that may progress to apnoea. In the author's experience monitoring the ICP supratentorially does not provide an early, reliable indication of changes occurring in the posterior fossa. High-dependency or intensive care, without mechanical ventilation, may therefore identify problems before pupillary dilation or an increase in ICP occurs, allowing immediate tracheal intubation, transfer to the CT scan room and appropriate management of oedema or haematoma. The decision not to ventilate these patients postoperatively does not imply that high-dependency care is unnecessary.

When a decision to ventilate a patient mechanically has been reached, the latex armoured endotracheal tube, if one has been used during anaesthesia, should be changed to a plastic tube with a high-volume low-pressure cuff. Most patients should be ventilated to normocarbia postoperatively. Certainly the routine use of hyperventilation in neuro-surgical intensive care to reduce intracranial pressure is being questioned, and it has even been suggested that hyperventilation may be harmful if applied to patients with a low cerebral blood flow. Ward and colleagues (1989) compared two groups of patients with severe head injury and found that patients ventilated to a $PaCO_2$ of 35 mmHg had a significantly better outcome 3–6 months after injury than did patients electively hyperventilated to achieve a $PaCO_2$ of 24 mmHg. Hyperventilation should probably be reserved for patients with demonstrable cerebral hyperaemia or for use temporarily as an emergency measure to control an increased ICP. Oxygenation is maintained by adjusting the fractional inspiratory oxygen concentration (FIO_2) and if necessary adding positive end-expiratory pressure (PEEP). There can be no doubt that hypoxaemia is detrimental to poorly perfused cerebral tissue and to other organs. In patients with associated chest injuries, neurogenic pulmonary oedema, aspiration pneumonia or the adult respiratory distress syndrome PEEP may be the only effective way of improving the PaO_2. Concern about the effect of PEEP on ICP in this situation is inappropriate, particularly since PEEP levels of 10–12 cmH$_2$O have been shown to be well tolerated (Cooper *et al.* 1985). The increase in ICP in response to chest physio-therapy and endotracheal suction can be attenuated by careful positioning of the patient, manual hyperventilation prior to and immediately after suction, by increasing briefly the level of sedation, or administering lignocaine 0.5–1 mg kg^{-1} intravenously (Fisher *et al.* 1982, White *et al.* 1982). This last technique is not used very often in the UK.

Tracheostomy will be required for patients whose conscious level remains depressed and those at risk of recurrent aspiration. It is possible to leave an orotracheal tube in place for up to 3 weeks in patients requiring mechanical ventilation. If, however, the patient does not require ventilation and fulfils all the criteria for extubation, but does not have an adequate cough reflex and is likely to retain secretions or obstruct the airway on extubation, then it is the author's practice to perform a tracheostomy at an early stage. In the author's experience this is preferable to repeated unsuccessful 'trials' of extubation, with the attendant risks of airway obstruction, hypoxaemia, sputum retention and pneumonia. The introduction of percutaneous dilational tracheostomy has certainly changed the Bristol practice by encouraging earlier tracheostomy. The technique, which is being introduced in some neurointensive-care units at present, offers all the advantages of conventional surgical tracheostomy and can be performed easily at the bedside, at the convenience of the ICU staff, without exposing critically ill patients to the risks of transfer to the operating theatre. It is suitable for intensivists without formal surgical training, and appears to be a safe technique both in terms of early and late complications (Hazard *et al.* 1991, Ciaglia & Graniero 1992).

Posture

Once haemodynamically stable the patient should be positioned 15–30° head-up without undue cervical rotation. This posture ensures clear cerebral venous drainage, reducing the intracranial pressure. However it is possible for cerebral perfusion pressure to be reduced more than intracranial pressure if the patient is fluid depleted or if the degree of elevation is such that it reduces cardiac output and blood pressure (Rosner & Coley 1986). In general, provided the cerebral perfusion pressure is more than 60 mmHg, then cerebral blood flow is maintained with the head-up position (Feldman *et al.* 1992). Nursing ventilated patients in the head-up position has the added advantage of preventing microaspiration of colonized gastrointestinal contents (Torres *et al.* 1992), thereby reducing the incidence of pneumonia from 100% in those who aspirate to 8% in patients without microaspiration (Kingston *et al.* 1991).

Monitoring

In addition to monitoring cardiorespiratory function, the level of consciousness using the Glasgow Coma Scale (Teasdale & Jennett 1974), pupillary size and responsiveness to light, and limb movement should be recorded regularly. A deteriorating level of consciousness, pupillary dilatation, bradycardia and hypertension or the development of focal neurological signs are indications for an urgent CT scan. Continued monitoring of patients is important during movement of patients to and from the CAT scanner. Intrahospital transport of patients with head injuries is, like interhospital transport, associated with a high incidence of adverse incidents (Andrews *et al.* 1990). The indications for other cardiorespiratory and neurological monitoring are discussed in appropriate sections of this chapter.

Postoperative analgesia

The Report of the Working Party on 'Pain after Surgery' (1990) has drawn further attention to the problems of inadequate postoperative analgesia. Opioids remain the mainstay of treatment of acute postoperative pain, but are used sparingly after intracranial surgery to avoid respiratory depression and the effects of hypercarbia. Following intracranial surgery the opioid of choice has been traditionally codeine phosphate, because there is a ceiling to its respiratory depressant effects and it does not mask pupillary signs. It is usually administered by intermittent intramuscular injection but adequate doses must be prescribed if postcraniotomy headache is to be relieved (Gabbott 1991). The opioid agonist—antagonist drugs have not fulfilled their original promise. They have no particular advantage over the pure agonists since they have comparable side-effects, the same potential for abuse, and a ceiling analgesic effect (Hoskin & Hanks 1991). Non-steroidal anti-inflammatory drugs (NSAID) may enhance analgesia and reduce the postoperative opioid consumption although, in general, side-effects, including respiratory depression, are not reduced. While their efficacy has been demonstrated after spinal surgery (McGlew *et al.* 1991), their safety after craniotomy remains to be established. There are three main concerns at present: the first is whether their use will increase the risk of postoperative haematoma formation as a result of their effect on platelet function. The second concern is the demonstration of a reduction in cerebral blood flow by as much as 30% when assessed by internal carotid artery flow velocity (Seideman & Von Arbin 1991). While the relevance of these data to patients following craniotomy is unknown, further study is required before their use can be recommended, particularly in patients with cerebrovascular disease. Finally NSAID are now recognized as the most common cause of drug-induced renal failure, and have been shown to impair renal function postoperatively (Power *et al.* 1992). This is not surprising in view of the recognized role of prostaglandins as local vasodilator hormones maintaining renal blood flow. Indeed renal blood flow can become 'prostaglandin-dependent' in the presence of conditions such as hypovolaemia or congestive cardiac failure which are associated with large concentrations of circulating vasoconstrictors (Carmichael & Shankel 1984). The administration of NSAID to neurosurgical patients being fluid-restricted postoperatively, or to patients with other risk factors for renal dysfunction receiving intensive care, must be considered to be contraindicated.

Sedation

In general intensive-care practice most patients receiving mechanical ventilation will need sedative and analgesic drugs to relieve anxiety and pain, allow sleep and permit therapeutic procedures. It is accepted generally that these aims can be achieved without inducing prolonged periods of unconsciousness, but by maintaining patient cooperation and comprehension (Wallace *et al.* 1988). In neurosurgical intensive care a deeper level of sedation is required to prevent coughing, Valsalva responses, agitation and pain, which increase the intracranial pressure and may cause intracranial venous bleeding. Admission to a neurosurgical ICU for mechanical ventilation is needed for patients with severe head injuries, cerebral oedema or following intracranial surgery. In these patients the sedative regimen is also therapeutic in that it should control ICP without influencing cerebral perfusion pressure, and it should reduce cerebral metabolic rate for oxygen ($CMRO_2$), thereby providing cerebral protection (see Chapters 3 and 14).

Many different sedative and analgesic agents have been used with or without muscle relaxants. Intravenous opioids, benzodiazepines and intravenous anaesthetics are most commonly used, the choice of agent frequently being dictated by the pharmacokinetics of the drug, those with a shorter duration of action allowing easier neurological assessment of the patient. The opioids are safe when the patient is ventilated, having no effect on ICP, $CMRO_2$ or CBF, although there have been isolated reports of phenoperidine raising ICP and alfentanil being a cerebral vasodilator. Morphine is useful, having sedative as well as analgesic properties. The opioids will also suppress cough reflexes and depress respiration, aiding mechanical ventilation.

The water-soluble midazolam tends to be the benzodiazepine of choice, since it has a shorter half-life than other benzodiazepines, and like them, reduces CBF and $CMRO_2$. It may be administered as an infusion or by intermittent injection. Accumulation may occur in slow metabolizers of the drug and in critically ill patients with sepsis (Shelly *et al.* 1987). Midazolam appears to reduce patient cooperation, which may make neurological assessment difficult in that drug effects may be ascribed to 'cerebral irritation', resulting in unnecessary patient transport for CT scans (personal observations).

Propofol, like other intravenous anaesthetics, reduces ICP, CBF and $CMRO_2$ (Vandesteene *et al.* 1988). It also has the theoretical advantage of having antioxidant properties (Murphy *et al.* 1991); since free radicals contribute significantly to postischaemic cerebral damage, it is possible that free radical scavengers may be useful in brain resuscitation. Its attractions include an easily controllable level of sedation, excellent recovery characteristics and a lack of accumulation. It is important to include the volume and fat content in calculations of fluid balance and nutritional requirements when propofol is being infused for sedation. It is the practice in Frenchay to use a combination of propofol and morphine infusions for most head-injured or other neurosurgical patients requiring sedation and mechanical ventilation. The combination provides good-quality sedation and control of ICP while allowing neurological assessment shortly after temporarily stopping the propofol infusion. Only rarely are muscle relaxants required.

Isoflurane reduces $CMRO_2$ and low concentrations have been used successfully for sedation in general intensive care (Kong *et al.* 1989). Concerns about its cerebral vasodilator properties have to date prevented its use in neurosurgical intensive care.

Cerebral oedema

Generalized cerebral oedema may follow head injury or ischaemic brain insults; more localized oedema tends to surround tumours or haematomas. Two main types of cerebral oedema are recognized. Vasogenic oedema results from the loss of intravascular fluid into the brain extracellular space as a result of a deficient blood—brain barrier. Cytotoxic oedema is the intracellular accumulation of fluid that follows cerebral ischaemia and subsequent impairment of cellular pump mechanisms. Other recognized types include hydrostatic oedema, which often follows surgical evacuation of large intracranial haematomas, and osmotic oedema, which is the result of reductions in plasma osmolality.

Cerebral oedema is one of the more common causes of raised ICP postoperatively and after head injury. It can be differentiated from other common causes of raised ICP only by its appearance on CT scan. Oedema appears as a radiolucent area with shift of surrounding structures.

The value of steroids in the treatment of oedema surrounding cerebral tumours or abscesses is well established, and it is possible that they may be of value in oedema surrounding cerebral contusions. Their use in generalized cerebral oedema following severe head injury may actually increase mortality.

Patients with generalized oedema causing a decrease in the level of consciousness or other pressure effects should be intubated, ventilated and sedated. Attention should be paid to fluid balance. These patients may benefit from ICP monitoring, osmotherapy and some forms of cerebral protection. The pathophysiology of cerebral oedema formation is discussed further in Chapter 2, and its management is discussed in Chapter 14.

Temperature control

It is common for patients to cool spontaneously during neurosurgery, and to be hypothermic in the immediate postoperative period, particularly after prolonged procedures. Spontaneous rewarming is easily achieved by nursing the patient in a warm environment and using a 'space-blanket'. Shivering and vasoconstriction may occur, increasing oxygen requirements and causing hypertension. Inducing hypothermia has been recommended as a method of cerebral protection by reducing CMRO$_2$ by approximately 5% for every 1°C reduction in body temperature, but is seldom used in clinical practice at present. However, allowing the patient to cool spontaneously to 34–35°C may have some beneficial effect (Berntman *et al.* 1981). There is further reference to this in Chapter 10.

Pyrexia is common following head injury, especially in children, and increases the CMRO$_2$ and the ICP. It is also common when blood is present in the cerebral ventricles and in injuries to the brainstem or hypothalamic region. Any infectious cause of pyrexia should be sought actively and treated appropriately, but frequently none is present. In this case the temperature should be reduced by tepid sponging and fanning. Rectal paracetamol is a simple and effective measure to treat pyrexia, as are small intravenous doses of chlorpromazine.

Infection

Prophylactic antibiotics should be used only for specified indications, since their use does not prevent infection but encourages colonization and infection with more resistant organisms. Their use in neurosurgical practice is being questioned increasingly, with many units abandoning their use even for such traditional indications as cerebrospinal fluid (CSF) otorrhoea or rhinorrhoea, preferring to treat infection only as it arises, and then using an antibiotic with the narrowest appropriate spectrum of activity. The possibility of meningitis, shunt infection or ventriculitis from an external ventricular drain should always be borne in mind in postoperative neurosurgical patients, and should prompt microscopic and biochemical examination and culture of CSF when the source of sepsis is in any doubt. Microbiological advice is invaluable in the treatment of individual patients with proven or suspected infection.

All patients receiving intensive care are at an increased risk of developing sepsis, which may progress to the development of organ failure and increased mortality. Many host defence mechanisms are breached: skin by intravascular and urethral catheters; coughing and ciliary function are depressed by sedative drugs; the filtering function of the nose bypassed with an endotracheal tube; the gastric acid barrier removed by using antacids or histamine-receptor antagonists. In the meantime the patient may be immunosuppressed by drugs such as steroids or sedatives, by the disease process itself, and by malnutrition. Finally the patient is being nursed in a microbiologically hostile environment. Infections in the ICU can be divided into exogenous, primary endogenous and secondary endogenous infections. Exogenous infection is derived from the patient's environment or his carers and relatives. Endogenous infection is derived from the patient's own flora: primary endogenous infection is caused by the patient's normal commensal flora whereas secondary endogenous infection usually follows carriage of potentially pathogenic microorganisms (PPM) such as enterobacteria, pseudomonads, *Staphylococcus aureus* and yeasts. These organisms initially colonize the gastrointestinal (GI) tract and spread retrogradely along the oesophagus to the oropharynx. Aspiration of colonized oropharyngeal or gastric secretions past the endotracheal tube cuff will then result in pneumonia, the most common nosocomial infection in the intensive-care population. It is also believed that endotoxin derived from Gram-negative organisms colonizing the gut can be absorbed into the portal and systemic circulations by a physiological breakdown in GI mucosal barrier function caused principally by GI ischaemia. Endotoxinaemia is the primary trigger of the cascades that lead to the development of the sepsis syndrome, septic shock and multisystem organ failure, all associated with depressingly high mortality rate, prolonged hospitalization and increased cost. For this reason recent attention has focused on methods of reducing the incidence of sepsis and endotoxinaemia. Regular microbiological screening and surveillance is essential.

Exogenous infection should be controlled by proper infection control procedures guided by an infection control nurse. Hand washing before every patient contact, adequate space between beds, appropriate care and handling of intravascular and urinary catheters, daily sampling of all external drains and catheters (and CSF if appropriate) for bacteriological examination, regular cleaning of the ICU equipment and environment, changing ventilator tubing, humidifiers and giving sets at specified intervals, and isolation of patients when required are all important. These simple and effective methods of reducing exogenous infection must be enforced, especially in medical staff visiting the ICU, who are notorious culprits when it comes to hand washing!

Avoiding the use of histamine antagonists will help to maintain a low gastric pH and reduce the incidence of nosocomial pneumonia (Fiddian-Green & Baker 1991). If ulcer prophylaxis is required then sucralfate is just as effective as histamine antagonists and does not effect gastric pH. Sucralfate delays the absorption of orally administered warfarin, certain antibiotics and phenytoin, and this may be important in the ICU. However, if the patient is in such a condition that he or she is requiring sucralfate, then he or she is unlikely to be taking oral preparations. Indiscriminate use of antibiotics will encourage colonization and potentially infection with more resistant organisms. One approach to limit the risk of secondary endogenous infection in ICU patients is the use of selective decontamination of the digestive tract (SDD). The goal of SDD is to prevent oropharyngeal and gastrointestinal colonization with PPM. This is achieved by administering non-absorbable antibiotics with selective activity against PPM. A mixture of polymyxin, tobramycin and amphotericin is applied topically as a gel to the oropharyngeal mucosa, and administered enterally as a suspension four times a day. This encourages colonization with obligate anaerobic organisms which in turn limit colonization by, or overgrowth of, PPM. Most clinical trials show a significant reduction in infection, including pneumonia and septicaemia, but a reduction in mortality has been demonstrated only in trauma and cardiovascular patients (Van Saene & Mostafa 1991). In addition SDD reduces the faecal endotoxin pool. ICU-related infection is only one cause of mortality, and it is unreasonable to expect SDD to have an impact on mortality in patients with severe head injuries or any other disease process with a poor prognosis in its own right. However, the precise role of SDD remains controversial (Fink 1992). In European intensive-care practice the technique is used for all patients in 2% of ICU, for selected patient groups by another 23% of units, and not at all by the remaining 75% (Rennie 1993). It is the author's current practice to prescribe SDD only for patients with multiple trauma, including head injuries, with an injury severity score greater than 16 and expected to require mechanical ventilation for at least 3 days.

In patients with multiple trauma, early stabilization of fractures will reduce the mortality from sepsis from 35% (if surgery is delayed) to 7.4%. In patients with head injuries surgery for associated injuries should therefore be delayed for as short a time as possible.

Fluid balance

Postoperative fluid restriction, avoiding crystalloid infusions for intra-vascular volume expansion, is believed commonly to reduce or prevent the formation of cerebral oedema. However, it is equally important to maintain intravascular volume to prevent haemodynamic instability. Recent studies indicate that even small reductions ($4\,mosmol\,kg^{-1}$) in plasma osmolality can lead to increased cerebral oedema formation, while large and prolonged reductions in colloid osmotic pressure ($>50\%$) have little effect as long as osmolality is maintained (Todd & Warner 1989). If the blood–brain barrier is intact there is no evidence that crystalloids will increase oedema formation. If the blood–brain barrier is disrupted then neither osmotic nor oncotic gradients can be produced, and oedema formation is determined by hydrostatic forces. Therefore altering the colloid oncotic pressure has little effect on oedema formation in damaged or normal brain. Altering the osmolality will, however, influence the water content of normal brain, but has no effect when the blood–brain barrier is disrupted. Therefore increasing the plasma osmo-lality will have no effect on brain water content around an injured area of brain, but may still reduce the ICP by reducing the water content of the remaining normal brain.

The aim of postoperative fluid management should be to maintain intravascular volume and a stable or slightly elevated plasma osmolality. This should reduce the water content of the brain and help to prevent an increase in ICP. Excess free water in the form of dextrose solutions should be avoided, as such solutions are likely to exacerbate any cerebral oedema. Intravenous fluids may be restricted to 1.5 litres of dextrose-saline over the first 24 h or until the patient is drinking or absorbing nasogastric feeds. Some units give saline in preference to dextrose–saline to avoid the administration of any dextrose in the postoperative period, but care must be exercised to avoid overloading the patient with sodium. Intravascular volume can be maintained using crystalloid or colloid solution, the osmolality of the solution being more important than its oncotic pressure. Fluid balance in patients with head injuries or cerebral oedema is based on similar principles of fluid restriction to achieve a slightly elevated plasma osmolality and maintenance of intravascular volume.

Endocrine

Hyperglycaemia in non-diabetic patients is a common feature of any critical illness. The worrying feature of hyperglycaemia in neurosurgical practice or following head injuries is that it augments ischaemic neuronal damage, probably as a result of enchanced tissue lactic acidosis (Fitch 1988). Fluids containing glucose are therefore avoided peroperatively, and hyperglycaemia treated with insulin in the usual way.

Diabetes insipidus may complicate severe head injuries, intracranial surgery or intracranial infections. It is a common finding in patients who are brainstem dead. It is heralded by the sudden onset of marked polyuria in the absence of diuretic administration. The diagnosis is confirmed by finding hypernatraemia, an increased plasma osmolality and an inappropriately low urinary osmolality and specific gravity. The hypernatraemia may cause irritability, an altered level of consciousness and convulsions. Conscious patients with an intact thirst mechanism should be able to compensate for the extra losses by increasing their oral intake. If not, and in unconscious patients, urinary losses should be replaced with dextrose saline, fluid balance being carefully monitored to avoid water intoxication or cerebral oedema. With large urinary losses deamino-D-arginine vasopressin (DDAVP) 1−4 µg should be administered intravenously or intramuscularly. The problem usually resolves spontaneously after 72 h.

The syndrome of inappropriate antidiuretic hormone (ADH) secretion frequently accompanies bronchial carcinoma, but is also a recognized complication of head injury, encephalitis and cerebral tumours. The increased secretion of ADH results in water retention and hyponatraemia, with a high urinary sodium concentration. The urinary osmolality is inappropriately high for a low plasma osmolality, which should differentiate the syndrome from hyponatraemia due to excessive water administration. The hyponatraemia may lead to confusion, tremor, convulsions and coma. If the hyponatraemia is not accompanied by neurological dysfunction, then rapid correction with hypertonic saline is unjustified since it may result in acute or permanent brain damage (Swales 1987), and simple water restriction will suffice. If the hyponatraemia is symptomatic then treatment with a diuretic and hypertonic saline is indicated, aiming to increase the sodium concentration by no more than $2\,mmol\,l^{-1}\,h^{-1}$ (Narins 1986).

Finally, patients may require physiological replacement of cortisol and thyroxine after hypophysectomy.

Nutrition

Debilitating disease, trauma or major surgery can result in a rapid deterioration in the nutritional state of the patient by inducing hypermetabolism and negative nitrogen balance. This is exacerbated by the presence of infection. Nutritional support should provide adequate nutrients to allow healing or replacement of damaged tissue, and to sustain visceral protein levels and immunocompetence. All patients need to be fed, and those unable to feed themselves should be supported nutritionally. In neurosurgical practice this is usually patients with severe head injuries or other causes for a prolonged depression in the level of consciousness. Occasionally patients with bulbar palsy or following posterior fossa surgery have swallowing dysfunction, and will require a nasogastric tube both to allow enteral nutrition and to prevent aspiration.

Severe head injuries are associated with increased energy expenditure and increased protein catabolism. This response diminishes after a week unless complicated by infection, seizures, decerebrate posturing or steroid administration (Deutschman 1987). Most patients will have an intact GI tract and should be fed enterally, since enteral nutrition is associated with less risks than parenteral nutrition and may protect against stress ulceration and maintain the integrity of GI mucosal barrier function. It has been suggested that enteral nutrition should not be used for the first 2–3 days after severe head injury if the ICP is raised, since the free water provided may further increase the ICP (Bell & Brown 1987). This should not, however, be a problem if the water content of the feeds is included when considering the patient's overall fluid balance, and enteral nutrition should be started as soon as practical. This may be administered via a nasogastric tube, or an orogastric tube in the presence of basal skull fractures. Gastric emptying is a frequent problem resulting in large nasogastric aspirates, and is occasionally improved with regular metoclopramide or cisapride. Continuous enteral feeding increases gastric pH significantly, and leads to a corresponding increase in the incidence of nosocomial pneumonia (Jacobs *et al.* 1990). This may be decreased by simply interrupting continuous enteral nutrition for 6 h daily (overnight) aiming to achieve a gastric pH < 3.5 at the end of the fasting period. While enteral nutrition is preferable to parenteral nutrition, the latter is better than no nutrition. If enteral nutrition cannot be established then parenteral nutrition should be commenced early (after the first 48 h) as this may have a favourable effect on outcome in patients with head injuries (Rapp *et al.* 1983).

Nitrogen requirements should be estimated by daily 24 h urinary urea nitrogen output measurements and calculated from the formula

$$\text{Nitrogen output (g)} = [\text{Urinary urea mmol} \, 24 \, \text{h}^{-1} \times 0.035]$$
$$+ \, [\text{change in plasma urea}$$
$$\times \text{ body weight (kg)} \times 0.046]$$

A sudden increase in urinary nitrogen output can be the first indication of the onset of sepsis. The calorific requirements are more difficult to assess unless calorimetry is used. Alternatively tables can be used to estimate calorie requirements, but can be inaccurate. Assessing nitrogen requirements and providing calories in a ratio of 100–120 kcal per gram of nitrogen administered is a simple and safe way of calculating energy requirements for most patients. Overfeeding with too many calories can result in an undesirable rise in body temperature, often difficult to explain unless this cause is considered (Henneberg *et al.* 1991).

Convulsions

Epileptic fits cause a considerable increase in both cerebral blood flow and metabolism, the CMRO$_2$ increasing two- to three-fold during status epilepticus, while airway obstruction and secondary physiological effects tend to reduce oxygen delivery to the brain. The increased oxygen and glucose demand and reduced delivery lead rapidly to an increasing cerebral acidosis. The cerebral blood flow and ICP increase and eventually cerebral oedema may develop. Prolonged fitting will cause hypoglycaemia, hyperthermia, dehydration and hypertension followed by hypotension; continued muscle contractions may lead to rhabdomyolysis, myoglobinuria and renal failure. Clearly convulsions should be prevented where appropriate, and treated aggressively when they occur.

Approximately 12% of patients will fit within the first week of intracranial surgery, the incidence increasing to 35% in patients with a preoperative history of seizures (Matthew *et al.* 1980). Anticonvulsants may be prescribed prophylactically in certain procedures associated with a greatly increased risk of seizures postoperatively. It is standard practice at Frenchay to administer prophylactic anticonvulsants during removal of meningiomas, particularly those affecting the cortical convexity, and during removal of intracerebral haematomas. The indications for prophylactic anticonvulsants vary from centre to centre; some would include middle cerebral artery aneurysm surgery, which has a 25% risk of postoperative convulsions, in their list and some do not use prophylactic anticonvulsants at all. The duration of treatment also differs between centres, and will influence the time when the resumption of driving is allowed. At Frenchay anticonvulsants are usually stopped 3 weeks after operation.

A single isolated convulsion postoperatively is usually easily controlled with diazepam. This should be followed by investigation and treatment of the underlying cause. Fitting in patients with head injuries should be treated with phenytoin rather than benzodiazepines, because they depress the level of consciousness further and increase the risk of respiratory depression.

Status epilepticus is a medical emergency associated with a mortality of 10%. It can be defined as the rapid, repetitive recurrence of any type of convulsion persisting for more than 30 min without recovery of baseline neurological function between attacks. The patient must be protected from injury and if necessary an oral airway inserted. Endotracheal intubation may be necessary to secure the airway. Oxygen is administered and intravenous access secured. Blood is taken for the investigations necessary to establish the underlying cause and treat it. These will include urea and electrolytes, blood glucose, arterial blood gases, plasma calcium and magnesium, and concentrations of anticonvulsant drugs if appropriate. Intravenous fluid is given if the patient is hypotensive. A CT scan will usually be required to exclude a structural cause of the fits.

Diazepam is the drug of choice to stop the convulsions. Incremental intravenous 2 mg doses are administered to a total of 20 mg and can be followed by an infusion titrated to a maximum of $3 \, mg \, kg^{-1}$ in 24 h. If intravenous access is difficult midazolam $0.2 \, mg \, kg^{-1}$ is effective when administered intramuscularly (Ghilain *et al.* 1988). At the same time a loading dose of phenytoin is administered, $15-20 \, mg \, kg^{-1}$ intravenously at a rate not exceeding $50 \, mg \, min^{-1}$ to avoid hypotension or arrhythmias; the ECG and blood pressure should be monitored. The therapeutic effect may be delayed for up to 30 min but this dose should produce therapeutic serum concentrations for the first 24 h and can be followed by a maintenance dose of 100 mg every 6–8 h. If the fits are not controlled with diazepam and phenytoin then a bolus dose of thiopentone should be given and followed by a continuous infusion titrated to control the fits. The required dose is usually in the range of $1-3\,\mathrm{mg\,kg^{-1}\,h^{-1}}$. Endotracheal intubation and mechanical ventilation are almost always required at this stage. Chlormethiazole is an effective anticonvulsant agent, but its use in neurosurgical practice may be limited because of the large volume of hypotonic fluid administered. Other drugs that may be useful in status epilepticus include clonazepam, paraldehyde, propofol and the recently introduced intravenous preparation of sodium valproate. Refractory status epilepticus may respond to isoflurane anaesthesia (Ropper *et al.* 1986). Vigabatrin is a newer gamma aminobutyric acid (GABA) transaminase inhibitor which is useful for refractory complex partial seizures, particularly if inadequately controlled with conventional medication (Tartara *et al.* 1989).

There is little place for the use of muscle relaxants in the management of status epilepticus, since they only mask the peripheral manifestations of the seizures without treating the seizures themselves. They should be used only if the fits are proving refractory to treatment and are causing secondary physiological effects such as pyrexia or myoglobinuria, or are interfering with ventilation. If relaxants are given then the use of a CFM is mandatory to determine if seizure activity is being controlled. Indeed, a case can be made for such monitoring in all cases of severe status epilepticus even if muscle relaxants are not being used. In general the anticonvulsant infusions are continued until seizure activity has been suppressed for at least 24 h. The dose may then be reduced gradually as guided by the CFM. In the meantime blood levels of maintenance anticonvulsants (phenytoin, carbamazepine, valproate) should be measured to ensure that therapeutic levels have been achieved before the anticonvulsant infusion is withdrawn.

It is important to diagnose and treat the secondary physiological effects in their own right, as well as the fits themselves. This may include the specific treatment of hypotension, metabolic acidosis, hypoglycaemia, hyperthermia, cerebral oedema and myoglobinuria.

Vasospasm

The two principal causes of morbidity and mortality in survivors of a subarachnoid haemorrhage as a result of a rupture of an intracerebral artery aneurysm are rebleeding and cerebral ischaemia from vasospasm. The recent trend in neurosurgery to clip intracranial aneurysms within the first 72 h of the bleed, to reduce the risk of rebleeding, means that patients are undergoing surgery before vasospasm becomes a problem. Therefore delayed cerebral ischaemia from vasospasm remains a risk after successful aneurysm surgery, usually presenting as increasing confusion, drowsiness and focal signs between 3 and 9 days following the initial bleed. Vasospasm is essentially a diagnosis of exclusion — other causes of deterioration in neurological function such as rebleeding, hydrocephalus, cerebral oedema or haematoma having been excluded. Nimodipine reduces significantly the incidence of delayed ischaemia and of poor outcomes when administered prophylactically after a subarachnoid haemorrhage from a ruptured aneurysm (Pickard *et al.* 1989). It also reduces morbidity and mortality in patients with established vasospasm (Jan *et al.* 1988). Other measures to increase cerebral perfusion pressure, blood volume and cardiac output may be used in patients developing vasospasm after the aneurysm has been clipped, and are achieved by the practice of 'hypervolaemic hypertension' (Archer *et al.* 1991). The aim of this therapy is to increase blood flow through the vasospastic vessels, but its value has yet to be proven. It is the author's practice to admit these patients to the ICU and monitor arterial and central venous pressures directly. They are then volume-loaded with a combination of crystalloid and colloid solution, to achieve and maintain a given central venous pressure. The arterial systolic pressure is increased to 160–200 mmHg using an infusion of metaraminol. Other centres prefer to increase the cardiac output with the use of dobutamine or similar agent, to volume expand with colloid, and to monitor pulmonary artery wedge pressure in addition. The patient is observed for any improvement in orientation and focal signs, and the pressure at which improvement occurs is noted and used as a guideline for continued treatment. A marked diuresis may make it difficult to maintain the hypervolaemic hypertension.

Haematoma

In the postoperative period, or in patients with head injuries, a deterioration in the level of consciousness or the development of focal neurological signs may indicate the development of an intracranial haematoma. The physical signs may indicate the site of the haematoma, but not reliably, and a CT scan will be required to confirm the diagnosis. After surgery in the posterior fossa many neurosurgeons prefer to observe their patient's breathing spontaneously, since a change in respiratory pattern may be the first sign of brain stem compression by a haematoma.

Neurogenic pulmonary oedema

Neurogenic pulmonary oedema is a rare complication of head injury with an incidence of only two out of 2100 patients, but may also occur with other CNS insults such as subarachnoid haemorrhage, cerebrovascular accidents, intracranial tumours and epilepsy. It usually develops extremely rapidly. Theodore and Robin (1975) speculated that a catecholamine surge in response to the intracranial insult causes a sudden increase in systemic vascular resistance, resulting in a shift of blood volume from the systemic to the pulmonary circulation. The increased pulmonary arterial pressure leads to hydrostatic pulmonary oedema and also damages the endothelium of the pulmonary vasculature, causing a sustained increase in capillary permeability. Thus protein-rich oedema fluid may continue to accumulate after the pulmonary artery pressure has returned to normal. Increased ICP may cause ischaemic myocardial damage, and focal myocardial necrosis has been reported in approximately 40% of patients dying of pathology causing raised ICP (Heinrich & Muller 1974). Catecholamines are again considered to be the most likely cause of this damage. While clinical evidence of myocardial damage following head injury or subarachnoid haemorrhage is usually limited to ECG changes resembling myocardial ischaemia, left ventricular dysfunction or life-threatening arrhythmias may also occur (Marion *et al.* 1986) (Fig. 15.1).

Treatment of neurogenic pulmonary oedema should be directed at the cause of increased ICP and should aim to reduce ICP rapidly, if necessary by early surgical intervention. Mechanical ventilation with PEEP and a high FIO_2 is usually required. Alpha-adrenergic antagonists have been advocated as adjunctive treatment as a result of animal work which demonstrated that neurogenic pulmonary oedema can be prevented, or considerably attenuated, by pretreatment with alpha-antagonists. However, vasodilators must be used with caution as they may jeopardize cerebral perfusion pressure further (Loughnan *et al.* 1980). More invasive monitoring using a pulmonary artery catheter may be helpful in guiding treatment, particularly if neurogenic pulmonary

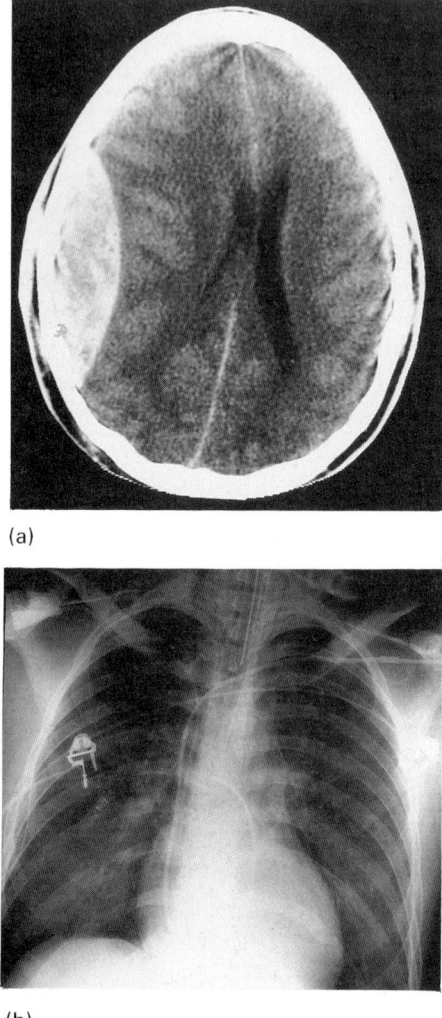

(a)

(b)

Fig. 15.1 Neurogenic pulmonary oedema and myocardial dysfunction. A 16-year old previously fit male sustained a head injury. CT scan of the head demonstrated a right-sided extradural haematoma (a). Plain supine chest X-ray showed marked pulmonary oedema throughout both lung fields (b) and a 12-lead ECG showed typical widespread T-wave inversion that may accompany raised ICP (c). Echocardiography documented left ventricular dilation with an end-diastolic diameter of 5.5 cm (normal 3.5−4.6) (d). A pulmonary artery catheter was useful in the management.

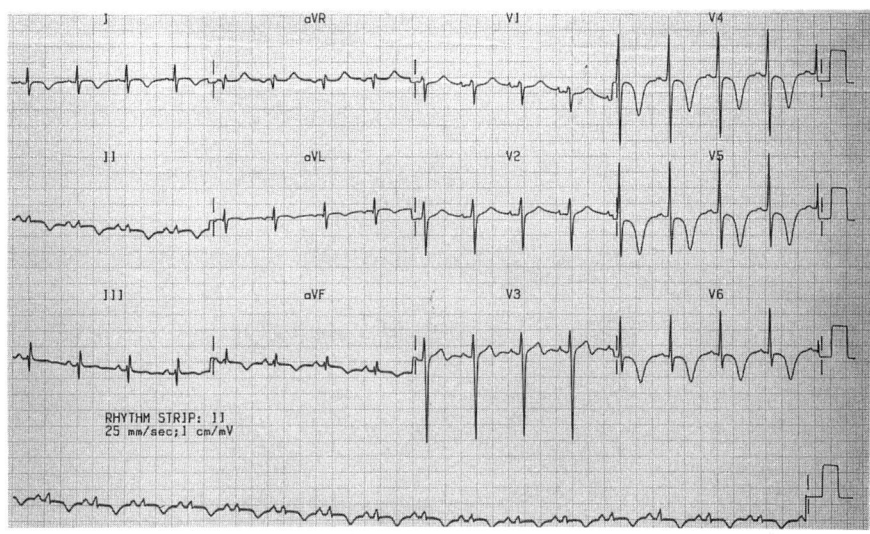

(c)

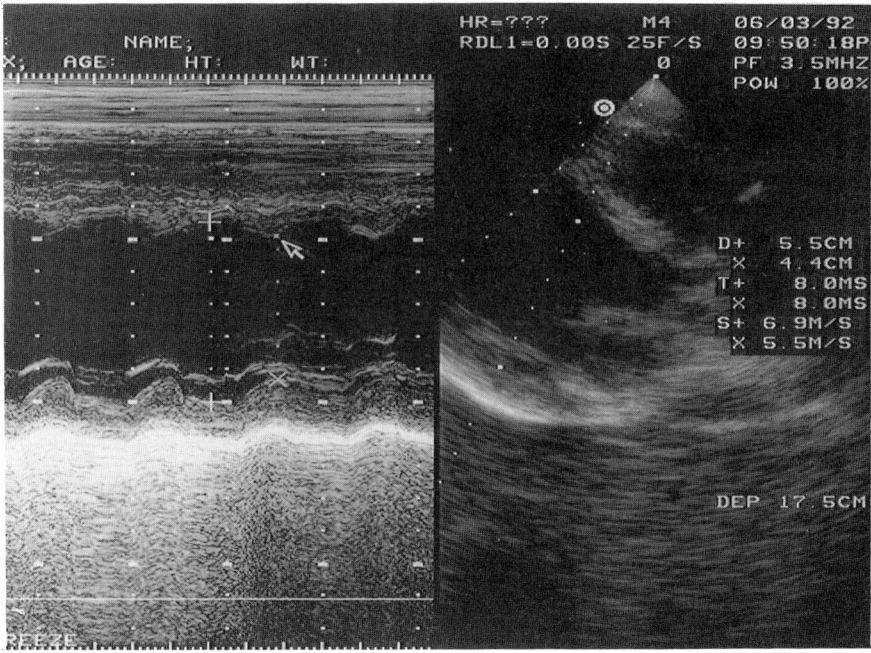

(d)

Fig. 15.1 (*Continued*)

oedema and left ventricular dysfunction are both present (Warwick *et al.* 1993).

Renal failure

Acute renal failure remains a frequent and important contributing factor to mortality in any intensive-care setting. The four most important risk factors in the development of acute renal failure are hypotension, sepsis, aminoglycoside antibiotics and radiocontrast media (Menashie *et al.* 1988). Developments in techniques of renal replacement therapy allow easier control of the patient's clinical, metabolic and biochemical status (Rylance 1990), but the overall mortality from acute renal failure has remained greater than 50%, although the pattern of patients appears to have changed (Cameron 1986). Prevention of renal failure therefore remains important. Measures designed to reduce the risk of the development of renal failure should include meticulous attention to the maintenance of intravascular volume and renal perfusion, measures to reduce the incidence and severity of sepsis, avoiding nephrotoxic agents (particularly aminoglycosides, NSAID and loop diuretics), and using safer radiocontrast media whenever possible. It is particularly important to avoid hypotension as patients developing acute renal failure due to sepsis or nephrotoxic agents but without hypotension have a better prognosis than patients developing renal failure due to hypotension. An infusion of a dopaminergic agent such as dopexamine or low-dose dopamine may prove to be beneficial in patients at risk of developing renal failure, by improving renal flow. These agents also improve mesenteric blood flow and may help maintain the GI mucosal barrier function, potentially reducing the incidence of translocation of bacteria and endotoxin from the gut and the subsequent development of sepsis and multiple organ failure.

Brainstem death

While death is defined conventionally as the cessation of the heart beat and respiration, it may also be medically and legally defined in terms of brainstem death. Cardiorespiratory death is easier to assess than, and will always follow, cerebral death. With the widespread use of ventilatory support it was soon recognized that, as long as respiration was supported, cardiovascular function could be maintained for some time, although invariably progressing to cardiovascular failure and asystole. It may be argued, therefore, that there is no need to diagnose brainstem death, since the cardiovascular criteria of death will be fulfilled eventually anyway. However, accepting this argument means continuing with futile treatment, prolonging unnecessary distress to the family and staff, denying the patient a dignified death, and utilizing health-care resources ineffectively. For these reasons it is desirable to diagnose brainstem death when it has occurred, to allow discontinuation of mechanical ventilation. Finally, not diagnosing brainstem death may deny the patient an expressed wish to be an organ donor, and will also deny many other patients with end-organ failure the chance to improve their quality of life and survive longer, since the number of organs for transplantation would decrease.

Data from the UK transplant service indicate that the two most common causes of brainstem death in this country are subarachnoid haemorrhage and severe head injury. Cerebrovascular accidents and hypoxic brain injury account for most other cases. Anaesthetists practising in neurosurgical centres are most likely to be faced with the condition in the ICU.

The clinical criteria for the diagnosis of brainstem death have been published by the Conference of Royal Medical Colleges and their Faculties (1976). The diagnosis depends on:

1 *Preconditions* The cause of the coma must be known to be an irreversible structural cause of brain injury in an apnoeic patient dependant on ventilatory support.

2 *Exclusion criteria* The body temperature must be over 35°C to ensure that hypothermia is not contributing to the coma. Reversible causes for brainstem depression must be excluded: sedatives, muscle relaxants, alcohol, metabolic or endocrine disturbances.

3 *Absence of brainstem responses* Tests of the brainstem reflexes should be performed only once the preconditions and exclusion criteria are fulfilled.

(i) The pupils are fixed and do not respond to light. The direct and consensual responses should be observed. The pupils are usually dilated but this is not essential for the diagnosis.

(ii) The corneal reflex is absent.

(iii) The oculovestibular reflex is absent. There is no eye movement in response to the injection of 20 ml ice-cold water into the external auditory meatus, direct access to the tympanic membrane having been verified using an auroscope. The eyes should be observed for at least 30 s after the injection.

(iv) There are no motor responses within the cranial nerve distribution to painful stimuli applied centrally or peripherally. It is recognized that spinal reflexes may persist in brainstem-dead patients, and may even return after an initial absence (Ivan 1973).

(v) There is no gag reflex or cough reflex in response to a suction catheter passed into the pharynx or down the endotracheal tube.

(vi) Apnoea is present on disconnection from mechanical ventilation. This test is done last, to avoid unnecessary hypercarbia should any of the other reflexes be present. The patient should be preoxygenated by ventilating with 100% oxygen for 5 min prior to disconnection from the ventilator. The patient is then disconnected and observed for any spontaneous respiratory movement for 10 min. The Pa_{CO_2} should be measured at the end and should be above 50 mmHg to ensure an adequate stimulus to ventilation. Hypoxia during disconnection can be prevented by passing a suction catheter down the endotracheal tube and supplying $6-10$ litres min^{-1} of oxygen. Oxygen saturation should be monitored continuously using pulse oximetry.

The diagnosis of brainstem death should be made by two medical practitioners who have experience in the field, one of whom must be a consultant. One must be the consultant in charge of the patient or the consultant in charge of the ICU. The second must be one of the above or his deputy, who must be another consultant or senior registrar. If a deputy is involved in establishing the diagnosis he must have been involved in the patients' management, been registered for more than 5 years, and have had previous experience of the procedures involved. Both must satisfy themselves that the preconditions have been met, and neither should be a member of the transplant team. They may carry out the brainstem tests together or separately and, if the tests confirm brainstem death, they should be repeated at a time decided by the doctors. An adequate interval should be allowed to reassure all concerned. The diagnosis should not normally be considered until at least 6 h after the onset of coma or, if cardiac arrest was the cause of coma, until 24 h after the circulation has been restored. In the UK there is no requirement for any other confirmatory tests. In other countries EEG, measurement of CBF, carotid angiography, brainstem evoked potentials or an atropine test may be required before the diagnosis can be made. The procedure is recorded on a form designed for this purpose, and death is certified at the time of completion of the second set of criteria. Figure 15.2 shows the form in use at Frenchay Hospital. If organ donation is being considered it is essential to inform the coroner and obtain his consent. This is particularly important when brainstem death is the result of a head injury. Authorization for the removal of organs should also be documented on a specific form (Fig. 15.2).

Management of the multiple organ donor

Advances in immunosuppression, surgery and intensive care mean that transplantation of abdominal and thoracic organs is a lifesaving procedure for many patients with end-organ failures. Those caring for patients in a neurosurgical ICU will be involved frequently with the management of organ donors prior to the surgical procurement of the organs. At a time when the annual number of transplant procedures is not sufficient to keep pace with the demand, it can be argued that intensivists have two obligations in this respect. The first is to try to increase the number of organs available for donation by maximizing the rate of organ retrieval from brainstem-dead patients (Gore *et al.* 1991). The proposal of increasing organ donation by transferring patients with incipient brainstem death from a general ward to the ICU specifically with the purpose of providing ventilatory support until organ donation can be organized is interesting, but has yet to be accepted widely (Feest *et al.* 1990). Our second obligation is to the organ donors (to respect their wishes) and to the organ recipients to provide organs for transplantation in the best possible condition, optimizing graft survival and function. To achieve this aim meticulous intensive-care management of organ donors is required to sustain organ perfusion. This requires adequate monitoring of organ donors, appropriate cardiovascular, respiratory and renal support, and management of endocrine changes, coagulopathy, hypothermia and infection (Timmins & Hinds 1991). A study from a level 1 trauma centre in the USA indicated that the incidence of complications likely to jeopardize the function of donor organs was as follows: hypotension 81%, multiple transfusion 63%, diabetes insipidus 53%, disseminated intravascular coagulopathy 28%, arrhythmias 27%, cardiac arrest and cardiopulmonary resuscitation 25%, pulmonary oedema 19%, hypoxia 11%, acidosis 11% and seizures 10% (Nygaard *et al.* 1990). The incidence of these complications increases progressively after brainstem death, and unnecessary delays in organ procurement should be avoided once the diagnosis has been confirmed.

Finally, appropriate care of the patient's relatives is an equally important part of the process of organ donation. The involvement of an experienced transplant coordinator at an early stage is highly desirable.

F.581

Affix Patient Identification Label or Complete		
Surname	Date of Birth	Unit No.
First Name	M.S.W.	
Address	Consultant	

Name and Address of Next of Kin . . . .

. . . .

FRENCHAY HEALTH AUTHORITY

CODE OF PRACTICE

Instructions on Completion of Procedural Check List

for A   **CERTIFICATION OF BRAIN DEATH**

     B   **AUTHORISATION OF REMOVAL OF CADAVERIC ORGANS**

Introduction:

1)   Part A of this form should be completed by two medical practitioners who have expertise in this field, one of whom must be a Consultant.

2)   One should either be the Consultant in Charge of the patient or the Consultant Anaesthetist for the I.T.U.

3)   The second may be one of the above or a deputy, who may be another Consultant or Senior Registrar. If a deputy is involved in the procedure, he must:—

      a)   be involved in the patient's management.

      b)   have had previous experience of the procedures involved.

      c)   have been medically registered for five years or more.

4)   Both must satisfy themselves that all preconditions have been met. Neither of those diagnosing Brain Death should be a member of the transplant team.

5)   They may carry out the procedures separately or together and, if the tests confirm Brain Death, they should nevertheless be repeated at a time decided by the Doctors but an adequate interval should be allowed to reassure all directly concerned. Double entry columns are included on the check list for this purpose.

Fig. 15.2 Frenchay Health Authority code of practice for (A) certification of brain death and (B) authorization of removal of cadaveric organs.

PART A   **BRAIN DEATH**

I   CRITERIA FOR DIAGNOSING BRAIN DEATH

Nature of brain damage

	Dr A	Dr B
PLEASE CONFIRM WITH A SIGNATURE THAT Date		
APNOEIC COMA IS **NOT** DUE TO: Time		

1   Depressant drugs
     Name of drug . . . .
     Dosage. . . . .
     Time given . . . .

2   Neuromuscular blocking drugs (relaxants)
     Name of drug . . . .
     Dosage. . . . .
     Time given . . . .

     State whether peripheral
     nerve stimulator used

3   Hypothermia
     Record temperature in degrees centigrade . . . .

4   Metabolic or endocrine disturbances

PLEASE CONFIRM WITH A SIGNATURE THE FOLLOWING

1   Pupils both fixed and unreactive to light

2   No eye movements with cold caloric test

3   No cranial nerve motor responses

4   No respiratory movements on disconnection from ventilator for 10
     mins. with intratracheal O_2

COMMENTS: (e.g. Biochemistry values, EEG report, Angiography report, etc.)

II   CONFIRMATION OF BRAIN DEATH
    DIAGNOSIS OF DEATH

    Date and Time Diagnosis is made   . . . .

    Name of Doctors: A   . . . .
    (BLOCK LETTERS)   B   . . . .

Signature and status of Doctors Making Diagnosis:

A . . . .   Status. . . . .

B . . . .   Status. . . . .

Fig. 15.2 (*Continued*)

PART B

REMOVAL OF ORGANS FOR TRANSPLANTATION

**Has the Form "CRITERIA FOR DIAGNOSING BRAIN DEATH" been completed   YES/NO
Now complete Section I or II as indicated.**

I   **To be completed if the patient had requested Removal of Organs after Death.**

  a   How was the request made?
     Donor Card ....
     Other (Specify) ....

  b   Which, if any, organs were specified? ....
     ....

  c   Views of relatives, if known (state relationship) ....
     ....

     (Provided this is not a Coroner's Case and no objection has been raised, authorisation may now be given)

II   **To be completed if there is no evidence that the patient had requested Removal of Organs after Death.**

  a   Name and status of person(s) making enquiries ....
     ....

  b   Name and relationship of person(s) approached ....
     ....

  c   Date, time and nature of approach (personal/phone) ....
     ....

  d   Views of those approached (specify any organs to which objections are raised) ....
     ....

     If such reasonable enquiry as may be practical was made but views could not be obtained, state reason:
     ....
     (Provided this is not a Coroner's Case, authorisation may now be given if there is no reason to believe that
     there is a relevant objection.)

N.B. Where the patient has requested removal of **ONE ORGAN** and additional or alternative organs are required,
SECTIONS I AND II SHOULD **BOTH** BE COMPLETED.

III   CORONER'S CASE

     In all cases which come into this category, no organs may be removed without the coroners specific
     consent.

     Name and Status of person approaching Coroner ....
     ....

     Organs specified for removal ....
     ....

     Date and Time consent given ....
     If consent withheld, state reasons ....
     ....

IV   AUTHORISATION FOR REMOVAL OF ORGANS

     If organs are to be removed, the relevant sections above must be completed prior to authorisation being
     requested.
     Date and time authorisation given ....
     How given (telephone, orally, etc.) ....
     Name of designated person ....
     (Sector Administrator or Deputy)

     Signature of person to whom
     Authorisation communicated ....

Fig. 15.2 (*Continued*)

References

Andrews P.J.D., Piper I.R., Dearden N.M. & Miller J.D. (1990) Secondary insults during intrahospital transport of head-injured patients. *Lancet* **335**, 327−330.

Archer D.P., Shaw D.A., Leblanc R.L. & Tranmer B.I. (1991) Haemodynamic considerations in the management of patients with subarachnoid haemorrhage. *Canadian Journal of Anaesthesia* **38**, 454−470.

Bell T. & Brown J. (1987) Effect of nasogastric feeding on intracranial pressure in severe head injury. *Anaesthesia and Intensive Care* **15**, 243.

Berntman L., Welsh F.A. & Harp J.R. (1981) Cerebral protective effect of low-grade hypothermia. *Anesthesiology* **55**, 495−498.

Cameron J.S. (1986) Acute renal failure in the intensive care unit today. *Intensive Care Medicine* **12**, 64−70.

Carmichael J. & Shankel S.W. (1984) Effects of nonsteroidal anti-inflammatory drugs on prostaglandins and renal function. *American Journal of Medicine* **78**, 992−1000.

Ciaglia P. & Graniero K.D. (1992) Percutaneous dilatational tracheostomy. Results and long term follow-up. *Chest* **101**, 484−487.

Conference of Medical Royal Colleges and their Faculties in the United Kingdom. (1976) *British Medical Journal* **2**, 1187−1188.

Cooper K.R., Boswell P.A. & Choi S.C. (1985) Safe use of PEEP in patients with severe head injury. *Journal of Neurosurgery* **63**, 552−555.

Deutschman C.S. (1987) Physiology and metabolism in closed head injury. *World Journal of Surgery* **11**, 182−193.

Feest T.G., Riad H.N., Collins C.H., Golby M.G.S., Nicholls A.J. & Hamad S.N. (1990) Protocol for increasing organ donation after cerebrospinal deaths in a district general hospital. *Lancet* **335**, 1133−1135.

Feldman Z., Kanter M.J., Robertson C.S. *et al.* (1992) Effect of head elevation on intracranial pressure, cerebral perfusion pressure and cerebral blood flow in head injured patients. *Journal of Neurosurgery* **76**, 207−211,

Fiddian-Green R. & Baker S. (1991) Nosocomial pneumonia in the critically ill: product of aspiration or translocation. *Critical Care Medicine* **19**, 763−769.

Fink M.P. (1992) Selective gut decontamination: a gut issue for the nineties. *Critical Care Medicine* **20**, 559−561.

Fisher D.M., Frewen T. & Swedlow D.B. (1982) Increase in intracranial pressure during suctioning−stimulation vs rise in $Paco_2$. *Anesthesiology* **57**, 416−417.

Fitch W. (1988) Hyperglycaemia and ischaemic brain damage. In: Kaufmann L. (Ed.), *Anaesthesia: Review* 5. Churchill Livingstone, Edinburgh.

Gabbott D.A. (1991) A survey of postoperative pain. *Anaesthesia Points West* **24**, 34−36.

Ghilain S., Van Rijckevorsel-Harmant K., Harmant J. & DeBarsy T.H. (1988) Midazolam in the treatment of epileptic seizures. *Journal of Neurology Neurosurgery and Psychiatry* **51**, 732.

Gore S.M., Ross Taylor R.M. & Wallwork J. (1991) Availability of transplantable organs from brainstem dead donors in intensive care units. *British Medical Journal* **302**, 149–153.

Hazard P., Jones C. & Benitone J. (1991) Comparative clinical trial of standard operative tracheostomy with percutaneous tracheostomy. *Critical Care Medicine* **19**, 1018–1024.

Heinrich D. & Muller W. (1974) Focal myocardial necrosis in cases of increased intracranial pressure. *European Neurology* **12**, 369–376.

Henneberg S., Sjolin J. & Stjernstrom H. (1991) Overfeeding as a cause of fever in intensive care patients. *Clinical Nutrition* **10**, 266–271.

Hoskin P.J. & Hanks G.W. (1991) Opioid agonist-antagonist drugs in acute and chronic pain states. *Drugs* **41**, 326–344.

Ivan L.P. (1973) Spinal reflexes in cerebral death. *Neurology* **23**, 650.

Jacobs S., Chang R.W.S., Lee B. & Bartlett F. (1990) Continuous enteral feeding: a major cause of pneumonia among ventilated intensive care unit patients. *Journal of Parenteral Nutrition* **14**, 353–356.

Jan M., Buchheit F. & Tremoulet M. (1988) Therapeutic trial of intravenous nimodipine in patients with established cerebral spasm after rupture of intracranial aneurysms. *Neurosurgery* **23**, 154–157.

Kingston G.W., Phang P.T. & Leathley M.J. (1991) Increased incidence of nosocomial pneumonia in mechanically ventilated patients with subclinical aspiration. *American Journal of Surgery* **161**, 589–592.

Kong K.L., Willatts S.M. & Prys-Roberts C. (1989) Isoflurane compared with midazolam for sedation in the intensive care unit. *British Medical Journal* **298**, 1277–1280.

Loughnan P.M., Brown T.C.K., Edis B. & Klug G.L. (1980) Neurogenic pulmonary oedema in man: aetiology and management with vasodilators based on haemodynamic studies. *Anaesthesia and Intensive Care* **8**, 65–71.

Marion D.W., Segal R. & Thompson M. (1986) Subarachnoid hemorrhage and the heart. *Neurosurgery* **18**, 101–106.

Matthew E., Sherwin A.L., Welner S.A. *et al.* (1980) Seizures following intracranial surgery: incidence in the first postoperative week. *Canadian Journal of Neurological Science* **7**, 285–290.

McGlew I.C., Angliss D.B., Gee G.J., Rutherford A. & Wood A.T.A. (1991) A comparison of rectal indomethacin with placebo for pain relief following spinal surgery. *Anaesthesia and Intensive Care* **19**, 40–45.

Menashie P.I., Ross S.A. & Gottlieb J.E. (1988) Acquired renal insufficiency in critically ill patients. *Critical Care Medicine* **16**, 1106–1109.

Murphy P.G., Myers D., Webster N.R. & Jones J.G. (1991) The anti-oxidant potential of propofol. *British Journal of Anaesthesia* **67**, 209P–210P.

Narins R.G. (1986) Therapy of hyponatraemia. Does haste make waste? *New England Journal of Medicine* **314**, 1573–1574.

Nygaard C.E., Townsend R.N. & Diamond D.L. (1990) Organ donor management and organ outcome: a six year review from a Level 1 trauma centre. *Journal of Trauma* **30**, 728−732.

Pickard J.D., Bailey S., Sanderson H., Rees M. & Garfield J.S. (1990) Steps towards cost−benefit analysis of regional neurosurgical care. *British Medical Journal* **301**, 629−635.

Pickard J.D., Murray G.D., Illingworth R. *et al.* (1989) Effect of oral nimodipine on cerebral infarction and outcome after subarachnoid haemorrhage: British aneurysm nimodipine study. *British Medical Journal* **298**, 636−642.

Power I., Cumming A.D. & Pugh G.C. (1992) Effect of diclofenac on renal function and prostacyclin generation after surgery. *British Journal of Anaesthesia* **69**, 451−456.

Rapp R.P., Young B., Twyman D. *et al.* (1983) The favourable effect of early parenteral feeding on survival in head-injured patients. *Journal of Neurosurgery* **58**, 906−912.

Rennie M.J. (1993) EPIC: Infection in intensive care in Europe. *British Journal of Intensive Care* **3**, 27−36.

Ropper A.H., Koofke A., Bromfield E.G. & Kennedy S.K. (1986) Comparison of isoflurane, halothane, and nitrous oxide in status epilepticus. *Annals of Neurology* **19**, 98−99.

Rosner M.J. & Coley I.B. (1986) Cerebral perfusion pressure, intracranial pressure, and head elevation. *Journal of Neurosurgery* **65**, 636−641.

Report of the Working Party on 'Pain after surgery'. (1990) Royal College of Surgeons of England & the College of Anaesthetists' Commission on the Provision of Surgical Services.

Rylance P.B. (1990) Renal replacement therapy for acute renal failure. *Clinical Intensive Care* **1**, 268−273.

Seideman P. & Von Arbin M. (1991) Cerebral blood flow and indomethacin drug levels in subjects with and without central nervous side effects. *British Journal of Clinical Pharmacology* **31**, 429−443.

Shelly M.P., Mendel L. & Park G.R. (1987) Failure of critically ill patients to metabolise midazolam. *Anaesthesia* **42**, 619−626.

Swales J.D. (1987) Dangers in treating hyponatraemia. *British Medical Journal* **294**, 261−262.

Tartara A., Manni R., Galimberti C.A., Mumford J.P. & Iudice A. (1989) Vigabatrin in the treatment of epilepsy: a long term follow up study. *Journal of Neurology Neurosurgery and Psychiatry* **52**, 467−471.

Teasdale G. & Jennett B. (1974) Assessment of coma and impaired consciousness. A practical scale. *Lancet* **ii**, 81−83.

Theodore J. & Robin E. (1975) Neurogenic pulmonary oedema. *Lancet* **ii**, 749−751.

Timmins A.C. & Hinds C.J. (1991) Management of the multiple organ donor. *Current Opinion in Anaesthesiology* **4**, 287−292.

Todd M.M. & Warner D.S. (1989) Perioperative fluid management in neurosurgery. *Current Opinion in Anaesthesiology* **2**, 559−563.

Torres A., Serra-Batiles J., Ros E. *et al.* (1992) Pulmonary aspiration of gastric contents in patients receiving mechanical ventilation: the effect of body position. *Annals of Internal Medicine* **116**, 540−543.

Vandsteene A., Trempont V., Engelman E. *et al.* (1988) Effect of propofol on cerebral blood flow and metabolism in man. *Anaesthesia* **43** (Suppl.), 42−43.

Van Saene H.K.F. & Mostafa S.M. (1991) The place of selective decontamination in intensive care. *Current Opinion in Anaesthesiology* **4**, 247−252.

Wallace P.G.M., Bion J. & Ledingham I.M. (1988) The changing face of sedative practice. In: Ledingham I.M. (Ed.), *Recent Advances in Critical Care Medicine*, pp. 69−93. Churchill Livingstone, Edinburgh.

Ward J.D., Choi S., Marmarou A. *et al.* (1989) Effect of prophylactic hyperventilation on outcome in patients with severe head injury. In: Hoff J.T. & Betz A.L. (Eds), *Intracranial Pressure*, vol. VII, pp. 630−633. Springer, Berlin.

Warwick J.P., Greenslade G., Carter J.A. & Manara A.R. (1993) Neurogenic pulmonary oedema and left ventricular dysfunction. A case report. *British Journal of Intensive Care* **3**, 92−96.

White P.F., Schlobohm R.M., Pitts L.H. & Lindaner J.M. (1982) A randomised study of drugs for preventing increased intracranial pressure during endotracheal suctioning. *Anesthesiology* **57**, 242−244.

16
Anaesthesia in the neurosurgical management of chronic pain

PAUL R. NANDI

Introduction

The management of chronic pain has, over the past few decades, evolved from a generally neglected area of medical practice to an increasingly recognized specialty in its own right. Painful disorders may involve any organ system; moreover since pain is in the ultimate analysis an emotional experience, there is a current trend of increasing emphasis on the affective and behavioural, as opposed to the purely sensory, aspects of pain. It is therefore hardly surprising that the consensus view of an ideal Pain Management Service is that it should draw on a wide range of skills. It is seldom within the capacity of any one individual to possess all these skills, and thus the concept of the multidisciplinary Pain Management Team has evolved, with input from psychologists and physical therapists in addition to physicians and surgeons with an interest in chronic painful conditions. This chapter is not intended to explore the now-established role of the anaesthetist as pain specialist, but rather to focus on the role of the neurosurgeon in the management of chronic pain; to discuss the special demands that neurosurgical pain procedures make on the neuro-anaesthetist; and to highlight those areas where surgical and anaesthetic practice merge in the treatment of certain disorders.

Limitation of neurodestructive procedures

There is no doubt that there has been a decrease in recent years in the popularity of neurodestructive procedures for chronic pain management. Despite the attractive simplicity of the concept that 'cutting the wiring' will abolish the pain, clinical experience has shown the shortcomings and complications that may arise from this approach. However, at the same time the still-important role of the neurosurgeon has become more clearly defined, while a better understanding of the physiology of pain has led to the development of new procedures, often involving either the production of more selective lesions, or the use of stimulatory

435

rather than ablative techniques. There are three basic limitations to the use of neurodestructive procedures: impermanence, deafferentation and neurological deficit.

IMPERMANENCE

Clinical experience has shown that neurodestructive procedures, whether surgically or chemically induced, frequently fail to provide long-term relief of pain (Turks 1988). The reasons for this are incompletely understood, and almost certainly multifactorial, but include the capacity for regeneration in the peripheral nervous system, and plasticity in the central nervous system. The transience of neurodestructive procedures is often most obvious with sectioning of peripheral nerves or nerve roots. Clearly if life expectancy is very limited (for instance by malignant disease) the transience of peripheral nerve lesions need not be a deterrent.

DEAFFERENTATION

Examples abound in non-iatrogenic clinical practice of conditions in which severe pain may arise from interruption of normal neural pathways. Traumatic damage to peripheral nerves may give rise to causalgia, a burning pain in the distribution of the injured nerve which may be excruciating. Spinal cord injury may result in extensive dysaesthesia. Infarctive or other injury to the thalamus or other deep brain structures may give rise to widespread hemicorporeal pain which is notoriously intolerable and resistant to treatment. The mechanisms underlying these syndromes are beyond the scope of this chapter, but it should come as no surprise that surgically inflicted injury in these territories may, by the same mechanisms, give rise to new pain problems which are both more severe, and more difficult to eradicate, than the original problem. There is, however, a (variable) latent period between the neurolytic procedure and the emergence of neuropathic pain, which may again increase the justification for such procedures in the preterminal patient.

NEUROLOGICAL DEFICIT

In general terms it is difficult to inflict selective injury on elements involved in nociception within the nervous system without causing coincidental damage to other structures, and thereby impairing function. In some cases the extent of the problem is self-evident (e.g. surgical section of a peripheral nerve will result in a complete motor and sensory deficit in the distribution of that nerve in addition to any effect on pain). The risks of neurological deficit when lesions are made within the central nervous system will obviously be determined by the anatomical site, which involves considerations not only of important adjacent neural structures but the risk of complications such as haemorrhage. In contradistinction to the previous two limitations on ablative therapy, the projected life expectancy of the patient may in this situation be less of a consideration than the degree of function already present — for example a patient with a brachial plexus injury that has already rendered the arm effectively useless will not be further disadvantaged by a procedure that selectively damages the upper limb innervation but abolishes pain; conversely a fit young patient with pancreatic cancer whose pain is reasonably controlled with systemic drugs will probably not be grateful for a neurodestructive procedure which removes the dependence on opioids but leaves the patient paraplegic.

Classification of neurosurgical procedures for the relief of pain

Neurosurgical procedures for pain relief may be broadly classified under the categories of destructive, augmentative (or stimulatory) and miscellaneous (see Table 16.1). These categories will now be considered

Table 16.1 Classification of neurosurgical procedures for pain relief

1 *Neurodestructive*
   (a) Peripheral
   (b) Spinal cord
   (c) Intracranial

2 *Neurostimulatory*
   (a) Peripheral nerve stimulation
   (b) Spinal cord stimulation
   (c) Deep brain stimulation

3 *Miscellaneous*
   (a) Spinal infusion devices
   (b) Intravenous infusion devices
   (c) Intrathecal saline or barbotage

in more depth. The list of individual procedures is not by any means exhaustive, but is intended to illustrate representative examples, with greater emphasis being placed on those procedures which are either relatively common, or which give rise to particular anaesthetic considerations beyond those of general neuroanaesthesia.

Neurodestructive procedures

Peripheral

The role of surgical lesioning of the peripheral nerves and nerve roots in the management of chronic pain is increasingly recognized as very limited, and will therefore not be discussed here in detail. The reasons for the poor results obtained from most studies have already been outlined in the Introduction. Peripheral neurectomy will not only inevitably give rise to sensory and motor deficit in the distribution of the sectioned nerve, but may (as a consequence of regeneration of the proximal end of the sectioned nerve), give rise to neuromas which can produce pain of greater severity than that which was present before the procedure. The incidence of deafferentation pain is high; moreover if rhizotomy is performed for a painful peripheral lesion, dermatomal overlap demands that several nerve roots are divided to ensure denervation of the territory of the lesion. This involves multilevel laminectomy; in the debilitated cancer patient this is likely to be poorly tolerated, and in the patient with non-malignant disease the likelihood of rapid emergence of the problems listed above provides a relative contraindication.

SYMPATHECTOMY

It is now clear that in a number of chronic pain syndromes the sympathetic nervous system is involved in the maintenance of pain, classically in the conditions of causalgia and reflex sympathetic dystrophy, and that interruption of the sympathetic outflow can be highly efficacious in pain relief. In contrast to procedures involving section of mixed peripheral nerves or nerve roots, selective sympathetic denervation does not give rise to problems of dysfunction or deafferentation. Chemical neurolytic destruction of the sympathetic nerves may also be undertaken percutaneously by the anaesthetist at a number of sites with an acceptably low risk of somatic nerve injury. Neurolytic block of the coeliac plexus for pancreatic cancer is perhaps the prime example of this. Sympathetically maintained pain in the lower limb may be effectively treated by lumbar sympathetic block, initially with local anaesthetic, proceeding to neurolytic block with phenol if the response is favourable. For comparable conditions of the upper limb a diagnostic cervicothoracic sympathetic block (stellate ganglion block) may be performed, but it is generally agreed that the risk of injury to adjacent structures precludes the use of neurolytic agents by this route. Surgical cervicothoracic sympathectomy may be performed for intractable upper limb causalgia if the response to diagnostic stellate ganglion block is favourable. It should be noted, however, that repeated local anaesthetic block of the sympathetic nerves may give rise to prolonged or permanent remission of causalgia, and therefore destructive procedures—either surgical or neurolytic—should never be undertaken lightly.

A recent study (Mockus *et al.* 1987) suggested 61% complete pain relief from causalgia following surgical sympathectomy with careful patient selection.

Spinal cord

PERCUTANEOUS CORDOTOMY

The treatment of intractable pain by open surgical division of the anterolateral quadrant of the spinal cord was described by Spiller and Martin (1912). This procedure has been almost entirely supplanted by percutaneous cordotomy (Rosomoff *et al.* 1965) which, while retaining the efficacy of the original procedure, is relatively safe, and sufficiently atraumatic to be employed even in severely debilitated patients of very limited life expectancy. The preferred means of producing the lesion is thermocoagulation using a radiofrequency generator incorporating a thermocouple so that the temperature of the probe tip can be precisely controlled.

The procedure

Percutaneous cordotomy is most commonly performed at the C1/2 level. The patient is placed supine on an X-ray table and the side of the neck contralateral to the pain is prepared. Under guidance of a C Arm fluoroscope, and following local anaesthesia of the skin and subcutaneous tissues, the lesioning needle is inserted using a direct lateral approach to pierce the dura just anterior to the dentate ligament, which may be identified by the injection of contrast medium. The electrode for producing the lesion is advanced through the intradural needle into the spinal cord; the appropriate depth depends on the site of pain, and electrical stimulation of the electrode should produce paraesthesiae in an area corresponding to the patient's pain.

Once the optimum position has been located a radiofrequency current is applied, raising the temperature of the probe to 70−80°C for a variable period of up to 3 min. Repeated testing for motor function and the presence of analgesia may be required during the production of the lesion.

Anaesthetic considerations

Controlled sedation rather than general anaesthesia is required, since the conscious cooperation of the patient during the procedure is mandatory. Preoperative sedative premedication is permissible provided that it does not impair the ability of the patient to cooperate. Intravenous access should be established before the commencement of the procedure. The patient should be fasted as for routine general anaesthesia. Basic monitoring should consist of ECG, pulse oximetry, and non-invasive blood pressure recording (sympathetic denervation may occur as a result of the lesion). Initiation of the lesion may produce pain and the patient should be warned of this and reassured that it is only transient.

The patient's usual dose regimen of opioid analgesia should be maintained up to the time of the procedure, since abrupt withdrawal may give rise to severe pain, which is likely to hamper patient cooperation in addition to the risk of withdrawal syndrome. Additional sedation may be unnecessary, but if it is required small incremental doses of propofol will permit a high degree of control over the level of sedation with a rapid return to full consciousness in order to allow motor and sensory testing to be carried out.

It is also possible to perform percutaneous thermocoagulation lesioning at a lower cervical level; this procedure is more involved (although the anaesthetic principles are similar) but may be indicated if bilateral lesions are contemplated, as bilateral high cervical cordotomy carries a high risk of producing severe central respiratory depression.

Postoperative management and complications

The patient should be monitored for signs of respiratory depression, hypotension, and delayed development of motor impairment. Urinary retention may occur. Abrupt withdrawal of opioid analgesia may result in withdrawal symptoms and the unmasking of pain, both at the site for which the lesion was produced and elsewhere; opioid withdrawal should therefore be gradual and progressive, and if the patient should develop pain during withdrawal from systemic opioids these drugs may need to be continued at a lower dose. It will be evident that the regimen for opioid withdrawal must be tailored to the patient's individual requirements. Sympathetic explanation and discussion with the patient before the procedure will do much to allay needless anxiety.

DORSAL ROOT ENTRY ZONE (DREZ) LESIONING

This novel procedure was pioneered by Nashold & Ostdahl (1979). The procedure entails the production of a selective lesion of the superficial laminae of the dorsal horn adjacent to the dorsal nerve roots (possibly also involving Lissauer's tract). The rationale for the procedure is based on the observation that, in cases of deafferentation pain, there is increased spontaneous activity in dorsal horn neurones. The place of this procedure is now generally regarded as being restricted to intractable deafferentation pain—classically the pain associated with brachial plexus avulsion. It is performed under general anaesthesia and involves multilevel laminectomy; the preferred means of producing the lesion is by radiofrequency thermocoagulation. Loss of sensation induced by the procedure should not be a deterrent in appropriately selected cases, since gross sensorimotor deficit should already be present.

Trigeminal neuralgia

INTRODUCTION

The management of this condition, characterized by lancinating pain in the distribution of the entire trigeminal ganglion or any of its branches, is currently based on systemic drug therapy. Carbamazepine is the first-line drug of choice, and if unsuccessful or poorly tolerated it may be substituted by phenytoin or other anticonvulsants, tricyclic antidepressants or baclofen. Nevertheless there remains a proportion of patients in whom control is not achieved by this means. There are essentially two neurosurgical approaches to the management of such patients; neurolysis and open microvascular decompression.

MICROVASCULAR DECOMPRESSION

A possible causal relation between trigeminal neuralgia and an aberrant contact of the trigeminal ganglion with adjacent blood vessels was postulated by Dandy (1934). Janetta (1985) pioneered the procedure of moving the offending vessel or vessels away from the nerve via a posterior craniotomy. The anaesthetic considerations for this procedure are those of any posterior fossa surgery. Morbidity is relatively low, and the procedure avoids the complications of postprocedural corneal anaesthesia and anaesthesia dolorosa, which may occur in trigeminal thermocoagulation. However, as the procedure entails open posterior craniectomy it is best reserved for patients at low surgical risk and is therefore usually restricted to patients under 60 years of age.

PERCUTANEOUS THERMOCOAGULATION

The treatment of trigeminal neuralgia with injection of neurolytic drugs into the trigeminal ganglion is now largely of historical interest, although glycerol injection may be effective (Hakanson 1981). Percutaneous thermocoagulation of the trigeminal ganglion or its branches as described by Sweet and Wepsic (1974a) permits much greater control over the extent of the lesion and reduces the distressing complication of anaesthesia dolorosa.

The procedure
Under fluoroscopic guidance and local anaesthesia to the skin of the cheek, the hollow needle of the radiofrequency probe is advanced into the foramen ovale. The lesioning needle is then inserted through the lumen of this needle and electrical stimulation is performed to produce paraesthesiae in the distribution of the patient's spontaneous pain. Once the needle has been demonstrated by this means to be appropriately sited, a radiofrequency current is applied to heat the needle tip in the order of 70°C, for a period of 1–3 min. Immediately following this, the extent of cutaneous hypoaesthesia is tested.

Anaesthetic considerations and complications
As in percutaneous cordotomy, the patient is required to be awake and cooperative during the precise locating of the lesioning needle. Withdrawal of opioid medication should not be a consideration, since it is usually ineffective and therefore not prescribed in the management of

trigeminal neuralgia. However, patients with this condition are typically elderly and may therefore be frail and suffering concomitant illness. The procedure should be discussed with the patient beforehand.

Intravenous access should be established before the commencement of the procedure. Percutaneous insertion of the radiofrequency probe usually requires insertion of the operator's finger into the patient's mouth to guide the direction of the needle, and injudicious sedation at this point is likely to result in airway obstruction. Infiltration with local anaesthetic should minimize discomfort during initial needle insertion, but penetration of the foramen ovale may be painful. Use of a short-acting opioid such as fentanyl or alfentanil may be helpful at this point, and (if unsupplemented by other CNS depressants) is unlikely to compromise patient cooperation or upper airway patency. It is advisable to administer oxygen enrichment to the gas mixture that the patient is breathing (via a nasal mask or catheter) in order to protect against periods of airway compromise.

During electrical stimulation of the lesioning needle the patient will be required to indicate whether the distribution of paraesthesia corresponds to that of the spontaneous pain. This may be accomplished by asking the patient to point to a diagrammatic representation of a face held above the patient; this procedure will clearly require both the conscious cooperation of the patient, and that he or she should have a free hand (unencumbered by monitoring devices, etc.) with which to point. Lesioning is usually painful at its commencement; a deepening of sedation or increase in systemic analgesic is generally required, but the pain is usually short-lived (less than 1 min) and therefore the agents chosen to cover this period of the procedure should be short-acting; otherwise once the pain subsides, the residual sedation may give rise to central hypoventilation or airway obstruction whilst the radiofrequency lesion is still being applied.

Complications

The complications of microvascular decompression are essentially those of any posterior fossa craniectomy, although the limited extent of surgery renders these lower than, for example, craniectomy for tumour.

The complications of trigeminal thermocoagulation include intracranial haemorrhage, meningitis, corneal anaesthesia (with the risk of subsequent corneal ulceration), and anaesthesia dolorosa. The last of these has a reported incidence of 8.9% in the series of Mittal and Thomas (1986); it is a dysaesthesia in the distribution of the lesion which is very distressing (sometimes intolerable) and extremely resistant to treatment. Major complications appear otherwise to be rare; a review by Sweet (1986) of 14 000 cases reported only one death (from intracerebral haemorrhage). Postprocedure withdrawal of carbamazepine (or other drug therapy) should be gradual, as abrupt discontinuation may result in the re-emergence of symptoms. There is a relapse rate following thermocoagulation for trigeminal neuralgia of about 25% over a 3–5-year period, but the procedure may be repeated successfully.

Stereotactic procedures

The broad indications for stereotactic surgery are covered in Chapter 12. The application of this technique in pain management may involve stereotactically controlled radiofrequency lesioning of various nuclei within the thalamus, or the implantation of electrodes for deep brain stimulation, or catheters for drug infusion (particularly opioids).

ANAESTHETIC CONSIDERATIONS

Stereotactic procedures for pain control generally have in common the requirement that the patient should be conscious for at least part of the procedure, in order to report whether stimulation produces sensation or analgesia in the appropriate territory. While it is possible for a patient to tolerate the application of a stereotactic frame under local anaesthesia, the bulk of the frame may render the procedure uncomfortable, particularly if precise localization of the thermocoagulation probe or stimulating electrode takes a considerable period of time, as is sometimes the case. Moreover lesioning may need to be repeated for optimal results, and this requires reapplication of the frame. A refinement of the technique (particularly for radiofrequency lesioning of the thalamic nuclei) involves a staged procedure in which the targeted area within the brain is first located approximately with a standard stereotactic frame under general anaesthesia, a burr-hole made at the appropriate entry site and a Bennett Ball inserted. This device consists of a small disc, multiply perforated in a grid arrangement and adjustably mounted in a ring frame which is fixed to the skull (Fig. 16.1).

The scalp wound is closed over the device and the patient is allowed to recover from anaesthesia; following full recovery the wound is reopened under local anaesthesia, at which typically little or no sedation is required, and the grid arrangement of the perforations in the ball

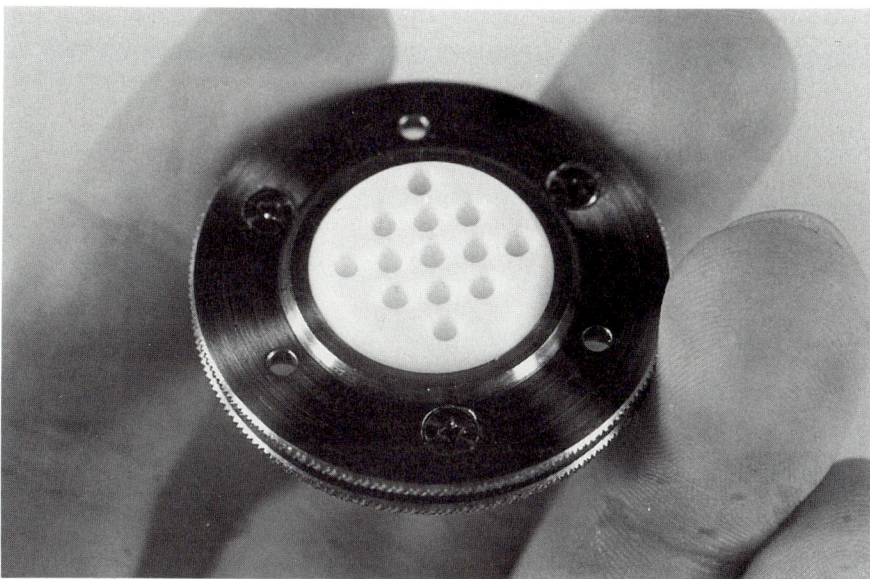

Fig. 16.1 The Bennett Ball.

permits the lesioning probe to be withdrawn and readvanced at different points in the grid until stimulation produces sensation in the optimum distribution. Having located the ideal point a radiofrequency lesion is produced as in percutaneous cordotomy. The wound is then closed; should the need for repeat lesioning become apparent after a day or so it is a simple matter to reopen the wound under local anaesthetic and repeat the process. Once a satisfactory result has been achieved the Bennett Ball is removed under general or local anaesthesia.

The quality of analgesia produced by this technique is generally good but of limited duration (typically 6–12 months). The technique is therefore best reserved for patients of limited life expectancy.

Frontal lobe surgery

Through the 1940s there was a considerable vogue for destructive oper-ations to the frontal lobes for patients with intractable pain. The success rate of these procedures is generally agreed to be low; there is a sub-stantial incidence of the development of seizures, and personality changes are inevitable. These procedures influence the behavioural and affective aspects of pain, rather than the sensory and discriminative aspects;

indeed pain threshold may be actually lowered by such procedures, although patients display an apathy towards the pain. Such operations are now almost entirely of historical interest, although there are some who consider that they may still have a place in the management of pain resistant to all other treatment modalities.

Neurostimulatory procedures

Introduction

The gate control theory of Melzack and Wall (1965) proposes that second relay neurones in the spinal cord concerned with pain transmission receive input from both slowly and rapidly conducting fibres, and that increased firing of the fast-conducting fibres inhibits input from the slow-conducting fibres (Fig. 16.2).

This theory, which has now gained wide acceptance, forms the basis for the use of electrical stimulation as a treatment for pain. The now

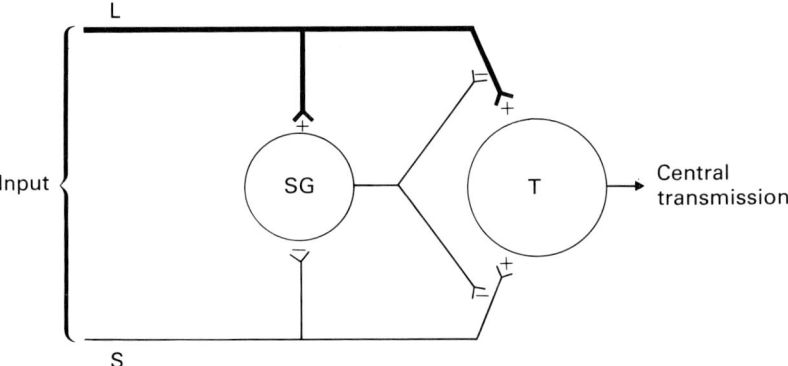

Fig. 16.2 Simplified schematic diagram of gate control hypothesis. Both large and small diameter primary afferent nerve fibres terminate at central transmission cells in the spinal cord. Interneurones in the substantia gelatinosa inhibit their input and additionally receive input from the primary afferents — excitatory in the case of the large diameter fibres and inhibitory in the case of small diameter fibres. It will be apparent that a relative preponderance of activity in the large diameter fibres will reduce activity in the central transmission cells. The system is additionally under higher central control (not depicted here). L, large diameter fibres; S, small diameter fibres; SG, substantia gelatinosa cell; T, central transmission cell; +, excitation; −, inhibition.

firmly established technique of transcutaneous electrical nerve stimulation was devised on the basis of gate control theory. Surgical implantation of neurostimulatory electrodes may involve placement at discrete peripheral nerves, or in the epidural space in the technique of spinal cord stimulation (dorsal column stimulation). Electrical stimulation of certain target areas within the brain may also have a beneficial effect on pain; the mechanisms for this will be discussed in the relevant sections.

Peripheral nerve stimulation

This technique has been reviewed by Nashold (1980). The electrode may be inserted percutaneously or at open operation (in which case it can be performed under local anaesthesia). This procedure has a limited place in the management of non-progressive injury to discrete peripheral nerves. The electrode needs to be sited proximal to the point of injury.

Spinal cord (dorsal column) stimulation

This procedure has particular relevance for the neuroanaesthetist as initial electrode placement is commonly carried out by anaesthetists. It has been advocated for a wide range of intractable chronic pain problems, and its place in a number of these remains to be clearly defined. The best results so far seem to be in patients with radicular pain in association with low back pain, often with previous surgery and in pain associated with peripheral vascular disease (De La Porte & Siegfried 1983, Fiume 1983). The epidural electrode may be sited by the neurosurgeon at open operation, in which case the anaesthetic considerations are very much those of any laminectomy. It is, however, now increasingly commonplace for a wire to be placed percutaneously via a Tuohy-type needle advanced into the epidural space under local anaesthesia. The electrode is advanced under X-ray control into the epidural space and stimulated with a pulse generator until paraesthesiae are reported by the patient in the distribution of his spontaneous pain. At this point the Tuohy needle is withdrawn leaving the electrode *in situ*. It is usual to subject the patient to a trial period of stimulation using an external pulse generator for a period of perhaps a few days, so that if the procedure is unsuccessful, the epidural wire may be removed without subjecting the patient to the full implantation procedure. If the patient derives significant symptomatic benefit, the second stage of the procedure is then carried out under general or local anaesthesia. This entails tunnelling the electrode subcutaneously (this may be undertaken at the time of the original insertion to anchor the electrode and preserve sterility) and then implanting either a battery-operated pulse generator or a receiver designed to be used in conjunction with an external pulse generator. The former has the advantage that it is fully internalized; it suffers, however, from the disadvantage of fairly short battery life, needing frequent surgical revisions. Recent advances in technology have increased the inherent reliability of the equipment, and the use of multichannel percutaneous electrodes has reduced the likelihood of technical failure as a consequence of migration of the wire once implanted.

There is little doubt that short-term pain relief from spinal cord stimulation considerably exceeds favourable long-term outcome. There is almost certainly an element of placebo effect involved in this, but probably also technical failures of the device and perhaps also compensatory changes within the nervous system. A study by Sweet and Wepsic (1974b) following 100 patients over a 2-year period suggested a good result (i.e. substantially increased activity and discontinuation of opioid analgesics) in one-third of patients, with a further third attaining a lesser degree of benefit. However, some other studies employing longer periods of follow-up suggest a less optimistic long-term outcome (Long *et al.*, 1981, Young 1985).

Complications of the procedure include infection, spinal cord injury, cerebrospinal fluid (CSF) fistula, epidural haematoma, and new pain related to the implant. With the exception of the last of these, the incidence of these complications should be very low with careful attention to technique.

Deep brain stimulation

Electrical stimulation of deep brain structures is a relatively recent development. Broadly speaking there are two target areas, and the mechanisms for the production of analgesia are different in these two sites.

PERIVENTRICULAR AND PERIAQUEDUCTAL GREY STIMULATION

Stimulation in these sites is associated with endorphin release into third ventricle (Akil *et al.* 1978). Analgesia is reversed by naloxone, providing further evidence that the analgesia is mediated via endogenous opioids; tolerance may occur with chronic stimulation. Analgesia is characteristically diffuse and may therefore be particularly appropriate for the patient with widespread pain involving both sides of the body. Periventricular and periqueductal grey stimulation has been reviewed by Young and Brechner (1986).

INTERNAL CAPSULE AND THALAMIC STIMULATION

Stimulation of these regions may have a role in the management of central pain disorders. The mechanism of analgesia is incompletely understood, but it is restricted to the contralateral side of the body, not associated with evidence of endorphin release and not reversed by naloxone. Anaesthetic considerations for such procedures are broadly similar to those involved in stereotactic thalamotomy. Studies such as that of Young *et al.* (1985) suggest long-term benefit in more than 50% of patients.

Miscellaneous

There is now available a wide variety of implantable controlled infusion devices for administering drugs intravenously, intrathecally within the spinal cord, or to selected intracranial sites, which may be dramatically effective in the short-to-medium term in alleviating pain. The longer-term value of such devices remains to be established. A detailed review of the options available is inappropriate to a volume such as this, but the technological advances of the past decade have done much to reduce the local complications associated with earlier devices. Broadly speaking contemporary drug-delivering implants consist of a subcutaneous reservoir from which a catheter leads to the desired site of administration; the reservoir is replenished by periodic percutaneous injections via a septum designed to withstand repeated needling without leakage. The early implants utilized electrically operated pumps to deliver the contents of the reservoir; a recent refinement has been the development of externally programmable pumps utilizing microprocessor technology. More recent developments include a bellows arrangement in which the motive force is gaseous expansion (Fig. 16.3), and intermittent limited-dose bolus devices in which drug delivery is patient-controlled.

The anaesthetic implications for implantation are fairly straightforward, as contemporaneous monitoring of the effect of drug administration is not usually a consideration.

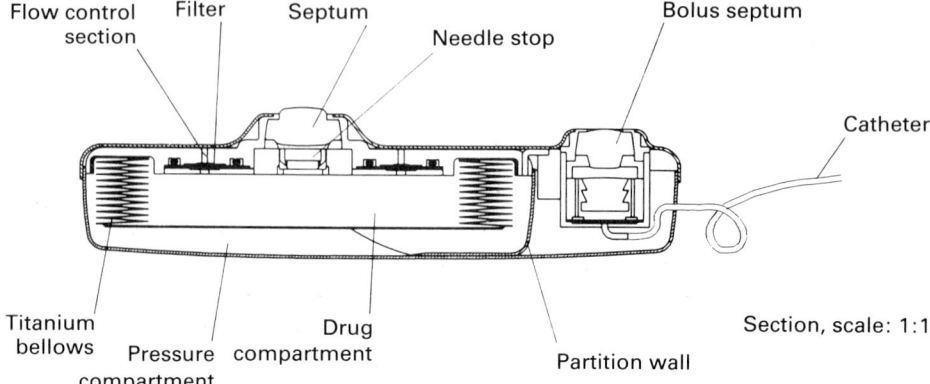

Fig. 16.3 A gaseous-expansion driven infusion pump. This example has two chambers permitting independent continuous infusion and bolus drug administration. From Anschütz.

Intrathecal saline/barbotage

Hitchcock (1967) described the alleviation of intractable pain by withdrawal of spinal CSF followed by intrathecal infusion of cold saline. Subsequent modification of the technique has entailed replacement of withdrawn CSF by hypertonic normothermic saline, and repeated withdrawal and reinjection of CSF (barbotage) which is better tolerated (Lloyd 1976). The initial incidence of pain relief is high, but recurrence of pain is common; the mechanism of analgesia is unclear but possibly related to brainstem demyelination.

References

Akil H., Richardson D.E., Hughes J. & Barchas J.D. (1978) Enkephalin-like material in elevated ventricular cerebrospinal fluid of pain patients after analgetic focal stimulation. *Science* **201**, 463−465.

Anschütz. *The New Generation of Implantable Infusion Pumps.* Publication Aco 680.03 e/N 9202. Anschütz−Medizintechnik, Zeiss-Gruppe, Kiel, Germany.

Dandy W.E. (1934) Concerning the cause of trigeminal neuralgia. *American Journal of Surgery* **24**, 447−455.

De La Porte C. & Siegfried J. (1983) Lumbosacral spinal fibrosis (spinal arachnoiditis): its diagnosis and treatment by spinal cord stimulation. *Spine* **8**, 593−603.

Fiume D. (1983) Spinal cord stimulation in peripheral vascular pain. *Applied Neurophysiology* **46**, 290–294.

Hakanson S. (1981) Trigeminal neuralgia treated by the injection of glycerol into the trigeminal cistern. *Neurosurgery* **9**, 638–646.

Hitchcock E. (1967) Hypothermic subarachnoid irrigation for intractable pain. *Lancet* **i**, 1133–1135.

Janetta P.J. (1985) Trigeminal neuralgia: treatment by microvascular decompression. In: Wilkins R.H. & Rengachary S.S. (Eds), *Neurosurgery* vol. 3, pp. 2357–2363. McGraw-Hill, New York.

Lloyd J.W. (1976) Treatment of intractable pain with cerebrospinal fluid barbotage. In: Morley T.P. (Ed.), *Current Controversies in Neurosurgery*, pp. 520–525. W.B. Saunders, Philadelphia.

Long D.M., Erickson D., Campbell J. & North R. (1981) Electrical stimulation of the spinal cord and peripheral nerves for pain control: a 10 year experience. *Applied Neurophysiology* **44**, 207–217.

Melzack R. & Wall P.D. (1965) Pain mechanisms: a new theory. *Science* **150**, 971–979.

Mittal B. & Thomas D.G.T. (1986) Controlled thermocoagulation in trigeminal neuralgia. *Journal of Neurology, Neurosurgery and Psychiatry* **49**, 932–936.

Mockus M.B., Rutherford R.B., Rosales C. & Pearce W.H. (1987) Sympathectomy for causalgia: patient selection and long-term results. *Archives of Surgery* **122**, 668–672.

Nashold B.S. (1980) Peripheral nerve stimulation for pain. *Journal of Neurosurgery* **53**, 132–133.

Nashold B.S. & Ostdahl R.H. (1979) Dorsal root entry zone lesions for pain relief. *Journal of Neurosurgery* **51**, 59–69.

Rossomoff H.L., Carroll F., Brown J. & Sheptak P. (1965) Percutaneous radiofrequency cervical cordotomy technique. *Journal of Neurosurgery* **23**, 639–644.

Spiller W.G. & Martin E. (1912) Treatment of persistent pain of organic origin in the lower part of the body by division of the antero-lateral column of the spinal cord. *Journal of the American Medical Association* **58**, 1489–1493.

Sweet W.H. (1986) Treatment of trigeminal neuralgia (tic douloureux). *New England Journal of Medicine* **315**, 174–177.

Sweet W.H. & Wepsic J.G. (1974a) Controlled thermocoagulation of trigeminal ganglion and rootlets for differential destruction of pain fibres. *Journal of Neurosurgery* **40**, 143–156.

Sweet W.H. & Wepsic J.G. (1974b) Stimulation of the posterior columns of the spinal cord for pain control: indications, techniques and results. *Clinical Neurosurgery* **21**, 278–310.

Turks E. (1988) Psychological and social dimensions of chronic pain. *Current opinions in Anesthesiology* **1**, 372–377.

Young R.F. (1985) Surgical role in relief of pain. *Seminars in Anesthesia* **4**, 323–331.

Young R.F. & Brechner T. (1986) Electrical stimulation of the brain for relief of intractable pain due to cancer. *Cancer* **57**, 1266–1272.

Young R.F., Kroening R., Fulton W., Feldman R.A. & Chambi I. (1985) Electrical stimulation of the brain in the treatment of chronic pain: experience over five years. *Journal of Neurosurgery* **62**, 389–396.

Index